Profession.   terest

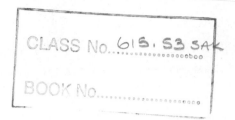
Do professions subordinate their own self-interests to the public interest? In *Professions and the Public Interest* Mike Saks develops a theoretical and methodological framework for investigating this question, which has yet to be analysed adequately by sociologists of the professions. The framework outlined here will be invaluable in future research on the professions.

To demonstrate how this innovative framework can be applied, Mike Saks focuses on health care and presents a case study of the response of the medical profession to acupuncture in nineteenth and twentieth century Britain. He argues that the predominant climate of medical rejection of acupuncture as a form of alternative medicine has not only run counter to the public interest, but also been heavily influenced by professional self-interest. He considers the implications of the case study for the accountability of the medical profession and makes broad recommendations about the direction of future research into this academically and politically important issue.

Professions and the Public Interest will be of interest to a wide readership, including sociologists of the professions and health care, and teachers and students of social policy, politics, social history and medical sociology. It will also appeal to orthodox health care professionals and to practitioners of alternative medicine.

Mike Saks is Professor and Head of the School of Health and Life Sciences at De Montfort University, Leicester.

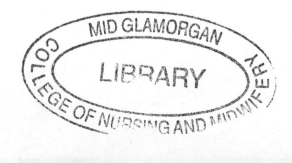

Professions and the public interest

Medical power, altruism and alternative medicine

Mike Saks

London and New York

First published 1995
by Routledge
11 New Fetter Lane, London EC4P 4EE

Simultaneously published in the USA and Canada
by Routledge
29 West 35th Street, New York, NY 10001

© 1995 Mike Saks

Typeset in Times by
Ponting–Green Publishing Services, Chesham, Bucks

Printed and bound in Great Britain by
TJ Press (Padstow) Ltd, Padstow, Cornwall

British Library Cataloguing in Publication Data
A catalogue record for this book is available from the
British Library.

Library of Congress Cataloging in Publication Data
A catalogue record for this book has been requested

ISBN 0–415–01805–6 (hbk)
ISBN 0–415–11668–6 (pbk)

10·4·95

Contents

Acknowledgements

This book could not have been completed without the assistance of many individuals and institutions too numerous to single out for thanks here. I would, however, particularly like to extend my appreciation to Michael Burrage from the London School of Economics for his support and to the Social Science Research Council for funding the initial research. I also owe a special debt of gratitude to my wife, Maj-Lis, and my children, Jonathan and Laura, for their forbearance throughout the enterprise. Finally, thanks are due to Anita Bishop, who assisted with the typing of the manuscript.

Abbreviations

AMA   American Medical Association
BAA   British Acupuncture Association
BMA   British Medical Association
BMAS British Medical Acupuncture Society
BMJ   *British Medical Journal*
CCAM Council for Complementary and Alternative Medicine
CFA   Council for Acupuncture
DoH   Department of Health
GMC   General Medical Council
ICM   Institute for Complementary Medicine
IROM International Register of Oriental Medicine
MAS   Medical Acupuncture Society
MRC   Medical Research Council
NHS   National Health Service
PMSA Provincial Medical and Surgical Association
PMSJ *Provincial Medical and Surgical Journal*
RCP   Royal College of Physicians
RCS   Royal College of Surgeons
RTCM Register of Traditional Chinese Medicine
SA   Society of Apothecaries
SMN   Scientific and Medical Network
TAS   Traditional Acupuncture Society
UKCC United Kingdom Central Council for Nursing, Midwifery and Health Visiting
WHO   World Health Organization

Introduction

In popular usage the term 'profession' has a wide variety of connotations, spanning from a highly skilled and specialized job to any full-time work from which income is derived (Freidson 1986). The boundaries of interpretation are narrower in sociology, but sociologists have also still to reach agreement about the meaning of the term 'profession' and the related question of which occupations are to count as professions. However, despite the absence of an unequivocal definition (Abbott 1988), most sociologists have for long acknowledged the growing importance of professions in Western industrial societies in the twentieth century. Millerson (1964), for instance, notes that roughly two dozen new qualifying associations were formed in each decade of the first half of the century in England, whilst Ehrenreich and Ehrenreich (1979) point to the rapid expansion in the range of professional occupations in more recent times on the other side of the Atlantic. This trend, moreover, is widely held to be paralleled by a major growth in the numbers of professionals in the work-force (Ben-David 1963; Goldthorpe 1982). Giddens (1981), indeed, has suggested that the proportion of professional workers in neo-capitalist societies has trebled since 1950, reaching as high a level as 15 per cent of the labour force in the United States – a pattern of expansion which is in part associated with the rise of the welfare, enterprise and information-based professions (Watkins *et al.* 1992). And, as if to underline the importance of what are assuredly some of the most privileged and prestigious strata in society (Portwood and Fielding 1981), Halmos (1970) claims that the political power of professionals has escalated too. To be sure, professions have sometimes come under political attack from Western governments in the contemporary era (see, for instance, Burrage 1992), but nonetheless they have increasingly insinuated themselves into positions of power since the turn of the century by becoming more directly involved in both national and local government.

The significance of these developments, though, has often been exaggerated, as is well illustrated by the work of prominent writers on the professions in the 1960s and 1970s. Parsons (1968: 545), for example, argues that the 'massive emergence of the professional complex . . . is the crucial structural development in twentieth century society', whilst Young (1963) holds that the new professional technocratic elite will become more secure in its position of leadership than any other historical dominant group. In a similar vein, Bell (1974) claims that in the post-industrial economy, services will outstrip manufacturing and theoretical knowledge will become the central basis for policy-making. In this new context he believes that the fast expanding technical-professional intelligentsia of Western Europe and the United States will supplant the controlling influence of the bourgeoisie; as Bell says, just as

> the struggle between capitalist and worker, in the locus of the factory, was the hallmark of industrial society, the clash between the professional and the populace, in the organization and in the community, is the hallmark of conflict in the post-industrial society.
>
> (1974: 129)

One problem with such accounts is that to imply that the occupational structure of contemporary Western nations is becoming predominantly composed of a growing number of professional service and technical elites is to engage in a sociological sleight of hand (Kumar 1978). The image of a society with a professional majority is soon lost once it is realized that this category consists of not only groups such as doctors, lawyers and accountants, but also large numbers of clerical employees, waiters, porters and other workers who would conventionally be seen as performing routine menial tasks. A further problem is that even the notion of a narrower band of higher, knowledge-based, professions emerging as a new ruling class cannot readily be extrapolated from more recent trends in the development of professions (Shaw 1987). Such a view also carries the dubious implication that the role similarities of the various segments comprising the 'knowledge class' will transcend the specific interests of each group based on jurisdictional claims and form the basis for a common consciousness (Abbott 1988). In addition, the related arguments concerning the supersession of capitalism and the convergence of the structures of industrial societies can be questioned (Davis and Scase 1985), even in the wake of the recent abandonment of socialism in much of Eastern Europe (Deacon 1992).

In fact, some sociologists have now begun to argue that professions are not so much in the ascendance in Western industrial societies as in the process of being proletarianized or deprofessionalized (see, for instance, Oppenheimer 1973; Haug 1973; McKinlay and Arches 1985; McKinlay and Stoeckle 1988). However, such theories are difficult to examine because of their loose formulation (Elston 1991). And whilst there is evidence for some of the associated claims about changes in the position of professional groups, their proponents also tend to err by overstating the currently depressed state of the professions (Murphy 1990). Although sociologists have at times inflated the contemporary significance of the professions, therefore, this author at least still believes that recent trends continue to endorse the view of Freidson (1973: 19) that these occupational groups are of 'very special theoretical and practical importance' – and thereby raise crucial questions about the nature and role of professions in modern Western societies. None of these questions is more pressing than that on which this book focuses, the issue of whether professional groups subordinate their own interests to the wider public interest in carrying out their work. Certainly, this broad altruism claim is made by most professions in the current Anglo-American context, alongside other central elements of their ideologies like the prescription that the occupation will encourage and maintain high standards of practice and give impartial service. As such, it can be seen as a core aspect of the majority of codes of professional associations today, to which even responsibility to the individual client tends to be subordinated.

The commitment of both established and aspiring professions to the public good can readily be illustrated. Town planners in Britain, for example, frequently claim that they take altruistic decisions in the allocation of land uses as a result of their political neutrality and technical expertise (Simmie 1974). The notion of a duty to serve the interests of the public is, similarly, a traditional component of veterinary codes in this country (Carr-Saunders and Wilson 1933), as well as of the codes of practice of groups such as pharmacists, social workers and nurses (Harris 1989; UKCC 1992). These trends are also clearly exemplified in the British context by the classic case of law where the Council of the Law Society has for long endorsed the general view that the legal profession is for the protection and advantage of the wider public (Council of the Law Society 1974). The altruism claim, moreover, figures no less heavily in the ideology of professions in the United States. Here the standards of conduct adopted by the legal profession, from the early *Canons of Professional Ethics* to the more recent *Code of Professional Responsibility*, have given increasing recognition to the limits imposed on lawyers' actions by the interests of the public

(Marks *et al.* 1972). It is interesting to note too that, as in Britain, such formal expressions of a public-interest orientation are by no means restricted to the highest ranking professional groups; a wide range of professional bodies in America, including the Institute of Chemical Engineers and the Society of Mechanical Engineers as well as the Institute of Professional Architects, have adopted the principle of serving human welfare as a central, codified professional objective (American Association of Engineering Societies 1987).

These tendencies, though, are nowhere more strongly in evidence than in the case of medicine. As early as the nineteenth century in Britain, the Royal College of Physicians (RCP) was defending corporate monopolism in medicine on the basis that the art 'should, as far as possible, be rendered both safe and useful to society' (Navarro 1978: 6). Such claims about the public duties of the profession have been reiterated very often in modern times. Sir Kaye Le Fleming, for instance, reminded doctors at the annual meeting of the British Medical Association (BMA) in 1938 about their responsibilities to 'the public as a whole' (Marshall 1963b: 165) and, as Jones (1981) points out, the BMA today will still argue – like any other professional association – that the ends it pursues promote the common good. On the other side of the Atlantic, meanwhile, the *Principles of Medical Ethics* which the American Medical Association (AMA) adopted in 1912 asserted that the profession 'has as its prime object the service it can render to humanity; reward or financial gain should be a subordinate consideration' (Duman 1979: 127). This theme has been reiterated in its modern code which states that the honoured ideals of the medical profession imply a duty to improve not only the well-being of the client, but also that of the wider community (Berlant 1975). The medical profession in both Britain and the United States, therefore, seems for a long time to have drawn strongly on the spirit of the Geneva Code of Medical Ethics, adopted by the World Medical Association in 1949, which involves doctors in a pledge to consecrate their lives to 'the service of humanity' (Campbell 1975).

The public service aspect of professional ideologies, however, has not always been so firmly emphasized. Gilb (1966) claims that nineteenth-century professional ethics in North America were more concerned with the relationship between individual professionals and their clientele. This view is reinforced in relation to such fields as law, where the early organized efforts of the private Bar placed greater explicit stress on the acquisition and improvement of the skill base for dealing with paying clients than ensuring responsibility to the public *per se* (Marks *et al.* 1972). The broader altruism ethos, though, appears to have been particularly slow to develop amongst professions in England – in large part because this country has historically been far more bound by traditional social distinctions than the United States (Stevens 1971). As a result, Elliott (1972) argues that in the later years of the pre-industrial period in English society, groups like the physicians, clergy and members of the Bar did not need to justify their position on the grounds that their learning was vocationally relevant or that they were oriented to the public good – for this was the period of 'status professionalism', in which such occupations were able to maintain a foothold in the ranks of gentlemen on account of their leisured and honourable life-style. However, such social superiority based on a status associated with the patronage of a small and wealthy group of landed aristocrats could no longer be sustained in the wake of industrialization. Accordingly, Elliott claims that it was only really at this stage, in the face of the decline of the landed gentry and the diversification of demand for services amongst the ascendant commercial and industrial classes, that the professions were forced to develop systematically professional training schools and, most importantly, to cultivate an ideology stressing the need for certified competence and public responsibility. In this shift towards what Elliott categorizes as 'occupational professionalism' in the nineteenth century, Duman (1979: 117) views the service ideal as the crucial aspect of the unique ideology which was being fashioned, for it 'provided professional men with a moral justification for their claim to high social status'.

This adoption of a chivalric code, contrasting with the business ethic which was seen to exhibit greed and selfishness (Perkin 1989), undoubtedly helped to provide an alternative platform for the defence of the established professions in England. From the outset, the new ideology contained references to the duty of professions to serve the wider, public interest; Percival's standard work on medical ethics published as early as 1803, for instance, informed doctors that they should only promote their occupational interests 'so far as they are consistent with morality and the general good of mankind' (Duman 1979: 118). Initially, however, the question of whether the duty of the profession to the client was more important than that to a wider public was much in dispute. But, with the drift away from a predominantly *laissez-faire* system dominated by private professional practice and the emergence of an age in which greater emphasis was placed on the fulfilment of broader public obligations, it was increasingly recognized that service to clients was insufficient in itself. As Marshall (1963b: 163) wrote in 1939: 'the professions are being socialized and the social and public services are being professionalized. The professions are learning . . . to recognize their obligations to society as a whole as well as those to individual clients'. This trend has, if anything, been accentuated over the last thirty years as the number of professional organizations with formal codes of conduct has mushroomed (Harris 1989).

Yet if professions in the Anglo-American context do now more resolutely and frequently claim to serve the public interest, notwithstanding the greater emphasis that has recently been placed on market forces by governments in Britain and the United States in areas previously regarded as the prerogative of the state (King 1987), do these elite occupational groups in fact embody a special moral standard based on the ideal of service? Or should such claims, which are often used in defence of professional privilege, be viewed with rather more cynicism? One of the main aims of the book is to develop an analytical framework for assessing the extent to which the altruistic ideologies of professions in modern Britain and the United States are translated into practice at the macro-level. This task is undertaken in Part I of the text, which highlights the fact that, despite the growing appreciation of the importance of professional groups in Western industrial societies, a rigorous examination of the degree to which professional self-interests are actually subordinated to the public interest is still awaited in the sociological literature on this subject. The reason for this unfortunate and important omission is located in the disturbing tendency of contributors in the field to substitute assertion for argument and to engage in research which is both inadequately formulated and insufficiently substantiated. Accordingly, an attempt is made to tackle the theoretical and methodological difficulties involved and develop a satisfactory research framework for investigating claims about the organized altruism of professions. The empirical applicability of this framework is then illustrated in its entirety in Part II, with reference to a novel case study of the response of the British medical profession to acupuncture in the nineteenth and twentieth centuries. This extensive case study of alternative medicine is centred on the analysis of the explanation for, and the implications of, the predominant climate of professional rejection of acupuncture established over the past two hundred years in Britain and raises important questions about professional accountability. These questions are taken up in the Conclusion, in which recommendations are also made about the future direction of research into the relationship between professions and the public interest.

It merely remains to say that, in discussing the issue of whether professions are 'simple monopolies whose anticompetitive effects distort the social and economic organization of a society or are . . .

institutions which have developed for public interest reasons and should be preserved' (Dingwall and Fenn 1987: 51), attention will be mainly restricted to Western industrial societies in general and the Anglo-American context in particular. Although the analysis of the structure and role of the professions in other parts of the world is no less crucial or interesting (see, for example, Bennell 1983; Heitlinger 1992), this constraint will tend to reduce, if not completely eliminate, the dangers of overgeneralization across national boundaries – especially given claims about the distinctive nature of professional organization in Britain and the United States (Collins 1990a). The book will also be primarily illustrated throughout with reference to examples drawn from the field of health care, ultimately culminating in the case study of acupuncture as a form of alternative medicine. Choosing to focus on one specific area in this way has the merit of increasing the overall coherence of the piece and bringing the main themes into sharper relief. The emphasis on health care in particular emanates not only from personal interest in an increasingly well-studied field, but also from more pragmatic concerns. For all the definitional disputes in sociology about which occupations deserve the title of 'profession', there is more or less universal agreement about the status of medicine in Britain and the United States. Alongside law, it is usually viewed as one of the most powerful classic professions (Morgan *et al.* 1985) and is widely used as a model on which theorizing about the genre has taken place (Moran and Wood 1993).

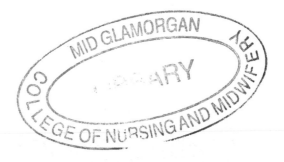

Part I

Sociology, professions and the public interest: a research framework

1 The sociology of professions and the professional altruism ideal

A critical review

As the Introduction to this book has indicated, the recognition given to the contemporary significance of professions in the Western occupational structure has certainly highlighted the pivotal question considered in this book – namely, that of whether professional groups act as altruistically as their own ideologies suggest. It is important to note, though, that this is not a new issue for sociologists in Britain and the United States. The relationship between the altruism ideal and professional practice has for long attracted considerable interest in the sociology of professions (Crompton 1990). Following Saks (1990), this chapter critically reviews the shifting form that this interest has taken in the Anglo-American setting in both the historical and contemporary context.

However, before proceeding further to document and appraise the diverse nature of the sociological contribution to the debate over the extent to which professions – or at least particular segments thereof – subordinate their own interests to the public interest, two points must be underlined. In the first place, it should be stressed that the discussion is centred on professional collectivities and not individual professional workers. These two levels of analysis are frequently confused in the literature, but the distinction is a crucial one for, as Ritzer (1973) points out, there is no necessary relationship between the attitudes and behaviour of practitioners and the institutional characteristics of the professional group of which they form a part. Although several contributors, therefore, have interestingly examined the altruism of professionals (see, for example, Blaikie 1974; Stacey 1980), such social-psychological questions are not the primary concern in this context. The second point which should be emphasized is that, within the macro-sociological focus on professional altruism adopted here, the notion of the public interest is taken to refer to the wider societal obligations of professions and not simply those involving the advancement of the well-being of individual clients. This point warrants reiteration because, as Marks *et al.* (1972) and Campbell (1978) have observed in relation to law and medicine respectively, action which is oriented towards the interests of the client may not always be compatible with the service of a more generalized public.

Having dealt with these preliminary conceptual issues, the direction and strength of the contributions from each of the mainstream macro-sociological schools of thought on the professional altruism ideal in Britain and the United States can now be evaluated. In this process greatest attention will be given to neo-Weberian and Marxist work which currently dominates the sociology of professions. The review will begin, however, by considering the traditional taxonomic approach that formed the previous orthodoxy in this field.

PROFESSIONAL ALTRUISM? THE TAXONOMIC APPROACH

The taxonomic approach, which held a position of ascendancy in the sociology of professions until the late 1960s and still continues to attract its adherents, is based on the assumption that professions can be intrinsically differentiated from other occupations, not least because of the positive and important part that they play in society (Klegon 1978). This approach takes two main forms. The first of these is the trait model of the professions which is based on the compilation of lists of theoretically unrelated sets of attributes, such as extensive knowledge and responsibility, that are seen to represent the central defining features of a profession. The trait account is distinguished by the singular lack of agreement amongst its proponents as to the precise combination of elements unique to professional occupations (Millerson 1964). This is a difficulty which the more theoretically refined, if ahistorical, functionalist perspective on the professions that constitutes the second major strand of the taxonomic approach has largely managed to avoid. For the functionalist, the central components of a profession are generally confined to those held to be of functional significance for either the wider social system or the professional–client relationship – on the basis of which professions are seen to have gained their privileged position in society (Rueschemeyer 1986).

For all their differences, though, the trait and functionalist variants of the taxonomic approach do share a benevolent conception of professions. It is not surprising, therefore, that sociologists of both these interlinked schools of thought have tended to view professions as being essentially altruistic occupations. Although Elliott (1972) has argued that the traditional emphasis on the relationship between altruistic service and professionalism did not continue after the Second World War, the contrary actually appears to be the case. Millerson (1964) discovered from his review of a wide range of Anglo-American literature on the professions – mostly produced in the two decades immediately following the War – that altruism, alongside such items as a lengthy period of training, the acceptance of an ethical code of conduct and skill based on a body of abstract knowledge, was one of the six most frequently mentioned elements of a profession. Freidson (1986) too notes that a collectivity or service orientation was still very commonly cited in definitions of professions deriving from the taxonomic approach in this period. Moreover, with the rare exception of the work of authors such as Moore (1970), these accounts continue to refer predominantly to the characteristics of professional groups rather than individual practitioners, and to service to the wider public as opposed to the client alone in the sense embodied in this book.

The continuing association of altruism with the professions in this regard within the taxonomic perspective can be even more firmly illustrated with specific reference to the trait variant of the approach. Here the subordination of self-interests to the public interest is usually seen as a core feature of the arbitrary and often inconsistent list of attributes which are held to provide an indication of the degree of professionalization of any given occupation. Wilensky (1964: 137) is fairly typical, stating that things like licensure and tenure arrangements are 'less essential for understanding a professional organization than the model of professionalism which emphasizes the service ideal'. Gross (1969) and Bennett and Hokenstad (1973) similarly highlight the centrality of the wider service ethos in professional behaviour – as, indeed, do Greenwood (1957) and Evan (1969) who also suggest that professions are more oriented towards the public welfare than their own parochial group interests. Such contributors can clearly be numbered amongst the many contemporary sociologists who belie Elliott's claims about the content of postwar studies of the professions. Far from diminishing in importance, therefore, altruism seems, if anything, to have become an even more customary feature of the trait model of professional occupations.

Durkheim (1964,1992) was one of the first to introduce this theme into the more developed functionalist variant of the taxonomic approach. Durkheim's conception of professions as a positive force in social development stemmed from his view of society as akin to an organism perpetually striving for equilibrium against pathological and disintegrative influences. He argued that the growing fragmentation of the division of labour in complex modern societies undermined mechanical solidarity, a primitive solidarity of resemblance based on shared values and beliefs. Although Durkheim felt that stability in the modern world would re-emerge in the form of organic solidarity, in which cohesion was rooted in functional interdependence and cooperation, he was concerned lest social order be subverted by the growing emphasis on self-interest. The solution was held to lie in the development of occupational associations which would provide moral authority, checking unhealthy, anarchic egotism and fostering a taste for selflessness. Such professional organizations would serve the public interest by acting as the source of a new moral order – restoring society once more to a condition of healthy equilibrium.

For Durkheim, therefore, the emergence of occupational corporations with a broader territorial basis of recruitment than the medieval guilds was in the interest of society because it would provide the necessary moral regulation to combat the pathological anomic conditions underlying social disorder (Parkin 1992). But, whilst Durkheim focused in detail on the beneficial role of professions as intermediary groups standing between the state and the individual, his comments on the specific content of the professional morality which was to serve as a kind of social cement are rather ambiguous. Most functionalist writers in fact have gone further here and argued that it is the altruistic ethos of professions rather than their integrative function which marks them off from other occupations in terms of the public interest. Thus, Tawney (1921) – who loosely deserves inclusion here in so far as a central theme of his work was that rights were derivative from function (Ryan 1980) – called in the interwar years for the expansion of professionalism into the acquisitive world of industry, so that private interests could be fully subordinated to the needs of the community in a functional society. Embedded in his vision was the image of a profession as 'a body of men who carry on their work in accordance with rules designed to enforce certain standards for . . . the better service of the public' (Tawney 1921: 107). He believed that a Christian conscience could be resurrected through the vehicle of the professions to harmonize the discords of human society and uphold the common good.

In more recent functionalist accounts the stress on altruism as an integral aspect of professionalism has been retained – usually being regarded as not only of functional relevance for society as a whole, but also of great importance in explaining the social and economic rewards of professions. Thus, Goode (1960), for instance, claims that a collectivity orientation is one of two pivotal characteristics of a profession from which, amongst other things, high levels of income and prestige and relative freedom from lay evaluation and control are derived. Barber (1963) similarly treats a primary orientation to the community interest as a key defining feature of professional occupations, arguing that, whilst self-interests are not completely neglected in professional behaviour, they are subserved indirectly. In his view, the existence of altruism in the professions is reinforced by the monetary and honorary rewards bestowed on these groups which function to ensure that the generalized and systematic knowledge in their possession is used for the benefit of the wider public.

The parallel between the legitimizing altruistic ideologies of professions and the work of taxonomic contributors should now be apparent. This parallel does not, of course, provide evidence in itself against the conclusions reached by those operating within the taxonomic approach (Rueschemeyer 1983). Taxonomic authors have, though, generally been guilty of accepting professional ideologies at face value, without seriously appraising the substance of the claims enshrined within them (Daniels 1975). Indeed, trait and functionalist writers have usually not only refrained from conducting rigorous empirical analyses of the relationship between professions and the public interest, but have also failed to provide an adequate theoretical framework within which such assessments might take place. This lacuna has arisen in part because of the self-fulfilling manner in which the service ideal has tended to be built into the definition of a profession by sociologists operating within the taxonomic perspective. The prospect of using this model of a profession as an 'ideal type' against which to examine empirically the altruism of professions, moreover, has hardly been advanced by the absence of satisfactory conceptualizations of crucial terms employed in the debate.

This is well illustrated by the notion of 'interests'. This concept plainly needs to be operationalized if a systematic evaluation is to be given of the extent to which professional egotism prevails over considerations of the common good in decision-making. Yet the notion of professional self-interests has generally been taken for granted as unproblematic and all too rarely explicitly defined by taxonomic writers. Many trait and functionalist accounts emphasizing the altruistic orientation of professions, though, seem to be underpinned by the belief that self-interests are best gauged in economic terms. Tawney (1921), for example, certainly stresses the pecuniary element in his view of private interests. And Barber (1963: 673) goes so far as to suggest that 'money income is a more appropriate reward for . . . self-interest', before contentiously downplaying the importance of such rewards in professional behaviour. Yet even in these instances problems remain.

Why should the advancement of the interests of an individual or group be conceptualized purely in terms of financial criteria rather than, say, indices of power and prestige, which are no less central aspects of the reward system in Western industrial societies? And, notwithstanding these limitations, who is to judge the relative balance of economic gains and losses associated with particular policies – the subject under scrutiny, or an external observer? But perhaps the main difficulty here is not so much that such vital questions have still to be satisfactorily resolved within the taxonomic perspective, as that so many of its proponents have failed to realize the importance of providing an explicit definition of the notion of 'interests' and a theoretical rationale for using this problematic concept in one way rather than another.

Much the same might be said about the employment of the even more controversial concept of the 'public interest'. The reader searches in vain for a clear definition of this term in the work of Greenwood (1957), Goode (1960) and Barber (1963), all of whom talk of professions as having a collectivity or service orientation. This deficiency is very common in the trait and functionalist literature. In fact of the sociologists so far considered, only Durkheim and Tawney – two of the earliest contributors to the taxonomic approach – offer fairly explicit definitions of the public interest. Both of their accounts, though, unfortunately have shortcomings. Tawney (1921: 228) bases his conception of the public good on the maintenance of 'the peculiar and distinctive Christian standards of social conduct'. Yet this yardstick appears outmoded in the light of claims about the growing process of secularization in industrial societies (Wilson 1966). Moreover, such a conceptualization is too vague to be successfully operationalized; although Tawney gives numerous illustrations of the principles Christianity would enjoin, this tradition of social ethics has been expressed in too many differing forms in both the historical and the contemporary context (Latourette 1975) to serve as a sufficiently precise indicator of policies compatible with the public interest. The view taken by Durkheim (1964; 1992) on the common good which is centred on the perpetuation of solidarity and integration in society is also vulnerable to attack. The major problem derives from his tendency to believe that sociology could provide a scientific diagnosis of health and social pathology in this respect (Cuff *et al.* 1990). As Giddens (1978) points out, this involves the tenuous assumption that values can be deduced unproblematically from analyses of 'fact'. The biological analogy which never appeared to be far from Durkheim's mind also creates other difficulties. His conception of the public interest is clearly grounded in the belief that the developing division of labour, like the functional differentiation of the organism, ultimately serves to foster integration in society. Such a notion has understandably not greatly appealed to sociologists who emphasize the analytical utility of viewing modern Western societies as based on inherently conflicting group interests (Rueschemeyer 1983). A more weighty final criticism, however, is that Durkheim tended to assert rather than substantiate empirically his claims about the function of professions in industrial societies. As Rex (1970: 49) comments: 'Instead of . . . seeking to verify statements about the operation of the "organic" elements by reference to social behaviour, the model provided by the analogy has been itself regarded as providing verification for sociological propositions.'

In light of the dearth of systematic empirical analyses of the extent of professional altruism, not to mention adequate and operational definitions of the central terms employed in the debate, it is hardly surprising that even some taxonomic authors have harboured doubts about the public service orientation of professions. Thus, Flexner (1915: 581), one of the pioneering advocates of the professional ideal, nonetheless suspected that organizations of teachers, doctors and lawyers 'are still apt to look out, first of all, for "number one"'. What, though, of the position of those who have been prepared to examine more critically the general function and behaviour of professions in the modern world?

PROFESSIONAL ALTRUISM? THE VIEWS OF THE CRITICS

Predictably enough, those writers identified as critics of the professions have tended to argue that such privileged occupational groups do not subordinate their interests to the common good. This has certainly been true of authors who launched early critiques from outside the realm of sociology. George Bernard Shaw, the famous playwright, for instance, was particularly cynical about what he saw as the pretensions of the professions in this respect (Shaw 1946). It is interesting to note, too, the tone of Sidney and Beatrice Webb in a piece on the professions written for the *New Statesman* at the beginning of the century with assistance from Shaw. Although they accepted that professionals fully catered for the interests of their well-to-do clients, the Webbs felt that they had ignored 'the question of how much professional service the nation as a whole requires, and how the work of the profession can be organized so as to best supply this need' (cited in Duman 1979: 128).

By far the strongest non-sociological critique of the professions, though, came from a much earlier and somewhat different vantage point – namely, that of the supporters of economic liberalism in Britain and the United States in the nineteenth century who shared a belief in the desirability of maximizing economic competition in the marketplace, maximizing the freedom of individuals to do as they pleased and minimizing state intervention in economic affairs. From this perspective, the 'unseen hand' of the market was held to provide a self-equilibrating system which would be fair to all and contribute to the larger community interest (Heywood 1992). Accordingly, economic liberals tended to see the professions as organizations collectively rigging the market in their favour at the expense of the wider public. As such, they concurred with Adam Smith, who had complained in the eighteenth century about the presence of corporate monopolism in English medicine (Berlant 1975). Milton Friedman is, of course, the most famous contemporary exponent of this position. He also argues that licensure is not in the public interest, even in the field of health care. State licensure underpinning professional privilege in this area in the United States has, he claims,

> reduced both the quantity and the quality of medical practice; ... it has reduced the opportunities available to people who would like to be physicians forcing them to pursue occupations they regard as less attractive; ... it has forced the public to pay more for less satisfactory medical service, and ... it has retarded technological development both in medicine itself and in the organization of medical practice.
>
> (Friedman 1962: 158)

These accounts of critics of the professions, though, are no less problematic than those of writers operating within the taxonomic tradition in sociology. Shaw, for example, again defines too narrowly the notion of professional self-interest which is weighed against the common good – in terms of financial criteria alone. Moreover, whilst one of the clearest and most explicit definitions of the public interest has been provided by the proponents of nineteenth-century liberalism, questions must be raised as to how far this is an appropriate philosophical yardstick against which to assess the altruism of the professions. In an age in which governments in Western industrial societies have generally sought to move away from a *laissez-faire* approach and foster the growth of a welfare state (Mishra 1981) – notwithstanding recent backsliding (Lane and Ersson 1991) – it must be asked whether classical liberalism furnishes a conception of the public interest which is any more applicable than the flawed notions of Durkheim and Tawney, who paradoxically view the common good in terms of the restraint, rather than the encouragement, of unfettered individualism.

The focus of this chapter, however, is on sociological perspectives on the altruism issue and it is to these that the analysis will now return.

A striking feature of the history of the sociology of professions is just how long it took for critical questions to be widely raised about the nature and role of professional occupations in general, and the degree to which professions displayed an altruistic orientation in particular. As Freidson says:

> Until recently, most sociologists have been inclined to see professions as honoured servants of public need, conceiving of them as occupations especially distinguished from others by their orientation to serving the needs of the public through the schooled application of their unusually esoteric knowledge and complex skill.
>
> (Freidson 1983: 19)

It is ironic that when a more critical approach to the professions did begin to emerge in sociological circles in the Anglo-American context in the period shortly after the Second World War, it was those operating within the predominantly micro-sociological frame of reference of interactionism who were the standard-bearers. Contributors employing this perspective, like Hughes (1951; 1963) and Becker (1962), refused to take professional ideologies on trust and treated the notion of professionalism as little more than a socially negotiable label. In this way, they were able to challenge several key assumptions of trait and functionalist writers on the professions – including claims about the widespread existence of professional altruism (Atkinson and Delamont 1990).

Interactionist accounts of the professions, however, are not only open to the accusation of being all too rarely based on a systematic consideration of evidence (Cuff *et al.* 1990), but are also of questionable relevance in this context because they are characteristically pitched at the micro-level. In the case of the altruism issue this is manifested in the focus on the orientation of individual practitioners towards clients rather than the interplay between the institutional features of professions and the wider public. Thus Becker (1962), for instance, argued that the symbol of a profession as an occupational group with codes of ethics to protect clients could not be taken as a realistic description of professional practice, for all professions contain unethical operators. Since this approach deviates from the macro-sociological concerns of this book, the remainder of the discussion about the contribution of the critics to the altruism debate will be centred on the broader-based work of neo-Weberian and Marxist authors which has become the new orthodoxy over the past two decades in the sociology of professions.

The neo-Weberian perspective

Sociologists adopting what is seen here as the neo-Weberian approach to the professions define these occupational groups primarily in terms of their monopolistic control over either the market for particular services (Parry and Parry 1976; Parkin 1979; Collins 1990b) or such related spheres as work organization (Freidson 1970) and the definition and satisfaction of client needs (Johnson 1972). This approach, which involves the direct or indirect application of the concept of social closure developed by Weber (1968) to the study of the professions, shares with interactionism the advantage over the taxonomic perspective of opening up more fully to empirical analysis questions concerning the nature and role of professional occupations in society, whilst at the same time avoiding its more obvious pitfalls – namely, the theoretical difficulties that interactionists have in dealing with, *inter alia*, the broader substance of professional privilege and the structural conditions underpinning successful strategies of professionalization (Saks 1983). This advantage is obviously no less applicable to the specific question of whether professional groups can be relied upon to subordinate their own interests to the common good, an issue on which neo-Weberian contributors in Britain and the United States have usually taken a highly sceptical line.

However, although sociologists working within this framework have conducted some useful empirical studies of particular professions on this basis (see, for example, Berlant 1975; Larkin 1983) and rightly avoided building formal assumptions about a public service orientation into their conceptualizations of a profession, doubts can be cast on the extent to which they have fully capitalized on their macro-sociological approach to the altruism issue. As has been observed by Halmos (1973), amongst others, the wave of public antipathy towards the professions since the 1960s has still far too frequently led writers in this school to make overly sweeping and unsubstantiated claims about the self-serving nature of professional groups. As such, existing neo-Weberian contributions to the consideration of the relationship between professions and the public interest may be said to represent little or no improvement on taxonomic accounts. This conclusion is borne out by a review of some of the more established literature in the field, which clearly illustrates that the neo-Weberian critics have also generally failed both to define adequately central concepts employed in the debate and to adduce convincing bodies of evidence in support of their characteristically more cynical case.

The relative absence of analytical rigour in this respect is epitomized by the early work of Johnson (1972), whose now classic book *Professions and Power* does not always adequately represent the standpoint of the taxonomic contributors he would condemn – particularly that of Parsons. Parsons is portrayed as holding that the professions, in contrast to business, 'are actuated by the common good' (Johnson 1972: 13). Yet in his analysis of the professions, Parsons stresses the similarities rather than the differences between the professional and commercial sectors in modern society, even going so far as to state:

> The typical motivation of professional men is not in the usual sense 'altruistic', nor is that of business men 'egoistic'. Indeed, there is little basis for maintaining that there is any important broad difference of typical motivation in the two cases, or at least any of sufficient importance to account for the broad differences in socially expected behaviour.
>
> (Parsons 1949: 196)

To the extent, moreover, that Parsons does associate a collectivity orientation with professional behaviour, he refers not to the service of the common good but of the client, and not to professions as Johnson suggests, but to professional roles. This point is thrown further into relief by the comments of Parsons (1952) on the medical profession in *The Social System*. As Ben-David correctly remarks, for Parsons, the apparent altruism of professional people

> is but an institutionally expected behaviour restricted to the professional–client relationship and is not necessarily generalized into broader social attitudes. The display of sympathy and understanding toward the client are only the requirements for the efficient performance of the service, just as good personal relations are the requirement of efficient work organization in a factory. Accordingly, Parsons did not see in the professional roles and associations indications of the rise of a new collectivist type of class. He interpreted them rather as structures adapted to the performance of certain functions characteristic of the existing modern type of society.
>
> (Ben-David 1963: 248–9)

This quotation also makes it clear that Parsons' account is pitched at the normative, as opposed to the descriptive, level in that it refers not so much to what professionals do as to what they should be doing. Although Parsons does not perhaps appreciate that deviations from his model of professionalism are anything more than peripheral phenomena in this respect, there is plainly evidence here of an additional misinterpretation by Johnson.

Nonetheless, it is true that many trait and functionalist writers do put forward community service claims on behalf of the professions in the sense which Johnson has in mind. Yet when he goes on to criticize such arguments, further problems arise. In brief, Johnson is sceptical of the claim that professions serve the public interest, because the application of professional codes does not have uniformly beneficial consequences for different sections of the community. Johnson may or may not be right to accept Rueschemeyer's argument that the legal profession, for example, provides services which are 'irrelevant to those groups in the society who seek radical change in the existing order' (Johnson 1972: 25) and that 'the values and organisation of that profession will vary in their consequences for different class or status groups' (Johnson 1972: 34). But to adopt a definition of the common good based on the view that applied knowledge should be of equal relevance to all sections of society – including advocates of Black Power and supporters of the Women's Liberation movement as well as those who wish to maintain the status quo – is not very helpful, because it is difficult to imagine any circumstances under which this requirement could ever be met. In other words, this criterion is far too stringent, closing off the possibility of any meaningful investigation into the question of professional altruism. To be fair, Johnson does suggest that the rationale for employing this conception is that it is the one which is embedded in taxonomic accounts. But this is not a watertight defence since, as has been seen, very few sociologists working within this framework actually articulate their definition of the public interest and, of those who do, Johnson's characterization surely only applies to the least refined trait and functionalist contributions (Saks 1985).

Johnson's early work, though, is not atypical of the genre. Many studies of the relationship between the professions and the public interest from the neo-Weberian perspective have proved deficient. Elliott (1972: 94), for example, seems very ready to accept the claim that, in the professions, 'no matter how lofty the ideals, given a choice between ideals and self-interest, the latter would prevail'. Yet he does not provide sufficient documentation to sustain this viewpoint, especially as far as the crucial issue of the service ethos is concerned. The main problem with Elliott's account in this respect is that the evidence he does adduce relates mainly to individual practitioners rather than professional organizations *per se*, and is largely limited to one particular profession in a single society – namely, lawyers in the United States. Krause (1971) fares little better in his discussion of this subject. To his credit, he does make an effort to state explicitly the meaning of the key concepts employed in the altruism debate, associating 'interests' with the gaining of benefits and the 'public interest' with a vaguely formulated version of egalitarianism oriented towards improving the position of the 'have-nots' in society. But even within this framework – which certainly requires much further refinement – he does not always appraise satisfactorily the extent to which particular policies serve professional self-interests rather than the public good. Thus, Krause specifically denies the altruism of the American legal profession on the grounds that its ethics committees are more interested in curbing the unauthorized practice of outsiders than checking serious abuse, but does not demonstrate that more stringent forms of self-regulation are necessarily beneficial to the public. This is problematic because tighter official control of individual deviance may well force lawyers to avoid undertaking risky, though well-advised, procedures at the expense of the public welfare. It is not without reason that Parsons (1952: 471), in another context, has suggested that the reliance on such informal controls as the colleague boycott in professional work 'may have its functional significance'. Part of the difficulty with the conclusions that Krause reaches may reside in his failure to distinguish adequately the wider public interest from the immediate interests of individual clients – a difficulty which also besets the more recent and otherwise incisive analysis by Mungham and Thomas (1983) that sheds doubt on the question of how far the response of the Law Society and its regional bodies to the duty solicitor scheme in England and Wales could be said to be altruistic.

The field of health care, however, will be used to provide the main illustrations of the deficiencies of neo-Weberian work on the altruism debate. In this respect, Robson (1973) has studied the implications of the control which he argues doctors have for long possessed over the health arena in Britain. After asserting that the medical profession in this society has always given priority to maintaining its own dominance rather than serving the interests of the public, Robson goes on to argue that this is exemplified by the opposition of the BMA to the National Health Service (NHS) in 1948, which contravened the 'needs of the population'. However, at no stage does Robson specify exactly how the nature and direction of the public interest in this sense is determined – although he does imply that he reached his more limited conclusions about the NHS because of the basic right of all persons to adequate health care. Yet this still does not fully establish his claim in this instance, even though state intervention in Britain in 1948 assuredly did establish a medical service available to all, and free at the time of use. What, for example, of those commentators who would argue that judgements about the public interest should embody not only a concern for equality, but also respect for individual freedom? It is on such grounds that Conservative politicians have subsequently sought to support their arguments for the expansion of the private medical sector in this country (Chandra and Kakabadse 1985). Indeed, some members of the Adam Smith Institute and the Centre for Policy Studies have put forward a case for wholesale private market-based solutions to the problems of the NHS (Mohan 1991), following the argument that 'the supply of goods and services, including medical care, should as nearly as possible be based upon individual preferences' (Lees 1965: 32). Robson's stress on adopting egalitarian principles in health care may also be further weakened by the fact that, although the NHS seems to command high levels of public support (Taylor-Gooby 1985), survey research has not consistently shown a majority of the population to be in favour of the preservation of universal state medical provision (see, for example, Lindsay 1973). Of course, there may well be good reasons for downplaying the importance of negative fluctuations in consumer preferences or for utilizing different criteria for assessing the public interest in health care in Britain. But the onus is on Robson to clarify the meaning of the term and carefully argue out his case; there is no room in this area for presupposing that any specific pattern of usage and application is unproblematic. Much the same comments also apply to Robson's discussion of the role of the professional self-interests which he sees as having deleteriously affected the public welfare in the health field. Here, Robson not only provides insufficient empirical evidence to sustain his far-reaching claims about the influence of such interests on the behaviour of the medical profession in general and on the BMA's opposition to the NHS in particular, but also predictably omits to define formally the meaning of this much-contested concept in the health context.

The difficulties surrounding the use of the notion of 'interests' in neo-Weberian accounts can be illuminated further with reference to the work of Jamous and Peloille (1970), whose study is often cited in the contemporary Anglo-American literature on the professions to high-light the challenge to more positive interpretations of the behaviour of such groups (see, for example, Roth 1974; Burrage 1990). Their inquiry questions Parsons' belief in the primacy of cognitive rationality in Western industrial societies, making reference to the resistance offered by the French University-Hospital Corps in the nineteenth century to the important discoveries of Pasteur in bacteriology and Bernard in physiology. Since these innovations threatened the elite by disputing the quality of what was then produced and transmitted, Jamous and Peloille argue that:

The valorization of the clinical orientation in medicine and the attachment to the norms and the balance of forces underlying it, which were to be responsible for the fame of the French school, were gradually to become ideological rationalizations and the instruments of defence of a sort of 'social caste' when faced with changes imposed by these expanding fields of study. The aim of this 'caste' was more to preserve its acquired positions and privileges and perpetuate its own identity than to open up and to share in the new stock of knowledge which was to be progressively built up outside itself.

(Peloille 1970: 131)

There is no denying that these authors go some way towards substantiating their claims, not least by noting that members of the professional elite stood to lose a considerable amount of income from private practice if they adopted the new research-oriented approach, and that they possessed the power to resist the threat through their control of the medical rewards system. But they do not go far enough in bolstering their argument for the centrality of professional self-interests in the defence of the clinic. In the first place, their account parallels that of Robson in that they fail to set out clearly and defend their notion of 'interests', even if their implicit definition of this concept in terms of the augmentation of income, power and prestige might not raise too many objections. They also neglect to examine rigorously potentially important alternative explanations for the rejection of the work of Pasteur and Bernard – such as the view that it was due to professional ignorance or client demand, rather than egotism. Indeed, they do not even provide any evidence to demonstrate that the replacement of the old paradigm was desirable from the standpoint of diminishing morbidity and mortality rates; questions regarding the superiority of the results obtained by employing the new knowledge and the relative therapeutic potential of the competing medical systems, then, are strangely left open, although the answers cannot be treated as self-evident in light of the growing critique of the efficacy of modern medicine (Illich 1976; Gould 1985; Pietroni 1991). In consequence, substantial doubt must be shed on their explanations of trends in medical science. While Jamous and Peloille (1970: 112) introduce their study by eschewing work based on preliminary conceptions of 'the social function *thought* to be performed by professions', their investigation, in the final analysis, must be vulnerable to precisely the same charge.

Admittedly, some neo-Weberian sociologists of the professions have exercised more caution in assessing the altruism claims of professional occupations. Freidson (1970), for instance, wisely shows an appreciation of the need for evidence in judging the extent to which the professional service ethos is translated into practice at the macro-level. He is, therefore, only willing to engage in a guarded critique of such occupations, suggesting that 'all that may be distinct to professions about a service orientation is *general acceptance of their claim*' (Freidson 1970: 82). For all this, however, Freidson still does not provide sufficiently rigorously worked out guidelines for investigating the altruism of professional groups in medicine and other fields in liberal-democratic societies. Although he develops an interesting interpretation of the public good based on such fundamental citizenship rights as equality and the self-determination of goals, he does not deal entirely satisfactorily with the problems involved in moving from these abstract, and potentially conflicting, principles to concrete evaluations of specific cases of professional decision-making. It is not enough for Freidson to rely as he does on the determination of the good of society by the courts, given the dangers in assuming that legal systems necessarily produce judgements based on rational reflection about the public interest (Tomasic 1985). Too little attention is also given to the discussion of the comparative theoretical merits of both this conception of the public interest and that of self-interests which Freidson views as a potentially countervailing influence on professional behaviour. This is disappointing in light of the important philosophical debates about the meaning of such terms (see Friedrich 1966 and Saunders 1983 respectively). But if even more sophisticated analyses of the altruism issue from the neo-Weberian school do not stand above criticism, what of the Marxist approach to professions?

The Marxist perspective

Marxist sociologists are no less sceptical about the altruism of professional groups than the neo-Weberians, but justify their claims on markedly different grounds – primarily because their accounts of the professions are based on the relations of production, rather than the relations of the market (Saks 1983). This distinctive common thread underpinning the Marxist literature on the professions in Western industrial societies should not, however, mask the diversity in Marxist thought about the ways in which such occupations are linked to what are seen to be the dichotomous and exploitative relations of production under capitalism. A minority view represented by Baran (1973) is that professions are lodged in an objectively antagonistic relationship with the bourgeoisie in the capitalist system of production, performing functions which would need to be multiplied and intensified in any future socialist society. More generally, though, Marxist writers regard the activities of professional occupations less favourably, viewing them as being either partially or wholly tied to the interests of the bourgeoisie (see, for example, Sibeon 1990). As the work of Braverman (1974), Carchedi (1975) and Poulantzas (1975) demonstrates, the precise nature of the linkage here much depends on where the line of class cleavage is drawn between the bourgeoisie and proletariat. Nonetheless, for all the variations within this more critical Marxist approach, its adherents are agreed that professional groups in one way or another play a significant role as agents of capitalist control in the contemporary Western world.

Marxist authors, then, share a predominant cynicism about the general nature and role of professions in countries like Britain and the United States – a cynicism which is clearly reflected in the position adopted by such contributors on the altruism ideal. In this respect, the public service ethos of professions is usually seen as a convenient myth which conceals not simply occupational self-interests, but also the supervisory and disciplinary tasks that professional workers perform for the dominant capitalist class. Thus, despite the prevalence of the altruism ethos in professional ideologies, Johnson (1977: 106) in his later, Marxist phase emphasizes the role played by professional elites in areas such as accountancy in carrying out 'the global functions of capital with respect to control and surveillance, including the specific function of the reproduction of labour power' and Picciotto (1979: 170) highlights the specific role of lawyers in 'reinforcing and maintaining the wage-labour relation in a way that is functional for capital'. Esland (1980a), moreover, is at pains to stress that personal service professions also serve as custodians of the capitalist system in seeking to diagnose and reshape people's behaviour under the auspices of scientific and humanitarian ideologies; for Esland, the essential contradiction in the work of welfare occupations like psychiatry, health visiting, child psychology and personnel management is that they claim to be mitigating the worst effects of monopoly capitalism and yet serve to uphold the very principles of social order on which it is based. It is important to note that Marxist sociologists regard this social control function as politically malevolent, as opposed to benign as in the structural functionalist perspective. The possibility of professions acting altruistically, therefore, is typically denied since the public interest is seen to lie in the transcendence of capitalism and the development of the higher phases of communism, not in bolstering an oppressive system. As a corollary, professions in this frame of reference are normally held to be self-serving; it is argued that such occupations are able to preserve their relatively highly rewarded position in society by maintaining the status quo and avoiding engagement in the kind of radical action on behalf of clients advocated by writers like Brake and Bailey (1980) and Langan and Lee (1989) in social work.

Such claims, though, just as those of the neo-Weberians, remain contentious. One major problem is that Marxist sociologists too often tend to assume, rather than demonstrate, that professional occupations operate in the interests of the dominant class in the Anglo-American context. Johnson (1977), for instance, seems to presuppose in his later work that the occupational control so characteristic of professions derives from the fact that they fulfil important functions for capital, without appreciating the need to provide systematic comparative evidence on the role of such groups in the occupational structure (Saks 1983). The deficiencies in Johnson's position here are thrown into relief by the lack of recognition he gives to the emergence of radical factions in the professions – which not only display awareness of the dilemmas of working within the structural limitations of advanced capitalism, but also see the solution of many of their clients' problems as lying in the establishment of a socialist system (Perrucci 1973; Watkins 1987; Senior 1989). It is, of course, true that organizations like the Socialist Medical Association in Britain and the National Lawyers Guild in the United States have never commanded more than minority support within their respective professions. Yet clearly the claims of any Marxist analysts of professional occupations should at least be tempered by the existence of such bodies. In this sense, it is encouraging to note that some Marxist studies of the professions – as, for instance, that of Esland (1980a) – do explicitly acknowledge these radical developments and sometimes endeavour to account for them from the standpoint of Marxist theory. Indeed, even Johnson (1980) more recently begins to follow this example when he draws attention to the new-found militancy of British junior hospital doctors and other professional groups and relates this to the tensions which occasionally occur between professions and the capitalist state in the continuous process of class formation.

However, in attempting to establish that the role of professions in Western industrial societies like Britain and the United States is largely compromised, many Marxist accounts run into a more important difficulty – namely, that of assuming that the state, which has increasingly acted as a formal employer of professionals and effectively underwritten the privileges of professions, is relatively autonomous of any particular fraction of capital and represents the long-term interests of the capitalist class as a whole. Such a conception plainly underlies the work of Castells (1978) who, in his structuralist Marxist analysis, sees the operation of the professions involved in urban planning as state intervention to regulate system contradictions within the limits of the capitalist mode of production. A similarly deterministic interpretation of the relationship between the state and capital, moreover, leads Cockburn (1977) to the conclusion that community work functions to reproduce the labour force and the relations of production under contemporary capitalism. However, as Saunders (1983) has convincingly argued, the structuralist notion of the state underpinning such accounts is not only teleological, but, more significantly, also effectively immune from falsification since every reform or policy introduced by the State and/or its agents must, by definition, be oriented towards the preservation and reproduction of capitalism. That this notion fails to square with the work of authors such as Abbott and Sapsford (1990) who accept the social control dimension of the operation of professions, but do not see this as irrevocably linked to dominant class interests, is an irrelevance for its Marxist proponents; for structuralist Marxists, the prospect of professions ultimately functioning in anything but the long-term interests of the bourgeoisie is theoretically precluded. Accordingly, much of the thrust of their implicit, and occasionally explicit, denials of professional altruism is, of necessity, based on assumption rather than carefully formulated and empirically grounded argument.

This weakness is no more apparent than in the work of Navarro in the health arena on which this book draws as a prime source of illustration. Navarro (1976; 1978) argues that the activities of the medical profession in both Britain and the United States are primarily influenced by capitalist class relations and that this is reflected in the contribution which the medical sector makes to capital accumulation by, *inter alia*, improving the productivity of labour and legitimating capitalism by dealing with the dislocation and diswelfare generated in the process of production and consumption in a capitalist system. Navarro (1986: 27–8) has recently reiterated this position, asserting that, from the viewpoint of capital, the 'medical profession is a stratum of trustworthy representatives to whom the bourgeoisie delegates some of its authority to run the house of medicine' and that the form of medical provision therefore changes 'according to the needs of the mode and social relations of production at each historical conjuncture.' Yet whilst this claim casts doubt on the altruistic orientation of doctors as a collectivity from a Marxist perspective, Navarro's analysis is predicated on two central assumptions which render his analysis self-fulfilling. The first of these is that the medical profession is inextricably bound up with the capitalist class and has little independent influence on the health field in its own right, a view which can be strongly challenged by a number of influential empirical studies of the part played by the medical profession in the development of health care in the Anglo-American context (see, for example, Eckstein 1960 and Starr 1982). The second major presupposition made by Navarro is that the state – which has had an important impact on the professional delivery of health care not just in Britain, but also to some degree in the United States – represents the interests of the capitalist class as a whole, a claim which seems to be largely based on the dubious belief that intent in policy-making can be inferred from the effects of policy as far as the house of medicine is concerned (Saks 1987). None of this, of course, is to deny that there may be some circumstances in which the medical profession could be seen as upholding the capitalist system. But it is necessary in this context to expose the pitfalls of analyses like that of Navarro which bring the integrity of professional groups into question by imposing a self-validating framework of assumptions on their subject matter.

Yet if Marxist work on the professions should be framed in such a way that there is at least the possibility of the state and, by extension, the professions acting independently of capitalist class interests, it is also worth stressing that the socialist conception of the public interest embedded in the accounts of Marxist contributors must be applied with great care if it is to be of any academic utility. In this respect, Marxist sociologists have very often been guilty of sweepingly judging professions in the Anglo-American setting directly against a distant conception of the common good completely alien to the prevailing liberal-democratic societies within which they operate. Irrespective of whether such societies are in fact dominated by the interests of capital, the abstraction of professions from their socio-political milieu in this way seems to be more obstructive than conducive to fruitful research into the extent to which professional groups fulfil their obligations to the wider public – a point which is highlighted by Brown's study of the division of labour in the health field in the United States. Brown concludes that the existing organization of American health care, in which physicians retain control over other subordinate health workers,

> is neither efficient nor favourable to the public interest. Medicine for profit leads inevitably to conflict over occupational territories, to distortion of the division of labor for the sake of income rather than service, and results in either the exploitation of workers through low wages or the exploitation of customers through high prices. Far

preferable would be a socialist division of labor among occupations whose cooperative interaction would serve everyone's needs.

(Brown 1973: 443)

This blanket condemnation of professional dominance in a society which is avowedly not guided by any form of Marxist philosophy raises questions about the relevance of applying a full-blown socialist notion of the public interest to the assessment of professional behaviour in such circumstances. Brown can also be criticized in the same vein as a number of other Marxist contributors for making no attempt to substantiate her contentious assertion about the virtues of a socialist division of labour in health care. This is a major source of omission for authors like Field (1957) who have argued that the situation in such self-proclaimed socialist societies as the Soviet Union, where it was possible for semi-professional health personnel who were party members to have power over fully-fledged physicians who were not, was actually a threat to the welfare of the population because it undermined authority based on skill, knowledge and competence. Admittedly, Bossert (1984) has drawn attention to some of the advantages of socialist policies in health care following the overthrow of the Somoza regime in Nicaragua, including the increased emphasis on prevention and the transfer of a considerable amount of responsibility to the community. But, unless the merits of socialism are to be taken as a pure article of faith, it must be said that Marxist contributors such as Brown do not do their position justice by treating claims about the nature of the public interest in such a superficial fashion.

It should finally be pointed out that Marxist sociologists have not always been successful in conceptualizing professional self-interests in such a way that the altruism issue can be profitably addressed within the perspective with which they operate (Sibeon 1990). These difficulties are in part bound up with the fact that in Marxist accounts the interests of individuals/groups and the public as a whole are both held, in the last analysis, to lie in overthrowing the capitalist state and building a communist social order in which human self-alienation will be abolished. This theme makes it difficult to develop an operational framework for assessing the altruism of professions, since empirical inquiry into possible conflicts between professional self-interests and the common good is seemingly ruled out *a priori*. This dilemma is readily apparent in the sometimes rather heavy-handed radical social work literature of the late 1960s and early 1970s (Langan and Lee 1989) – such as the critique by Cannan (1972) of trends in the health and social services field in Britain. In this study, the logic of Cannan's Marxist position leads her to argue that social workers in this area should openly take a political stand and 'recognize their *common* interests with clients, dropping the idea of the client–professional relationship' (Cannan 1972: 261). Having taken this stance, however, it is difficult for Cannan also to employ the concept of 'interests' in apparently contradictory fashion to explain why most social workers have not followed a more radical line. She therefore accounts for the persistent and heavy reliance of practitioners on casework skills simply by referring, in a conceptual vacuum, to factors like the risks to the jobs and careers of those involved in adopting alternative approaches, without mention of self-interests, even though this whole area seems potentially suitable for explanation in such terms. This should not be taken, though, to imply that Marxist analyses are inherently incapable of dealing with the notion of 'interests' in evaluating the extent to which self-interest prevails over the common good in professional behaviour. Clearly, an adequate conceptual framework for this purpose can be developed, providing a distinction is drawn between short- and long-term interests. But, unfortunately, writers like Poulantzas (1973a) who make this distinction are the exception rather than the rule. Consequently, many Marxist discussions of the professions follow Cannan in containing only implicit and indirect references to professional self-interests in the sense encapsulated in this book.

The work of Marxist contributors on the professions, therefore, has scarcely improved on that of the neo-Weberian school as far as the altruism issue is concerned. Like neo-Weberian accounts, Marxist studies in this area have far too frequently consisted merely of the uncritical reiteration of anti-professional beliefs. Key terms in the debate have been either inadequately conceptualized or, worse still, not defined at all. Empirical evidence has also only sporadically been used to sustain the positions maintained. In light of these shared failings, therefore, the Marxist and neo-Weberian critique of professional claims to subordinate self-interest to the common good is paradoxically little more firmly grounded than the more benevolent view of professions taken by the much castigated authors working within the taxonomic perspective.

CONCLUSION

On the one hand, then, sociologists have been prepared to take the altruistic ideologies of professions at face value. On the other, professional groups have been condemned for their lack of social responsibility. Johnson (1972: 17) has suggested that such inconsistent views which currently coexist in sociology 'may be explained by the fact that they relate to different professions at different points in time and also that contradictory processes may exist in the development of any single profession.' This proposed explanation for the Janus-headed profile which professions have presented to the sociologist in Britain and the United States, however, is, at best, highly partial in view of the imperfection of work conducted to date on the subject. This is not, of course, to say that the altruism debate can be resolved in a manner which is wholly without presupposition. But the fact remains that the problem has still to be satisfactorily formulated or researched within any of the mainstream sociological perspectives on the professions considered in this chapter. As such, existing sociological literature on the extent to which the altruistic ideologies of professional groups are translated into practice mirrors that on the nature and role of the professions more generally which has also been shown to lack empirical rigour across the spectrum of theoretical approaches on offer (Saks 1983).

If this deficiency is to be remedied, sociologists must develop means by which the altruism issue can be systematically investigated. Given the range of competing perspectives which exist in sociology, however, there is obviously more than one possible way of dealing with the fundamental theoretical and methodological questions involved. But this does not mean that no general guidelines can be provided for such an enterprise. As Saunders (1983) points out, although sociology is manifestly multi-paradigmatic, a major criterion of adequacy of all sociological theories claiming to go beyond the level of idealized classification is that they must be testable within the bounds of the paradigm from which they derive. It follows, therefore, that any viable research framework for assessing the degree to which professions pursue their own interests at the expense of those of the wider public must be capable of generating the counterfactual conditions required to subject theories about the altruistic orientation of professional groups to rigorous examination (Saks 1990).

This is a very important principle in this context, for it is precisely this task of specifying the conditions under which such theories would need to be abandoned or at least modified that sociologists of professions in Britain and the United States have not yet adequately undertaken. In this respect, it is clear from the review of the literature conducted here that any analysis will need to give particular attention to the problem of how the self-interests of professional groups are to be identified; how the relative importance of professional self-interests as opposed to other explanatory factors is to be assessed in particular decision-making situations; and how the compatibility of specific policies with the public interest is to be discerned. If these questions are not directly and judiciously addressed, the altruism issue will continue to be handled predominantly by theoretical fiat.

A major aim of this book is to tackle these central theoretical and methodological difficulties and to provide an acceptable framework within which the altruism claims of professions can be empirically examined. The task of developing such a research framework is taken up in the next two chapters, beginning with the formulation of an operational concept of the public interest against which to evaluate the behaviour of professional groups.

2 The development of a viable conception of the public interest

If a viable conception of the public interest is to be established for evaluating the extent to which considerations of the collective good prevail over occupational self-interests in professional behaviour, it is first necessary to explore the various interpretations of this term to date. In this respect, as was seen in the Introduction, the notion of the public interest employed by professions in the contemporary Anglo-American context has very little specific meaning, save for the fairly nebulous emphasis on a commitment to serving society as a whole. Even fewer clues can be picked up from its broader employment in everyday affairs – especially in the arena of politics where it is usually left totally undefined. Since contradictory policies are quite often supported by a common appeal to the public interest (Griffith 1985), it is small wonder that cynics have argued that the term means nothing more than the originator's own view of a desirable course of action. Certainly, politicians and civil servants seem to use it as a smokescreen to conceal decisions based on the interests of the groups that most effectively deploy their resources (Barry 1967a). And Marxists in particular tend to see the government's employment of the concept of the public interest in political debate as a component of the dominant ideology, since decisions defended in such terms are generally held to represent the interests of the ruling class (Hyman 1984).

Yet if popular usage has little to offer in the development of a rigorous concept of the public interest, can academic accounts clarify the picture? As will be recalled from the last chapter, sociologists of the professions writing on the altruism issue scarcely inspire an affirmative answer to this question, for they usually fail to specify the meaning of the 'public interest' and leave an implicit, undefended and often equivocal definition to be teased out by the reader. This situation is not just due to intellectual slackness, but also to the great difficulties involved in the undertaking. Hickson and Thomas (1969), for instance,

omitted altruistic service from their scale of the degree of professionalization of different occupations, as they found that they were
unable to operationalize the concept.

Some commentators, however, have despaired about the possibility
of formulating an analytically fruitful concept of the public interest, not
because of the absence of clear definitions of the term, but because it
has been employed in such diverse ways in scholarly accounts. This
diversity is illustrated, as was seen earlier, by the varied philosophical
bases of the definitions of the few social scientists prepared overtly to
explore this subject in the debate over the altruism of professional
groups – which span from the Christian social ethics of Tawney (1921)
to the economic liberalism of Friedman (1962). These exceptional
accounts, though, do not fully express the variety of hues and shades
assumed by the notion of the public interest in the academic literature
(Heywood 1992). The shifting usage of the concept can be traced
historically from Plato and Aristotle through Augustine, Locke and
others to the late nineteenth-century interpretation of Marx (Niemeyer
1966). Even in modern society, moreover, the term has been employed
in highly divergent ways in different academic disciplines; Colm
(1966), for example, notes the relativism of sociological definitions, the
stress on judicial interpretations in law and the emphasis economists
place on the satisfaction of individual wants in their delineation of the
public interest. But not all the divergencies are accounted for by
disciplinary boundaries. Frankel (1970), for instance, finds it conceptually helpful to distinguish 'objectivist' and 'subjectivist' yardsticks of the national interest, whilst Schubert (1960) classifies existing
views of the public interest into 'rationalist', 'idealist' and 'realist'
explications.

Such problems, though, do nothing to undermine the enterprise
engaged in here. It does not follow from the vague and misleading usage
of the concept of the public interest in everyday life that the term cannot
be precisely delineated and profitably applied. And whilst there are
extensive disagreements about the notion of the public interest amongst
academics, these do not entail, as Rosenau (1968) suggests, that it
should simply be viewed as a datum requiring analysis in political
action. In terms of such disagreements, it is difficult to see how the
'public interest' fundamentally differs from widely used and respected
concepts like 'class' and 'alienation'. Concepts are theory-dependent
and the fact that social scientists operate with a broad spectrum of
theoretical perspectives will inevitably lead to a divergence of view. Of
course, some particular notions of the public interest may be inadequately formulated in relation to the theoretical framework in which

they are embedded, but this does not mean that the concept in general should be dispensed with (Saks 1990).

The utility of a concept, then, cannot be divorced from the purpose for which it is intended. The specific purpose of this chapter is to develop an operational notion of the public interest against which the activities of the professions in Britain and the United States can reasonably be judged. Now that the main in-principle objections to this exercise have been countered, further progress can be made by critically appraising the relevance to the task at hand of three major explications of the public interest outlined by Held (1970) – the unitary, preponderance and common interest conceptions respectively.

UNITARY CONCEPTIONS OF THE PUBLIC INTEREST

Unitary conceptions of the public interest assert a frankly normative position for the public interest, which is seen as a moral concept, constituted by a unitary scheme of moral judgements that ideally guide decision-making in society. Importantly, too, arrangements which serve the public interest in these terms cannot validly conflict with individual claims of interest. Definitions falling within this compass are numerous, including those of Plato, Aristotle, Augustine, Aquinas and Hegel. Although there are distinctions to be drawn between the work of each of these contributors – according to the significance given, for example, to the religious, rather than the political, order in defining the public welfare (Niemeyer 1966) – they all crucially share the belief that what is good for the individual/group is compatible with the good of all (Held 1970). This normative unitary view, though, is no more clearly accentuated than in Marx's work. Whilst Marx objected to the modern bourgeois state, which Hegel had seen as representing a unity of human interests, he argued that the real interests of both individuals and the public as a whole coalesced, albeit in a communist system in which the free development of each would be the condition for the free development of all (Lukes 1985).

Before evaluating such accounts, however, it is worth briefly illustrating the implications to which unitary conceptions of the public interest can give rise in the health field in Britain and the United States. Marxists, for instance, argue that the public interest lies in the establishment of a communist health system which

> will imply a change not only in the distribution but, most important, in the production of health, where health, disease, and medicine will not be ontologically defined by a dominant class, and administered

by 'experts', but . . . will be defined and reproduced by a collectivity
of unexploited agents, within a division of labor in the production
of knowledge, practice, and institutions that will not be exploiting
nor exploited.

(Navarro 1986: 257)

Other unitary conceptions would, of course, see different policies as
being in the public interest. In a religious frame of reference, Roman
Catholics might claim that this would be best served within the existing
political structure of Western industrial societies by the adoption of a
range of moral principles including the prohibition of abortion under
any circumstances, as the foetus has an immortal soul and a destiny in
the eyes of God (Campbell 1975).

Nonetheless, however applicable particular unitary notions may
seem to be in the health field, the general approach raises difficulties
from the viewpoint of the research framework under construction here.
One major problem concerns the moral implications of unitary conceptions of the public interest. Totalitarianism can, for instance, be
justified by many of these conceptions in so far as they can be seen as
entitling the state to override individual rights and to sacrifice personal
development to the sovereign end of the body politic. This certainly
appears to have been the case in Soviet-style socialist societies (Raskin
1986), but is most starkly exemplified by the horrific medical experiments conducted on prisoners of war and those in concentration camps
in Nazi Germany (Phillips and Dawson 1985). Unitary views which
emphasize the moral authority of the Church as opposed to the state can
also carry similar abhorrent implications based on moral intolerance.
The persecution of female healers in the witch hunts of the sixteenth
century underlines this point (Oakley 1992). In such circumstances, it
must be questioned whether it is legitimate to employ a concept of the
public interest in research focused on countries like Britain and the
United States which would manifestly not be morally acceptable to
most people living in these societies.

Admittedly, it might be claimed that the above examples involve the
distortion of socialist and Christian ideas (see Navarro 1977 and
Poynter 1971 respectively). But whatever the merits of this view,
reservations must still be expressed about the relevance of these
particular notions of the public interest to an Anglo-American context
which, as seen in the previous chapter, has been interpreted as being
both capitalist and increasingly secularized in modern times. All unitary
conceptions of the public interest are also of questionable relevance in
this contemporary setting because they are, by definition, universally

rooted in a political principle that is alien to liberal-democratic countries – namely, the idea that irreconcilable or conflicting interests are unjustifiable (Hague and Harrop 1987). Nor can proponents of the unitary approach rescue their position by appealing to natural law, for so many incompatible principles have been put forward on this basis in areas ranging from blood transfusions to organ transplants that the force of the argument evaporates (Campbell 1975). However, some sociologists might contend that since fact and theory are inextricably linked, the inquirer is free to adopt any concept that accords with his or her own political standpoint. But this still does not resolve the dilemma. Any research into altruism in the professions in Britain and the United States is destined to be a singularly barren exercise if it is built around a concept of the common good rooted in moral values to which doctors and other professional groups could not be expected, nor indeed would purport, to subscribe. A crystal ball would hardly be needed to forecast the results of such an investigation for it would not be dealing with the problem in its own terms.

In sum, therefore, unitary conceptions of the public interest seem to suffer from a certain inapplicability to ongoing deliberations and decisions. Held amplifies and extends this criticism by stressing that in modern Western societies

> the appearances of conflict are so inescapable and overriding that, . . . as far ahead as one is likely to be able to see, one can predict that situations of conflicting interests are those which will have to be argued about and resolved. To assert that someone involved in such conflicts is always misguided, or that one of any two conflicting positions must be evil, is to close one's sensitivities to the actualities of human affairs.
>
> (Held 1970: 156)

In consequence, Held (1970: 156) concludes that 'to consign the concept of the public interest to an unforseeable time at which all such conflict can be called unjustified is to rob the concept of current utility'. The lack of utility to which she refers, though, is no more apparent than in the context of this book. If justifiable conflicts of individual interests are to be ruled out, it is clearly going to be conceptually difficult, if not impossible, to tackle the problem under consideration – an issue that was highlighted in relation to the Marxist treatment of the professional altruism debate in the last chapter.

Whilst unitary conceptions do have the virtue of underlining the normative content of the public interest, there must be grave doubts as to whether they can be used to assess the extent to which professional self-interests hold sway over the public interest in policy formulation.

A further set of explications of the public interest, therefore, will now be considered.

PREPONDERANCE ACCOUNTS OF THE PUBLIC INTEREST

Preponderance accounts of the public interest take the public interest to be represented by policies which satisfy the majority of individuals or, at least, increase aggregate individual satisfaction. There are a number of ways in which it is argued that these calculations should be made. But the obvious advantage of the preponderance approach is that, unlike the unitary conception, it does provide for the possibility that the public interest may not be in the interests of all individuals and groups.

This approach has roots which go back to Epicurus and is reflected in the work of Hobbes and Hume in British philosophy (Held 1970). Its most well-known and influential historical form, however, is undoubtedly that of utilitarianism, of which Bentham was a prime exponent and which, baldly stated, holds that the formula for determining the right decisions in any situation is to avoid pain and maximize happiness for the greatest number of people (Plant 1991). This equation, moreover, seems highly applicable to dilemmas in health care; as Campbell (1975) suggests, for instance, a contemporary Benthamite would probably favour increasing hospital staffing levels in a child psychiatric unit at the expense of a geriatric ward when resources are tight, given the greater potential long-term effects on the happiness of the majority.

Bentham's ideas still have an impact today, for economists often use arguments based on the interpersonal comparison of utilities to solve the problems of welfare economics (Musgrave 1966; Hill and Bramley 1986). Their endeavours usually go under the label of the cost–benefit approach which aims to enumerate and sum as completely as possible all the costs and benefits expected in particular situations, in order to provide a basis for decision-making. This technique for determining the public welfare – and a variant form called cost-effectiveness analysis, which is employed when benefits are difficult to measure and/ or render commensurate – has been regularly applied in the health sector to such issues as the treatment of rheumatism and kidney disease, the introduction of mass screening programmes and comparative methods of psychiatric care (Pentol 1983). The preponderance approach, though, has gained recent expression not only in the writings of economists, but also in the work of political scientists. Such contributors tend either to stress the importance of consulting public opinion directly through the ballot box to discover the common good

(Schubert 1966) or to argue that the public interest is equivalent to the interests of a preponderance of actual and potential interest groups in society (Dearlove and Saunders 1984). Both kinds of political science approach are illustrated in the health field by Lindsay (1973: 88), who observes that institutions like the British NHS can only be justified 'if a large segment of society believes that medical care should be distributed equally among men of all stations, and is willing to bear the costs of implementing these beliefs'.

However, such aggregationist views of the public interest do not stand above criticism. Despite the illustrations given, they would not be very easy to operationalize in the context of the professional altruism debate. This is indicated by the problems faced by the early utilitarian approach in taking account of factors like the quality of life as well as purely quantitative elements when evaluating the merits of different health policies (Campbell 1975) – problems which are strongly reflected in the controversy current surrounding the use of QALYs (quality adjusted life years) by health economists in assessing priorities in health care (Ashmore *et al.* 1989). A further classic dimension of difficulty in judging which course of action will result in the 'greatest happiness' relates to the frequently uncertain consequences of medical intervention (Phillips and Dawson 1985). Similar problems also apply to modern cost–benefit analysis, especially in pricing intangible elements like the patient's time and the relief of pain which cannot be conventionally costed (Culyer 1975). By far the most obvious item, though, to which it is hard to assign a monetary value – as a unique and irreplaceable good – is the much-debated concept of life itself (McGuire *et al.* 1988). Nor should it be imagined that political scientists working within the preponderance framework escape such operational dilemmas. Braybrooke (1966: 147), for example, notes that 'when there is no policy that would gain a majority over each of the other ones proposed . . . we are prevented from identifying social choice with the results of voting in any rationally satisfactory way.' This problem is particularly likely to occur when relatively unfamiliar subjects – such as the role of homoeopathy in the NHS, which has been discussed in the House of Commons in Britain on more than one occasion in the postwar years (Inglis 1980) – are approached without shared values. And given the shifting, uncertain and tentative character of most identifications of interest, there are also practical difficulties in ascertaining the direction of such interests at particular moments in time to compute the public interest equation (Bodenheimer 1966).

But although the complications involved in implementing preponderance accounts are substantial, they should not be overstated, for at least some of the difficulties can be circumvented. Probability theory could, for example, be used by utilitarians to resolve the problem of the uncertain consequences of action, whilst political scientists might argue that there are relatively few occasions in which a clear ordering of individual or group preferences fails to emerge. A more fundamental objection to employing a preponderance account of the public interest in this context, though, is that such accounts, like the unitary conceptions considered earlier, can carry implications which would not be morally acceptable within the confines of contemporary Britain and the United States. Conducting potentially harmful clinical trials without the consent of the patients involved, for instance, could be justified by utilitarians on the grounds that the data obtained would bring about 'the greatest happiness of the greatest number' through the development of more effective medical procedures (Campbell 1975). Equally, the emphasis placed by political scientists on majority opinion in decision-making in health and other fields opens the way for people to express selfish preferences in the process of resource allocation which could lead to the infringement of the protection given to minority rights in liberal-democratic societies (Dryberg 1992). Clearly, then, aggregationist notions of the common good run into similar difficulties as unitary conceptions, in so far as they tend to favour policies to which the population in general and professional groups such as doctors in particular could not be expected to adhere.

That the preponderance approach lacks moral applicability in the examination of the altruism claims of professions in the Anglo-American context is not surprising. As Held (1970) notes, any attempt to ground the concept of the public interest simply on a greater weight of actual opinion, a superior group strength or an aggregate gain in utility necessarily faces a familiar ethical problem – namely, that it is logically impossible to derive a normative judgement from a set of empirical statements. To the extent that the public interest is a normative notion, therefore, it cannot be based on empirical data about the capacity of the interests of some individuals or groups to outnumber, outweigh or overpower those of some other individuals or groups. Accordingly, there are further reasons for having serious reservations about the credentials of the aggregationist account.

Preponderance conceptions, then, seem no more viable than unitary views of the public interest in relation to the task at hand. Admittedly, they do permit individual and/or group interests to diverge legitimately from the common good which at least would enable the inquirer to assess the relative role of professional self-interests in decision-making.

But, since such notions of the public welfare are importantly flawed in other significant respects, a concept of the public interest applicable to the research framework being developed here must be found elsewhere.

THE PUBLIC INTEREST AS COMMON INTEREST

Definitions of the public interest in terms of common interest certainly seem worth exploring from the viewpoint of the professional altruism debate, if only because they at least appear to avoid some of the operational difficulties of aggregationist accounts, since they base judgements of the public interest on non-conflicting interests rather than on decisions between conflicting interests or preference scales. More specifically, the common interest approach equates the public interest with individual interests which are shared by all members of the polity. Unlike unitary conceptions, however, the common interest view acknowledges that what is in the interests of an individual or group may not always be equivalent to the public interest, and that individual interests may validly conflict.

Rousseau is the leading historical figure associated with this perspective. He felt that governments should meet the class of interests over which there was unanimity – that is, the 'general will', as distinct from private individual interests (Heywood 1992). But since Rousseau felt that the common good could only be established if the whole people could meet in assembly, his notion of the 'general will' can strictly be regarded as inapplicable to large, modern states such as Britain and the United States (Campbell 1978). Accordingly, the remainder of this section will focus on the appraisal of more recent conceptions of the common interest which are more in tune with the nature of the contemporary Western industrialized world.

One much-employed formulation fitting in with the common interest approach in economics is the well-known Pareto criterion of optimality, which asserts that the welfare of a group of individuals can only be considered to increase if at least one individual in the group is made better off without anyone being made worse off (Sugden 1981). This conception is certainly relevant to the contemporary context as Arrow (1973) illustrates. He suggests that the growth of state medicine in societies like the United States is in the public interest, since the market mechanism does not yield a Pareto-optimal allocation in medical care, primarily because of the non-marketability of the bearing of health risks and the imperfect marketability of information. Another type of common interest approach is represented by the philosopher Barry (1965), who highlights the interests people have in common as members of the public and divides these into negative and positive applications, according to whether they are aimed at the prevention of undesirable activities or the direct provision of benefits. Barry (1967b: 197) interestingly follows Arrow in citing government medical programmes as examples of policies which serve the common interest, for 'though the benefits and costs are always specific, nobody can know whether over the course of his life he will gain from them or not so it may be in everyone's interest to support such programmes and save worry'.

For all their apparent applicability to medical policy, however, these attempts to reduce the public interest to common interest ultimately face even more operational difficulties than conceptions deriving from the preponderance framework. The main problem arises because, as was made apparent in the discussion of the definition of the public interest adopted by Johnson in the last chapter, the common interest requirement is too stringent; as Held (1970) observes, if an individual's own estimates of his or her interests are to count for anything, then the judgement that particular decisions are in the public interest could never be made. Such difficulties in applying the common interest approach are very apparent in the case of the Pareto criterion, which, Musgrave (1966) suggests, overlooks gain or loss from change in relative position. Consider, for example, the philanthropic funding of medical research in the United States, the history of which has been documented by Berliner (1985). If money from a private benefactor was spent on investigating, say, possible cures for deafness, it may superficially seem that the deaf would gain and no other group would lose. But other categories of sick individuals – such as cancer sufferers – might need some convincing that they had not lost, since their comparative standing in the research expenditure hierarchy would have been altered. Similar comments might be made about Barry's contribution, which also seems at best to 'yield weak but not strong orderings of aggregated preferences' (Runciman 1970a: 228). Barry gives no indication of how to decide on the common interest in cases where some indeterminate persons are harmed as a result of the benefit to other indeterminate individuals. And even if common interests are identified in activities like increasing government intervention in health care and education, his account provides no more of a guideline than the Pareto criterion for resolving disagreements over the amount of resources that should be allocated to each. Indeed, these shared operational difficulties are accentuated by the so-called 'free-rider' problem which arises because, even when joint interests can be discerned, it is more in the interests of particular individuals that others apart from themselves bear the cost of the activities to which they relate (Boadway and Bruce 1984).

A second limitation of the common interest approach is that, like the preponderance and unitary conceptions, it can lead to the equation of policies which would widely be regarded as unjust in the Anglo-American context with the public interest. The utility of employing accounts such as that of Barry as yardsticks against which to assess the altruism of doctors and other professional groups must, therefore, be doubted. As Benn and Peters relate,

> even where the objective is of general benefit, a truly 'common good' it does not follow that it should therefore override all other claims . . . . For instance, the common good of defence might not be a good enough reason for uprooting a hundred families to make a rocket range. It might be better to compromise for the benefit of the few, and make do with a somewhat less efficient range elsewhere.
>
> (Benn and Peters 1959: 272)

Similar questions might be raised about the Pareto criterion, for a Pareto-optimal solution could widen, or at least condone, existing patterns of inequality in a manner opposed to the central political ideals of liberal-democratic societies. The strongly supported claim, for instance, that the disadvantaged position of women pursuing careers in medicine should be ameliorated on both sides of the Atlantic (Leeson and Gray 1978; Lorber 1984; Riska and Wegar 1993) would scarcely be permissible under the Pareto criterion since it would be likely to involve, amongst other things, a reduction in the number of male doctors in more prestigious and highly-rewarded medical roles. The common interest conceptions so far considered are therefore too restrictive in a moral as well as operational sense for the purpose at hand.

It might be argued, though, that such problems are not intrinsic to the general approach on the strength of the ideas put forward by Rawls who stipulates that:

> All social primary goods – liberty and opportunity, income and wealth, and the basis of social respect – are to be distributed equally unless an unequal distribution of any or all of these goods is to the advantage of the least favoured.
>
> (Rawls 1973: 305)

This is certainly a conception rooted in the common interest mould that largely accords with present Western moral and political ideas, as the latest work by Rawls (1993) on *Political Liberalism* underlines. It also seems to be operational, as McCreadie (1978) has illustrated in her analysis of the debate about the financing of the British health service. The view, however, that this theory of justice – which Rawls concedes may be only part of a vision of the good society – provides the basis for formulating a viable notion of the public interest is ultimately a chimera because it relies on a highly questionable heuristic device termed the 'original position'. More specifically, Rawls derives his theory from the interests people would allegedly share in a situation in which they are ignorant of their endowment as individuals, their social position and the state of development of their society. But unfortunately Rawls is only able to establish an apparently workable notion of the common interest which conveniently meshes with modern liberal ideas by introducing moral bias into his model – by assuming, *inter alia*, that people in the original position would not be prepared to gamble on where they might end up in a society with wide inequalities (Dworkin 1975), and that such individuals are unaware of the class identity which Marxists argue would cause them to seek an end to exploitation rather than merely to improve the lot of the disadvantaged piecemeal (Fisk 1975).

Yet if Rawls' much-acclaimed enterprise is crucially flawed because there is no Archimedian point for judging the basic structure of society, what of the functionalist form of the common interest approach which has been widely employed by taxonomic authors in the professional altruism debate? It is finally worth assessing how far the functionalist concept of the public interest escapes the dilemmas faced by other proponents of this general approach in the consideration of the extent to which professions serve the public good in Britain and the United States because of the frequency with which it too has been used to support dominant Western liberal moral and political ideas (Dunleavy and O'Leary 1987).

Although there are many variants of functionalism, its underlying theme is that societies are best conceived as social systems consisting of interdependent parts which adjust and adapt to meet general biological and/or social needs (Lee and Newby 1983). Within this framework it can be inferred that the public interest is served when these functional needs are met and society is maintained in a state approximating to equilibrium. This tenet certainly coloured the thinking of Durkheim, as has been seen in the previous chapter, as well as that of subsequent functionalist contributors – not least Parsons, whose implicit notion of the public interest rests on the need of every social system to ensure that the functional prerequisites of adaptation, goal attainment, integration and pattern maintenance are fulfilled (Rocher 1974). Parsons (1952) illustrates the application of his functionalist analysis to health care in this context by suggesting that the public interest is served when the pattern variables of affective neutrality, universalism, functional specificity and a collectivity orientation are adopted by doctors in their relationship with clients to foster the application of technically effective medicine, based on scientific competence and good faith, in the task of preserving, repairing and enhancing the ability of actors to carry out necessary social roles.

But despite the seeming relevance of the functionalist form of the common interest approach to health care, it has been prone to operational difficulties. The field is littered with examples of *a priori* theorizing and tautological arguments – including those relating to the functionalist theory of stratification (Cuff *et al.* 1990). Even Parsons fails to explore adequately his own claim about the functional value of affective neutrality in the doctor–patient relationship, given that this could be interpreted by the patient as disinterest and thus prevent system needs from being met (Berlant 1975). Notwithstanding such aberrations, though, Parsons' work shows that the functionalist concept of the public interest can potentially offer as much operational promise as that of Rawls in conducting meaningful empirical investigations into the altruism claims of professions. What ultimately condemns the functionalist approach, however, is that the rationale for establishing the public interest is rooted in the dubious idea that societies can be seen as reified entities, having certain needs as a whole (Mennell 1980). This leads Rex (1970) to observe that what functionalism passes off as the 'objective' functional needs of social systems rest in reality on an implicit scheme of goals and values. As such, functionalist contributors must be open to the same charge as Rawls of covertly introducing moral bias into their purportedly value-free conceptions of the public interest.

Since the functionalist account is no more convincing than that of Rawls, the public interest as common interest view would seem to be untenable. Indeed, the final blow to this type of conception is that the teleological functionalist position under discussion, which deals with the problem of system regulation without reference to the purposive actions of social actors, follows the formulations of Barry, Pareto and Rawls in not allowing justifiable conflict between the public and individual interests. This, by definition, accentuates the inability of common interest conceptions, like unitary accounts, to permit an adequate analysis of the relationship between professional self-interests and the public welfare.

TOWARDS A VIABLE DEFINITION OF THE PUBLIC INTEREST

Several notions of the public interest deriving from the unitary, preponderance and common interest perspectives have, therefore, thus far been rejected. But this does not mean that the discussion to date has been unproductive. On the contrary, a careful assessment of the shortcomings of the approaches so far considered allows the development of a list of minimum requirements for a viable notion of the public interest in the context of the research framework being constructed here.

In the first place, it is clear that any acceptable definition should be relatively easy to operationalize and apply to a wide range of situations. The operational dilemmas of the common interest and, to a lesser extent, preponderance conceptions must, as far as possible, be avoided. A second prerequisite of an applicable formulation of the public interest is that it should not follow common interest and unitary perspectives in ruling out justifiable conflicts between individual/group interests and the public good. The concept, therefore, must be defined in such a way that the extent to which decisions are shaped by the self-interests of professional groups rather than the common good is open to empirical assessment. As has been seen, the prime virtue of preponderance accounts is that they do allow for this possibility. Yet in basing the concept of the public interest on aggregationist principles, such formulations can be criticized for attempting to derive normative concepts from empirical statements. This gives rise to a third essential feature of any acceptable notion of the public interest – namely, that there must be recognition that the public interest is a normative concept, prescribing what people ought to do rather than simply reflecting a preponderance of opinion or utility. However, this still leaves open the question of how the choice is to be made between the whole range of potentially applicable normative concepts on offer. As was shown in the discussion of unitary conceptions of the public interest, it is not sufficient to invoke natural law as the basis for the selection. It is also evident that it is inappropriate to hold against professional groups notions of the public interest to which they would neither purport to, nor be expected to, subscribe; to employ definitions prevalent in alien cultures or at other points in time would turn research into the altruism of professions in Britain and the United States into a sterile and meaningless exercise. Accordingly, a fourth requirement of any adequate conception of the public interest is that it should be relative to the time and place with which the inquirer is concerned. This distinctly sociological feature of the concept of the public interest is important because it neatly extricates the researcher from all the problems faced by philosophers like Rawls who attempt to establish transcendental principles against which human conduct is to be appraised.

This statement of minimum prerequisites goes a long way towards resolving the difficulties of establishing a viable notion of the public interest. Yet not all concepts meeting even these criteria fit the bill. This is exemplified by the idealist view of the public interest set out by Schubert (1960), which relies on the wisdom of government officials like political leaders, administrators and judges to define the public good. Admittedly, this conception – which would interpret the general welfare in the health field as lying in such officially legitimated action as the introduction of Medicare and Medicaid in the United States in 1965 (Anderson 1989) and the reorganization of the NHS in Britain in 1974 and 1982 (Levitt and Wall 1992) – is simple to operationalize, allows individual/group interests to conflict with the public interest and is characterized by both relativity and prescriptive content. But the notion of reducing the public interest to the decisions of public officials is doubly flawed. First, it is an excessively limiting definition, in that it precludes the possibility of actions like the BMA's struggle to improve medical care in face of the money-pinching poor law authorities in nineteenth-century Britain (Vaughan 1959) from being considered as public interest endeavours because they lack official government sanction. The second weakness of the idealist account is that state-legitimated decisions may be a very poor indicator of the public interest, for, as the low priority given to the foundation of an adequate health prevention system by the Republicans in the United States indicates, officialdom does not always operate in the sugar-coated manner implied (Raskin 1986). The greatest problem with the idealist definition in this respect is the fact that government decisions may be based on the views of the most powerful factions, rather than rational reflections about the public interest (Simmie 1974). Since the substantial corporate power of a number of professional bodies – including doctors – has been widely accepted on both sides of the Atlantic (see, for instance, Wilding 1982; Freidson 1986), conceding that the public interest lies in whatever the public authorities declare it to be is likely to rob the inquirer of a good deal of analytical leverage in evaluating the degree to which professions act altruistically; the futility of employing the rulings of government officials as a bench-mark here is obvious if such decisions are heavily shaped by the power of dominant professions in their areas of presumed expertise.

For these reasons, the idealist position must be discarded as inapplicable to the problem at hand. It is now clear, though, that any viable notion of the public interest must be broader than the decisions of state agencies alone and must ideally have roots completely independent of government officials. A wider, more autonomous conception of the public interest would not only permit the evaluation of government policy itself, but, most importantly in this context, also avoid the adoption of a self-validating indicator of the altruism of professional groups. Such stipulations, together with the criteria set down earlier as minimum requirements for an adequate conception of the public interest, can, however, be met by defining the concept in terms of the established complex of common values prevalent at the time and place under consideration. As Cohen says, these basic values may

> relate to substance as well as to the rules of the game – to ideals of human well-being, to fundamental methods for achieving them, and to basic procedures for resolving disputes when disagreement and conflict concerning means as well as ends arise. They ultimately determine what satisfactions are to be sought, who are to be satisfied, and at whose expense. The basic values need not have originated from all or most of the members of the community; indeed, as is more likely, they spring from the more articulate and influential within it. What makes them community values is acquiescence in them by its members, either overtly, implicitly, reluctantly or by default.
>
> (Cohen 1966: 156–7)

It is argued here that only when a policy or decision meshes with such values can it be seen to be in the public interest.

In this sense, it should be stressed that since both contemporary Britain and the United States are liberal democracies – each possessing a representative and elected legislature, an executive accountable to this organ, a network of centres of private power serving as a brake on the activity of government and a system of political checks and balances (Finer 1974) – the social principles of the liberal-democratic state should form the basis of any yardstick used to appraise the public interest claims of professions in this context. The central principles in such political communities include the objectives of promoting the overall welfare, seeking justice, and securing the maximum amount of liberty compatible with these ends (Benn and Peters 1959). As they stand, though, these principles are not particularly meaningful because they do not sufficiently distinguish the moral ends of modern liberal democracies from other historical and current forms of society (Raphael 1990). This can be illustrated with reference to the concept of 'justice' which is as much appealed to by revolutionaries as upholders of the liberal status quo (Parsons 1952). It should be made clear, therefore, that the ideal of promoting the overall welfare in contemporary liberal democracies refers to the responsibility of the State for seeing that some measure of material support – as, for example, protection from unemployment, sickness, and old age – is available to all its citizens. Justice here defined, moreover, relates to claims for consistency, the removal of arbitrary inequalities and the provision of equal satisfactions of certain basic needs. Unless there are relevant grounds for making exceptions, this concept enjoins the pursuit of goals like equality before the law and equality of opportunity for self-development. The concept of liberty, on the other hand, embodies the notion of the absence of restraint from doing what one chooses; political and social institutions, in consequence, should be designed to preserve or achieve freedom unless there are good grounds, such as the defence of the state from external threat, for interfering in the affairs of particular people or groups. The ideal of liberty, then, is usually associated with, amongst other things, freedom of thought, freedom of discussion, freedom of assembly and association and freedom of the individual to own private property in the modern democratic state.

This is the broad normative framework, therefore, within which it is argued public interest claims should be evaluated in liberal-democratic societies like Britain and the United States. The distinctiveness and relativism of this notion of the public good can be highlighted by contrasting it with the conception of the collective interest that would, on this interpretation, prevail in such socialist countries as the previously constituted Soviet Union and China where – in contrast to the Western democratic model – responsibility rests with a single, dominant party for formulating and upholding the ideology that is the exclusive official creed of the state (White *et al.* 1990). From the standpoint of this socialist ideology, as Parkin (1979) comments, the rights sought and defended in liberal democracies are perceived as being merely formal in content because of the continuing existence of social classes. The claim to preserve freedom, for example, is seen as no more than the right of a small minority to exploit and trade on the labour of others (Campbell 1978), whilst the notion of equality is held to refer to equality of opportunity to compete in an already unfairly weighted contest, not equality of condition that would enable all individuals to develop freely (Gould 1981). Accordingly, as was apparent in the earlier discussion of unitary approaches, the public interest in socialist states is viewed as being furthered by the transcendence of a class society based on private property and the development of a communist order characterized, *inter alia*, by freedom from domination and the primacy of social need as a distributive principle (Heywood 1992).

If this comparison throws into relief the distinguishing features of the definition of the public interest for assessing the activities of professions in the Anglo-American context, a number of additional points also need to be made about the general nature of the conception of the common good advocated here. In the first place, it should be noted that the public interest is not a goal, since it cannot be attained, only protected or advanced within the confines of the social principles of the form of society in which the evaluation is taking place – be this liberal democracy, socialism or some other political variant. Nor can the concept be seen as fixing a unique optimum, for factors like technological capabilities are constantly changing; as Raskin (1986) suggests, the common good should be viewed as a fluid notion, rather than a compendious final objective. Moreover, no claim is made that there will be complete, or even large-scale, agreement amongst the population of any given community about the desirability of the broad moral principles encompassed in the notion of the public interest advanced here. There may in fact be overt conflicts over basic values – for competing moral conceptions of what is good and right can exist within the framework of a single social system along class, religious, racial and other lines. Indeed, as Mann (1982) has argued, even if there is social cohesion, this may owe more to a lack of commitment to core values on the part of the less privileged than a sharing of these values. But although a fairly high degree of accord is likely unless the system is purely based on naked coercion (Cohen 1968), it should be emphasized that the notion of the public interest put forward in this context does not formally hinge on the employment of the tenuous methods of preponderance theorists to calculate empirically the degree of acceptance of central moral values. The concept is also strengthened by the avoidance of the pitfalls of the teleological functionalist approach, as it is not assumed that the institutionalized values associated with the collective interest meet the needs of any specific social system.

OPERATIONALIZING THE CONCEPT OF THE PUBLIC INTEREST

This may all seem very convincing, but questions might still be raised about whether even this conception of the common good is too vague and general to be fully operationalized. Admittedly, consideration of the public interest in the sense outlined here would permit the identification of decisions showing a flagrant disregard for justice, liberty and the overall community welfare in the liberal-democratic societies of Britain and the United States on which this book focuses. But what of situations when these principles conflict, where there would appear to be no clear guidelines for discerning the meaning of the concept of the public interest to evaluate the behaviour of professional groups?

Benn and Peters (1959) deny that conflicts between the principles of the social democratic state pose a major problem in this respect.

Notwithstanding the possible tension between, say, aggregative and distributive principles, they argue that the morality of particular decisions will depend on the extent to which the needs and interests of people liable to be affected by them have been considered with no partiality towards the claims of those with needs and interests at stake. Yet this argument is difficult to accept, because they fall into a similar trap to Rawls in endeavouring to establish a higher principle by means of which political debates can be resolved – even though in their case this principle would only apply within the relativistic and limiting constraints of the moral framework of liberal-democracy. The problem is that there is no impartial way of determining the proper balance between the ends of freedom, justice and the advancement of the overall welfare where these goals conflict (Barry 1967a).

This point can be reinforced by considering the varying balance that has been struck between these social principles in differing liberal-democratic societies. As Raphael (1990) observes, in the *laissez-faire* days of the eighteenth and nineteenth centuries, freedom was usually given priority over notions of justice and welfare, with state intervention being kept to a minimum. Today, in contrast, most countries in the democratic world have taken a more positive view of the goals of ensuring equal rights and catering for the basic needs of the whole population at the expense of curtailing a certain amount of individual liberty. But even contemporary democratic societies display a considerable degree of variation in the way in which they handle the tensions between the social principles on which they are based. Different views prevail, for instance, as to what constitute the basic necessities of human existence that ought to be provided for all and that can be afforded; Mishra (1981) notes in this regard that the United States has not generally given such a high priority to the provision of a welfare state as Western European societies.

Such distinctions seem largely to relate not to variations in the extent to which the interests of various groups are considered impartially, but to important differences of values which exist within the political communities of liberal democracies. Donabedian (1973) sets out two polar views in this respect. On the one hand, he distinguishes the libertarian position which sees charity as the proper vehicle for social concern and freedom as the supreme political good. Proponents of this viewpoint place their faith mainly in the invisible hand of the market and limit considerations of equality to ensuring equality before the law. On the other hand, he highlights the egalitarian position which puts less stress on the political ideal of freedom and far more on meeting basic needs through collective provision and ensuring equal opportunities for

achievement. Donabedian goes on to illustrate this debate with reference to health care, asserting that whilst libertarians favour the private
medical system, egalitarians wish to remove medical care from the
reward system and to guarantee equal entitlement to all. As such, his
argument clearly endorses the view of Abel-Smith (1976) that there is
no value-free theory for resolving the problems of organizing and
financing health services – even within the broad political confines of
the liberal-democratic state.

The upshot of all this is that the definition of the public interest based
on the central values of liberal democracies can only provide a fairly
weak criterion for distinguishing altruistic endeavours in the Anglo-
American context. However, it is argued that such operational difficulties can be circumvented and acceptably strong guidelines for
discerning the public interest established if the concept is further
particularized by defining it in terms of the dominant values prevailing
at a specific time in the liberal-democratic state under scrutiny.

This can be illustrated with reference to the British democratic state
in the latter half of the twentieth century. Whilst there have often been
bitter conflicts over priorities in the period since the War – and
especially since 1979, when the Conservative government came into
office (Tivey and Wright 1989) – these have generally taken place
within an overriding and substantial area of political consensus lying
rather more towards the egalitarian than libertarian pole of Donabedian's spectrum. In this respect, for all the rhetoric which has issued
from the Conservative Party about the need to return to Victorian values
(Riddell 1991), the consensus in Britain has continued to embody a
significant element of egalitarianism coexisting with a growing political
emphasis on the market (King 1987). Notwithstanding obvious differences of political opinion over the past few decades about such issues
as the extent to which the ideal of fairness should outweigh that of
liberty and the public welfare, then, the Conservative and Labour
Parties have generally agreed in modern times that 'some weight should
be given to incentive for the sake of individual freedom and of a higher
national product and that some weight should be given to the reduction
of inequality for the sake of social justice' (Raphael 1990: 70). Clearly,
it would be naive to claim that the prevailing political consensus in the
British variant of social democracy – which is also sustained by parties
of the middle ground (George and Wilding 1985) – could furnish the
value-relevant framework for discerning one particular policy or decision that would best serve the public interest in every specific case.
But such a consensus does at least seem to permit the identification of

a range of options compatible with the common good as here defined, about which debate might legitimately occur.

It is instructive to contrast the weighting given to the various values of the liberal-democratic state in Britain with the balance arrived at in the United States. In this regard, contemporary American society differs significantly from Britain not just on account of its more fragmentary social structure and the absence of a traditional ruling elite (Finer 1974), but also because its dominant political ideology lies further towards the libertarian end of Donabedian's continuum (King 1987). In the United States there is a more substantial emphasis on individual initiative, self-help and the decentralization of decision-making. Government policies, therefore, traditionally have not focused as strongly as in Britain on the restriction of certain freedoms for some so that the freedom of other less privileged citizens may be preserved or enhanced. This was especially accentuated in the Reagan era in which the keynote, as McKay (1985: 189) observes, was 'the less government spending and control and the more market freedom, the better'. Indeed, it must be said that even the most moderate administrations in the United States since the War have upheld the essential value of market freedom to a greater degree than any British government in recent times – including that of the Conservative Party. The current web of values within which it is argued professional altruism claims should be assessed in the American context, then, places more stress on individual freedom and less on modifying the resulting structure of social inequality than in British society. Given the comparatively narrow band of ideological consensus over fundamental values which has for long existed between the Republicans and Democrats (Bowles 1993), the distinctive liberal-democratic principles underlying American political culture also appear to provide a sufficiently operational yardstick for discerning the main contours of the public interest in the United States.

The need to particularize the notion of the public interest proposed in order to make it more fully operational is not, of course, restricted to liberal democracies. Socialist societies can also be characterized by differing value systems deriving from diverse interpretations of Marxism. This is starkly demonstrated by the contrast between the Leninist political principles which underpinned much of the history of the former Soviet Union and the Maoist philosophy which was dominant in China during the Cultural Revolution. In the Soviet Union, the Communist Party – acting as the vanguard of the proletariat – viewed the establishment of communism in orthodox Marxist-Leninist terms as depending on the generation of the material conditions for such a transformation, including collective ownership and a well-developed industrial infrastructure (Lane 1985). Accordingly, the public interest was seen to lie in the high priority given to socialist industrial development in the Soviet context, which was ultimately manifested in the drive to re-equip, and increase labour productivity in, industrial concerns in the latter half of the 1980s in light of the scientific-technical revolution (McCauley 1986). In China, however, the industrial focus in the Soviet Union was attacked after the early 1960s as being based on too mechanical a version of Marxism, in the wake of the political rift that occurred between the two countries at this time. With the onset of the Cultural Revolution in 1966, an alternative set of Maoist political values emerged which emphasized the primary importance of inculcating socialist morality by breaking down the division of labour, stressing moral rather than material incentives and encouraging mass participation in decision-making, rather than simply engaging in rapid industrialization *per se* (Wheelwright and McFarlane 1973). Although the Cultural Revolution has now ended and the commanding role of economic production has been restored – signalling the demise of the so-called 'mass line', the re-emergence of a hierarchical party structure, a return to higher wage differentials and the growing disappearance of worker management groups (Chossudovsky 1986) – the differing framework which Maoism, as opposed to orthodox Marxism-Leninism, provided for the interpretation of the public interest in the socialist world is plainly apparent.

These differences underline the need to elaborate the meaning of the notion of the public interest beyond the bounds of broad political form, if the concept is to be satisfactorily operationalized. Examples will now briefly be given to indicate how the concept can be applied to specific issues drawn from the health field in the modern era.

THE APPLICATION OF THE CONCEPT OF THE PUBLIC INTEREST TO HEALTH CARE

Britain

In the case of Britain, the operation of the definition of the public interest sustained here can be illustrated by the fact that the existence of the NHS would be seen to be in the public good. This is because the provision of a health care system financed primarily from general taxation, making a range of health services available to the whole population on the basis of need rather than ability to pay, accords with the major aspects of the prevailing political ideology in modern British society. In so far as increased accessibility to such resources improves the overall health of the public, the NHS can be said to contribute to the general welfare (Butler and Vaile 1984). It also plays a large part in diminishing formal inequalities of opportunity and thus helps to increase social justice, a value which is still given particular emphasis in the British context (Allsop 1984). In addition, the parallel existence of a relatively small private health sector means that the principle of freedom is to some degree upheld because, although everyone is entitled to use the NHS, all citizens have the opportunity to seek treatment outside the state system (Levitt and Wall 1992). As such, the fact that the Conservative government has generally maintained the basic structure of the NHS intact is consistent with the public interest – notwithstanding the encouragement that it has given to the creation of the internal market with the reforms based on the White Paper *Working for Patients* (DoH 1989).

Against this, the commitment of the Conservative government to increasing privatization in the health field by, *inter alia*, fostering the growth of private medical facilities and expanding the role of the private health insurance sector (Higgins 1988) cannot so readily be identified as a public interest endeavour. This is highlighted by the detailed study conducted by McCreadie (1978) of a programme put forward by the BMA in the early 1970s for a national health system allowing people to contract out of a new, utility standard, health service funded by compulsory insurance and taxation and join a voluntary insurance scheme offering more attractive health benefits. This showed that whilst a minority of consumers might gain from the proposal by obtaining a superior level of health care, the move towards a more privatized system would be unlikely to further the general welfare by increasing overall resource availability and would almost certainly make justice a secondary consideration by encouraging an unequal distribution of scarce health resources between high and low income groups. Clearly, then, policies simply focused on increasing individual freedom through privatization do not necessarily serve the public interest in the health field in Britain, even when a substantial state-funded health sector remains. Much depends in this respect on the nature of the specific reforms proposed; further research may suggest that less far-reaching measures like sharing the costs of expensive medical equipment between the NHS and the private sector (Chandra and Kakabadse 1985) – and indeed collaboration over the distribution and use of health care facilities (Mohan 1991) – could play a more significant part in advancing the common good.

For the moment, though, it is enough to stress that the above conclusions about radical reform of the financial basis of the health service are also borne out by the recommendations of the Royal Commission on the NHS (1979), which was highly supportive of retaining a predominantly public system for the provision of health care, having been set up to assess the best use and management of NHS resources in the interests of both health service workers and patients. Documents such as the report of the Royal Commission are important publications in a wider sense here, because they can be seen to articulate the prevailing political values surrounding health care in Britain and hence provide fairly clear guidelines for evaluating claims about the altruism of the medical profession. This is particularly illuminating in relation to the reaffirmation by the Commission of the need for centralization and coordination in the NHS; in so far as it believes that the health system must be capable of providing services at the appropriate time and place and at the lowest reasonable cost, any unjustified impediment to planning and integration could be seen as contravening the public interest. Such obstacles militating against the public good would certainly include the perpetuation of the independence of teaching hospitals from regional control in the period up to the 1974 reorganization (Forsyth 1966). They might arguably encompass too the decision taken in the 1982 reorganization of the NHS to abandon the shared boundaries which had helped facilitate cooperation between the health and local authorities (Klein 1989). More topically, however, one of the key impediments today is arguably the move since 1989 to establish self-governing trusts and independent general practitioner fund-holders which threatens to fragment the service (Light 1990) and, if not properly controlled, to operate against the interests of the consumer (Strong and Robinson 1990). As Baggott (1994: 178) says, although there are potential benefits in employing market forces in the health sector, 'these tend to be asserted rather than demonstrated'.

The way in which the concept of the public interest might be operationalized in the health sphere in Britain can be illustrated further with reference to the distribution of general practitioners over the country. Butler *et al.* (1973) concluded from their classic study that family doctors tend to have larger list sizes in areas with the highest morbidity and mortality rates than those operating in locations with the healthiest population. This situation – also unfavourably commented on more recently in the *Black Report* (Townsend *et al.* 1988) – would plainly not be in the public interest on the definition adopted here, given the emphasis which is placed on the ideal of equality in contemporary British society. Indeed, the Royal Commission on the NHS (1979) formally acknowledged the desirability of generating a more equitable geographical distribution of family doctors, a priority that is also confirmed in *Working for Patients* (DoH 1989: 60), which notes that it is the responsibility of government 'to ensure that there is adequate access to family doctors across the country'. This does raise the question, however, of how this is to be achieved, in view of the possibility that any redistribution of general practitioners could detrimentally affect the general welfare by damaging the health of those currently living in areas with lower doctor–patient ratios to a greater extent than improvements in the mortality and morbidity rates of those who benefit from the redistribution would justify. As the Commission suggests, steps towards resolving this dilemma could be taken – at a time when significant additional resources are unlikely to be forthcoming – through research into optimum list size. Similarly, the problem of squaring the central value of equality with that of liberty could be resolved in a manner compatible with the public interest by ruling out attempts to coerce doctors to work in unpopular areas and relying primarily on methods based on moral, financial and other inducements.

A final detailed example of the application of the proposed concept of the public interest in Britain can be given in relation to the education of female doctors. In the period up to the late 1970s, there was strong evidence of discrimination against women applicants to medical school in this country – even if not quite on the scale of that documented by Witz (1990) in the nineteenth century. In 1978 females made up only around one-third of medical students and one-fifth of the medical profession; this seems to have had more to do with the informal quota system for women operating in some medical schools than the relative level of academic qualifications of women applying for places (Leeson and Gray 1978). Such discrimination can be seen to have militated against the public interest, in that it violated the meritocratic principle of equality of opportunity for women which has gained increasing political force in modern times (Charles 1993) and limited the individual freedom of women both to enter the profession and to choose a female doctor in their capacity as patients (Roberts 1985). Admittedly, this interpretation of the public interest could be challenged by the claim that women medical students are less likely than their male counterparts to remain in medical practice on qualification. But this is not a very convincing argument, as the differentials between the sexes in this respect not only are largely explained by the lack of suitable part-time employment opportunities in medicine, rather than the absence of motivation to work, but also are relatively small in nature (Royal Commission on the NHS 1979). In this light, the fact that quotas on female entry to medical school have now been abolished and the proportion of women students in medical schools has risen to some 45 per cent (Doyal 1985) is consistent with the public good as here defined, particularly at a time when the government is actively endeavouring to expand the participation of women in medicine and other key spheres of the NHS through Opportunity 2000. Continued vigilance is necessary, though, as women still only form around one-quarter of all medical practitioners in this country (Stacey 1985) and are even less well represented at senior levels (Macfarlane 1990); since it is also illegal for educational establishments to give less favourable treatment to female applicants under the terms of the 1975 Sex Discrimination Act, it would be in the public interest for any future cases of discrimination in this field to be acted upon and for medical schools to ensure that they operate in a suitably egalitarian manner.

United States of America

If these examples represent some applications of the concept of the public interest in British society, there are significant differences in the way the public interest would be interpreted in health care in the United States, the other liberal-democratic country on which this book is focused – differences which reflect the varying balance that has been struck between the core values of liberty, justice and the general welfare in the British and American context. This is certainly true of the financing of the health service. In the United States, in contrast to Britain, the majority of funding for health care comes from private sources in a system which is more heavily centred on the fee-for-service principle and voluntary health insurance schemes; although the government does make some contribution through public expenditure on such items as sanitation, control of communicable diseases and mental health, it does not act as in Britain to guarantee to all citizens the supply of basic medical care either completely free or at a nominal charge at the point of access (Stevens 1983). The continuing existence of this form of health provision, however, can broadly be seen to be in the public interest in American society, given the greater stress which is placed on preserving the freedom of individuals to pursue their own affairs and interests – including the freedom to choose what to spend on their own health care.

This is not, of course, to say that all aspects of the current system can be justified on the definition of the public interest advanced in this context. Notwithstanding the provision of the Medicare and Medicaid schemes – which have helped to improve access to medical care for disadvantaged groups in recent years (Aday *et al.* 1980) – one consequence of the present arrangement is that for financial reasons millions of Americans have for long had to go without adequate health care (Butler 1990). By the mid-1980s Navarro stated that the position was such that

> nowhere in the developed capitalist world are there as large sectors of the population without . . . limited health care rights as in the USA: 32 million citizens and residents of the USA do not have any form of health insurance coverage whatsoever, 88 million do not have any form of catastrophic sickness insurance, 1 million are refused care for not being able to pay for their services.
>
> (Navarro 1986: 7)

Although efforts have subsequently been made to extend the scope of 'catastrophic' insurance to the elderly population through the Medicare Act (Anderson 1989), even would-be liberal reformers of health care recognize that a system based on the British model of large-scale state financing of the health service would not be politically acceptable in the United States (Starr 1982). Nonetheless, with 37 million Americans now uninsured against health risks (Moran and Wood 1993), consideration of the public interest undoubtedly warrants more thoroughgoing action than the American government has as yet undertaken (Raskin 1986). In this vein, President Clinton's administration has recently produced plans to provide all Americans with health insurance on the basis of an amalgamation of market principles and government direction, under the oversight of a National Health Board (Berliner 1993). Whilst these proposals have been criticized for, amongst other things, providing insufficient control over health costs (Cockburn 1993), they do have the potential to enhance the public interest; as Stevens (1971) has noted, an extension of the national health insurance principle, coupled with limited additional federal intervention, is consistent with the public welfare in the United States in so far as it facilitates wider access to health care in times of need, whilst minimizing the threat to individual choice in the health system.

But if this highlights the deficiencies of American health policy in modern times in terms of the public interest, contrasts with Britain can also be drawn in relation to the extent to which a coordinated and centralized health system is compatible with the common good. In Britain, as has been seen, the health system has traditionally been based on a large degree of centralized planning and unification of services which – for all its residual shortcomings following specific reforms and reorganizations (Strong and Robinson 1990) – could generally be justified as a public interest concern on the grounds of its relative efficiency compared to the system in the United States (Light 1990). However, in the United States, as Fry (1969) has pointed out, the great suspicion of governmental bureaucracy and the emphasis on individual effort and self-help make a pluralistic and decentralized structure more politically acceptable. This ethos is certainly manifested in the existing form of the American health system which has been very significantly less coordinated and centrally directed than the NHS (Stevens 1983), even when compared with the situation following the recent de-velopment of the internal market in British health care (Saltman and von Otter 1992). Although a limited amount of planning does occur – as exemplified by the 1974 National Health Planning and Resource Development Act which, amongst other things, established state control over the supply and quality of hospital beds (Starr 1982) – it is common to find, for example, the duplication of expensive, yet rarely used, medical facilities in many localities in a health system in which there is no one organization committed to providing the best health service out of a given budget (Abel-Smith 1976). It is still clear, therefore, that introducing a higher degree of regulation and control to diminish inefficiency and waste within the prevailing framework of American political values – by, for instance, increasing cooperation between both federal government departments and the private and public sectors involved in the health field – would be consistent with the public interest. This conclusion is underlined by the currently rapidly esca-lating costs of health care in the United States which are increasingly seen as demanding regulatory attention at the state and local level in the decentralized American system (Hillman and Christianson 1985).

Interesting comparisons can also be made with Britain as regards the distribution of doctors. This is a far more significant issue in the United States, because of the vast disparities in doctor–patient ratios both between and within different states, reflecting the geographical, eco-nomic and social attractiveness of particular areas of practice rather more than the incidence of ill health (Roemer 1977). Needless to say, just as in the case of general practitioners in Britain, efforts to ensure a more equitable distribution of medical personnel would further the ideal of equality and thus be in the public interest (Anderson 1989). However, as even Navarro (1974) seems to recognize, measures to alleviate the situation in the United States may only be feasible in the current political climate if they are formulated on the basis of the prevailing market ideology and not an ethos of increasing public regulation – as in Britain where the Medical Practices Committee can refuse applica-tions from family doctors to practice in areas with extremely low average list sizes (Ham 1992). Although Daniels (1984) has called for American physicians to sacrifice at least some of their liberty in this respect, it may be more consistent with the public interest in the United States to decrease inequalities in the distribution of doctors by, for instance, providing financial resources to under-served groups to raise their consumption of health care, offering incentives to the medical profession to offset possible supply–demand imbalances and expanding the amount of supply of medical care to encourage surplus physicians in over-served areas to move to the under-served ones. Arguments have also been put forward for correcting the skewed distribution of doctors by influencing the type as well as the amount of supply of health care, such as by further increasing the number of health maintenance organ-izations based on prepaid group practice – a strategy which it has been claimed would considerably reduce the costs of medicine, particularly when generalized to the wider population within a system of open economic competition (Enthoven 1984). Admittedly, the effectiveness of schemes like these may be limited by the power of the medical profession to resist change (Fielding 1984) and the extent to which they are attractive in terms of costs in practice (Rayner 1988). But they do have the merit from the viewpoint of the public interest of being highly compatible with American values, because they involve only restricted government intervention and preserve a significant element of consumer choice, as their dramatic recent growth indicates (Robinson 1990).

Notwithstanding these differences between Britain and the United States, the substantive direction the public interest would take in relation to the distribution of doctors is broadly similar in both societies. This is even more true of the question of discrimination against women applicants to medical school. The fact that the United States has one of the lowest proportions of women in the medical profession in the whole of the Western developed world (Riska and Wegar 1992) and that women still only comprise some 25 to 30 per cent of American medical students (Stacey 1985) – despite the increase in this figure from 9 per cent in 1970 (Starr 1982) – suggests that discriminatory admissions policies may be even more evident than in Britain. Given that the sex stereotyping of doctors in the United States seems so resistant to change (Miles 1991), it would also be in the public interest for women to employ to the fullest extent the legal provisions which exist to ensure equal opportunities are available to all (Novarra 1980), should informal efforts fail to correct the situation.

That there are such similarities should not be surprising, since the two countries are both species of liberal-democratic society. Many other examples of parallels between these nations as regards the public interest could be given in the sphere of health care. One particularly tragic illustration in this context is the case of thalidomide. As the account by Sjöström and Nilsson (1972) of the development of the international distribution of thalidomide by Chemie Grünenthal in West Germany suggests, it was plainly against the public interest in both Britain and the United States for this drug to have been released and misleadingly advertised as safe for consumption by pregnant women in massive publicity campaigns launched on its behalf. According to these authors, the pre-clinical testing of thalidomide was more superficial than appropriate for new medications and the drug was known to have substantial risks when it was put on the market in the late 1950s. The release of this drug ultimately resulted in the malformations of thousands of infants throughout the world. As such, the introduction of thalidomide could scarcely be seen to have served the overall welfare, and there were therefore good grounds for restraining the liberty of the companies – Distillers in Britain and Richardson-Merrell in the United States – which had bought licenses from Chemie Grünenthal to sell the drug. The most ironic feature of the episode, though, was that thalidomide was widely used in Britain, with disastrous effects, whilst in America, for all its *laissez-faire* principles, the Federal Food and Drug Administration acted in the public interest by not only outlawing the drug at the outset for safety reasons, but also subsequently tightening up its procedures for drug approval (Bodenheimer 1985).

The Soviet Union and China

It is worthwhile outlining at this juncture the kinds of policies to which the concept of the public interest might give rise in the health field in socialist, as opposed to liberal-democratic, societies. The case of the former Soviet Union – which since 1989 has been transformed back into a cluster of independent states, along with its various former satellite countries in Eastern Europe (Deacon 1992) – has therefore been chosen alongside that of the People's Republic of China to clarify further the boundaries of interpretation of the notion of the public interest which it is proposed be employed to assess the altruism of professional groups in the Anglo-American context.

In the Soviet Union, Marxist-Leninist principles broadly legitimated a system in which health care was the sole responsibility of government, with all health facilities being owned by the state and all health services being made available to the population at no direct cost (Raffel 1984). This was certainly true until the coming of *glasnost* and *perestroika* and the associated attempts to expand the market elements of the health care system in the latter half of the 1980s and early 1990s (Lear 1989; Novak 1990). Throughout the period of the Soviet Union, however, the black market in medicine which had grown up outside the official state-based system in Soviet society must be seen to have run against the public interest, whatever the benefits to the patients involved in terms of speed of service and quality of treatment (Ryan 1978). This contrasts strikingly with the United States and, to a lesser extent, Britain where, as has been seen, the existence of private medicine is legitimated by the ideal of individual freedom. In socialist societies Marxist-Leninist philosophy decrees that unless such activity can be justified as a transitory form necessary for the establishment of socialism, it must be eliminated because it is rooted in capitalist social relations (Lane 1985). Although the provision of health services on the basis of need rather than the ability to pay in Britain and government intervention to supply a restricted range of health care at no direct cost in the United States are compatible with the public interest in these societies, therefore, the application of the concept in the Soviet Union supported more extensive programmes of action in this respect. This is also true of the related question of the centralization and coordination of the health service. Here the Soviet authorities established a highly centralized system in which the development of all health measures took place within the framework of a single plan under the direction of the Health Ministry. Whilst not without its imperfections, this distinctive system was generally justified by the need to facilitate the realization of the socialist commitments of the regime (Davis 1989).

Even further removed from the realms of political acceptability in liberal-democracies like Britain and the United States, though, is the idea that the industrial working class — which forms the bedrock of the socialist order in Marxist-Leninist theory — should be given priority over other groups in health care. In this sense, Soviet workers were favoured by having 'separate industrial medical services, which include special resort facilities for convalescent and chronically ill patients and periodic medical examinations' (Campbell 1978: 56) and a significantly lower doctor–patient ratio than in rural areas (Raffel 1984). Such discriminatory treatment on formal political grounds would not ordinarily be viewed as moral in liberal-democratic societies. This is not to imply, however, that the scope and nature of all inequalities in the former Soviet Union could be justified in terms of the common good. The manifest oversupply and underemployment of doctors in cities like Moscow (Field 1967), for instance, suggested that the extent of the uneven geographical distribution of physicians was not in the public interest – especially given the continuing importance of the peasantry to the Soviet economy, which helped to inspire the official policy of reducing differentials in health care between town and country (Venediktov 1973). It is difficult, too, to justify the unequal treatment of high-ranking Party officials who were served by a 'closed' network of superior health facilities not available to the population as a whole, as part of a wider system of privilege (Kaiser 1977), a point highlighted by Gorbachev's campaign in the 1980s against the existence of two nations in the Soviet Union (McCauley 1986). Admittedly, the use of health care in this way may have assisted the regime in enforcing ideological conformity amongst the elite of Soviet society. Yet the policy hardly seemed in keeping with Marxist-Leninist distributional principles – not least because the upper echelons of the membership of the Communist Party were drawn predominantly from the non-manual sector, rather than the ranks of the extolled industrial workers (Lane 1982).

Another pertinent difference between the public interest in the former Soviet Union and the liberal-democratic societies of the United States and Britain is that Marxism-Leninism legitimated more coercive strategies for attaining state objectives in health care. The ideological rationale for this lay in the party's exclusive role in interpreting the correct political line, which usually made dissent from official policies intolerable, in contrast to the formally pluralistic nature of liberal-democracies where individual liberty is held to be a more central political value (Gregory 1990). Thus, whereas it will be recalled that the public interest would be served primarily by searching for an appropriate balance of incentives to ensure a more equitable geographical distribution of doctors in Britain and the United States, the official stress placed on compelling doctors to work in the countryside for two or three years after qualification in the Soviet Union (Field 1967) was more compatible with prevailing political principles. It might, indeed, even be argued that the actual emphasis given to compulsion in this respect was insufficient, for the strategy did not meet with much success despite being supplemented by a package of material inducements; many newly qualified physicians exploited administrative loopholes to evade service in the countryside because of the poorer medical, cultural and living facilities in rural as opposed to urban areas (Raffel 1984). Against this, some coercive strategies can be seen to have gone too far, even by Soviet standards. A case in point is the forced labour of the chronically sick which formed part of Stalin's programme of socialist reconstruction in the 1930s (Field 1957). Although this policy appeared to be retrospectively justified by the survival of the Soviet Union in face of the powerful war machine of Nazi Germany in the Second World War, Nove (1964) has claimed that the harshness of such actions was counterproductive and unnecessary, since less severe measures more consistent with Marxist principles could have achieved the same objective.

Yet if these examples highlight the differing nature of the debate about health care and the public interest in socialist as compared to liberal-democratic societies, so too do illustrations drawn from the People's Republic of China, where the definition of the common good since the communist takeover in 1949 has, to varying degrees, paralleled that in the Soviet Union. In this respect China, like the Soviet Union, has for long attached great importance, amongst other things, to the prevention of illness and the need to set up a comprehensive public health care system in which treatment is free at the point of access (Hillier 1988). Significantly, though, while China has taken great strides in the area of prevention, the fee-for-service principle in health care is still widespread (Hu 1984). Accordingly, any further moves towards a more fully fledged socialist health system should be interpreted as being in the public interest – in contradistinction to Britain and the United States which, in differing ways, remain firmly wedded ideologically to the notion of a mixed economy in health care.

But it is the differences rather than the similarities between the former Soviet Union and China in the health field that are the most interesting. These differences were most apparent during the period of the Cultural Revolution in China from the mid-1960s onwards. At this time, Mao set the tone for the public interest in health care by attacking the hierarchical management structure of Soviet medicine and arguing for a greater degree of decentralized decision-making, with more involvement by the masses in policy implementation (Sidel and Sidel 1983). Although the idea of encouraging participation in community health was by no means alien to the Soviet Union (Field 1967), the scale and form of the mass campaigns that were instigated against such diseases as syphilis and schistosomiasis would not have been legitimated by Marxist-Leninist principles in the Soviet Union in the way they were by Maoism in China at this time (Horn 1971).

This point is reinforced by the fact that implicit in the mass line policies of the Cultural Revolution was the Maoist conception that the peasantry could be the backbone of the revolution, which fundamentally differed from the orthodox Marxist-Leninist stress on the exclusive role of the industrial proletariat (Furtak 1986). It should not, therefore, be surprising that the Chinese authorities regarded the skewed distribution of doctors between the urban and rural areas as a more significant political problem than their counterparts in the Soviet

Union (Hu 1984) and, indeed, one which required pressing attention in the interests of the common good. What most distinguished the interpretation of the public interest in Mao's China, though, was the means prescribed. During the Cultural Revolution neither the type of material incentives, around which strategies for diminishing such geographical inequalities tend to centre in liberal-democracies, nor the method of imposing decisions made by a remote, centralized bureaucracy employed in the Soviet Union, were felt to be politically acceptable (Chossudovsky 1986). Given this situation, only policies based primarily on the use of moral incentives and the diffusion of the ideology of 'serving the people' could be seen to advance the public interest in changing the pattern of distribution of health practitioners in China in this period (Sidel and Sidel 1974).

A further aspect of the distinctive framework which was employed to assess claims about the public interest in health care in China during the Cultural Revolution was the Maoist emphasis on the importance of putting socialist politics in command by destroying barriers between experts and the masses in the division of labour. On this criterion, the common good was promoted by both the introduction of 'barefoot doctors' – peasants with a short training who act as health care personnel whilst continuing to work in the fields with their compatriots – and the fulfilment of the requirement that fully qualified doctors undertake menial tasks in addition to their normal medical duties (Sidel and Sidel 1983). Such an approach contrasts with that of the Soviet authorities, who for many years used the notion of the public interest to elevate the virtues of narrow specialism in medicine and would happily have phased out the feldscher, a traditional grade of health personnel with four years of training, had there not been such severe shortages of fully qualified doctors in some parts of the countryside (Field 1967). It is also pertinent to note that judgements in liberal-democratic societies about the extent to which the employment of health workers with relatively short periods of training – like the assistant physician in the United States – is compatible with the public interest would be based mainly on their standards of competence in carrying out their duties rather than their ideological correctness as in the socio-political milieu of Maoist China in the late 1960s (Navarro 1986).

CONCLUSION

Despite the fact that the period of the Cultural Revolution has now been concluded – with such consequences as the recall of barefoot doctors for more intensive instruction and the lengthening of medical courses (Hu 1984) – the consideration of the politics of health care in both this unique phase in Chinese history and the recent past of the former Soviet Union has accentuated the web of values in which it is argued the altruism of professional groups should be evaluated in the Anglo-American setting. This comparison of bourgeois democratic and socialist versions of the public interest, though, might prompt objections to the conservative implications of the definition of the common good advocated in this context, which is firmly anchored to the existing liberal order. Marxists, in particular, might disagree with the formulation on the grounds that it bestows legitimacy on what they would view as an oppressive order based on the private ownership of the means of production and, by definition, that it appears perversely to categorize attempts to overthrow capitalism as activity militating against the public interest.

Such objections must be treated with some sympathy. It is, of course, very possible that the values on which the notion of the public interest proposed here is pivoted are not the result of the independent expression of the will of the members of the societies under discussion, but products of the political process relating to the power of dominant groups to impose their own definition of reality. Moreover, it is clear that the policies to which the concept of the public interest gives rise in liberal-democracies are ones that opt for relatively little interference in matters of private property, social class and personal income and can, therefore, have implications that might be regarded as detrimental. This is perhaps most starkly demonstrated in the health field in the United States, where the great shortage of doctors in the poorest areas and large income-based differences in access to health care referred to earlier can be rationalized, to some degree at least, in terms of ideals like 'freedom' and 'equality' which are integral to the concept of the public interest outlined in this study.

Nonetheless, although there may be more subjectively appealing notions of the public interest than those circumscribed by the social principles of particular liberal-democratic states, it should be recognized that the conception of the common good elaborated here is intended to be a relative concept. Indeed, it is the relativism of the term that is its most important virtue. In this context, the underlying formal complex of dominant values prevailing in Britain and the United States respectively appears to be the only set that can be realistically used to evaluate the activities of professions in each of these societies. Admittedly, these principles may vary in other places and at different times. And, of course, the fact that the content of the concept of the public interest set out here is necessarily restricted to a given political consensus and unable to go beyond it is unfortunate in light of the popular association of the notion with the universally desirable. But to define the public interest otherwise would be to mistake the nature of the enterprise.

A viable notion of the public interest which can be readily operationalized has therefore been developed for gauging the extent to which professional groups can be said to serve the common good. Attention must now focus on completing the remainder of the research framework for investigating professional altruism claims in the next chapter.

3 The role of professions
Power, interests and causality

A considerable amount of time has been devoted to the question of devising an operational concept of the public interest against which to appraise decision-making in the Anglo-American context. Two further problems, though, need to be dealt with if an adequate research framework for empirically examining the extent to which professions pursue their own interests at the expense of the common good is to be established. In the first place, criteria must be provided for identifying policies serving the self-interests of professional groups. Second, guidelines have to be laid down for evaluating the causal role of such interests, if any, in particular decision-making situations. As in the case of the public interest, these issues have yet to be satisfactorily tackled in the sociology of professions. But before outlining one way in which they may be resolved in what is again an essentially contested field, it is first necessary to comment briefly on a related question – namely, the meaning of the pivotal term 'profession' in the context of this book.

THE NATURE OF A PROFESSION

So far, the concept of a 'profession' has been loosely employed to cover the wide span of definitions encompassed by the various theoretical perspectives on offer in the sociology of professions. The range of interpretation, though, must now be limited so that the relationship between professional self-interests and the public interest can be ascertained without undue prejudgement. As was apparent from Chapter 1, this means avoiding taxonomic conceptualizations which reflexively equate professions with a collectivity orientation. Equally, there is no place for the more rigid Marxist classifications which assume that professions carry out oppressive social control functions for a dominant class in capitalist societies and have no real independent influence on decision-making. These categories of approach can at best only be used as ideal types against which to assess a complicated reality, not as definitional preludes to an open-ended analysis of the altruism of professional groups.

Within these boundaries, however, most other sociological definitions of professions will at least suffice from the viewpoint of the research enterprise at hand – although some are more useful than others. Thus, the interactionist conceptualization of a profession as an honorific label, for instance, may be excessively narrow in scope, but it does have the merit, as has been seen, of exposing the altruism issue to empirical scrutiny. So too do taxonomic definitions which exclude altruistic service from the categorization of the central elements of a profession (Hickson and Thomas 1969) and Marxist contributions which demarcate the established professions purely in terms of indices such as high levels of pay and security in employment (Parkin 1979). The neo-Weberian concept of social closure, though, provides the most helpful basis for the analysis of the collectivity orientation of professional groups in this context. The primary benefits of distinguishing professions from other occupations in terms of market control were, of course, discussed earlier. However, it is worth stressing that the preference displayed here for definitions like that of Parry and Parry (1977), who view professionalism as an occupational strategy involving colleague self-government and a monopoly over the provision of specific services in the marketplace, or Collins (1990b), who sees professions as being based on a combination of market closure and high occupational status honour, is not just related to the greater potential they offer for escaping the constraints of less refined taxonomic and Marxist accounts. An additional advantage over other approaches of defining professions as a form of exclusionary closure is that it provides a more direct key into crucial policy issues surrounding the professions. Once this restricted band of occupations is seen as commanding not simply greater prestige and/or material rewards, but also the state support which underwrites these privileges, then fundamental questions are raised about the virtues of this form of intervention by the body politic in the occupational structure – questions that are taken up in the Conclusion of this book.

In Britain, the occupations that have achieved professional closure based on legal monopolies gained by means of state licensure include groups as diverse as veterinary surgeons and patent agents (MacDonald 1985). The legally based privileges of such professional groups have, to be sure, come under recent government challenge (Burrage 1992). Nonetheless, the case of the English legal profession still provides one of the best illustrations of the notion of occupational closure. Both solicitors and barristers in Britain have for long enjoyed legal monopolies over a number of services under the regulation of the Law Society and the Bar Council respectively. Although solicitors have now lost their conveyancing monopoly, they continue to have the exclusive right, for instance, to undertake probate work for profit (Zander 1978). Barristers too have retained their monopoly of advocacy in the higher courts, even though the recent Courts and Legal Services Act has now created the potential for the extension of this right of audience to solicitors (Alaszewski and Manthorpe 1992). The existence of legally enshrined closure is not limited to Britain. Occupational licensing in the United States has become no less common in the modern era – extending not only to lawyers, but also to groups such as dentists and social workers – even though this mode of licensure was slower to emerge and takes a different form to that prevailing in Britain (Freidson 1986). Whilst themselves by no means exempt from the operation of the anti-trust laws in recent times (Krause 1992), American professions maintain a parallel position of substantial monopolistic control.

Given the focus of this book on health care in the Anglo-American context, however, it is important to emphasize that doctors themselves also constitute a classic example of a legally privileged group on both sides of the Atlantic. In Britain the origins of the notion of the medical profession as a privileged body in this sense can be traced back to the early sixteenth century, when the the Royal College of Physicians was granted a charter to oversee the practice of medicine within a seven-mile radius of the City of London (Stevens 1966). The most significant piece of legislation underpinning the closure of the profession, though, was undoubtedly the 1858 Medical Registration Act, which laid the foundations for the autonomous self-control so characteristic of the medical profession today (Moran and Wood 1993). Berlant (1975) notes that whilst this legislation did not transform the British medical profession into a legally restrictive group in relation to outsiders, it was monopolistic because, amongst other things, it only allowed the government to employ registered medical practitioners. In America, in contrast, he argues that the medical monopoly – as in other leading professions – was achieved later and in a more indirect and diffuse manner. Freidson captures the essence of the legally privileged position of the medical profession in the United States, which is based on licensure in individual states in the more fragmented American political system, when he observes that although

the state has ultimate authority in matters of licensing and prosecution of practitioners, much of its authority has either been given to the AMA or been based on the advice of the AMA. In the case of licensing, state officials are usually nominated by representatives of medical societies.

(Freidson 1970: 33)

Whilst the existence of a significant degree of state-sanctioned occupational control in such powerful professions as that of medicine in Britain and the United States vindicates the adoption of a neo-Weberian definition of professions in this context, one final observation needs to be made about such occupations in examining how responsibly this control is exercised – namely, that it may not always be appropriate to view professions as monolithic wholes for the purpose of analysis, since they usually contain sub-groups with different identities and missions. This can certainly be illustrated with reference to the medical profession in which there are significant divisions, for example, between generalists and specialists, those in different specialisms and junior and senior members of staff (Saks 1987). But if professions may need to be broken down into their component parts on occasion to facilitate analysis, this still leaves open the question of how the self-interests of professional groups – whether viewed as unified collectivities or segments thereof – are to be conceptualized. This issue can now be addressed.

THE CONCEPT OF PROFESSIONAL SELF-INTERESTS

It will be recalled that the explication of the public interest proposed in Chapter 2 was considered superior to unitary and common interest notions because it allowed individual and/or group interests not only to diverge from policies compatible with the common good, but also to conflict with them. Yet although this formally enables the inquirer to assess the relative influence on decision-making of professional self-interests as compared to the public interest in a manner other than by theoretical fiat, the extent to which this goal can be achieved depends on how the controversial concept of 'interests' is defined. Thus far, as has been seen, sociologists of the professions have made few inroads into this area; contributors from all sides of the theoretical spectrum have tended to treat the notion of professional self-interests as unproblematic, rarely articulating its meaning and still less defending their conception against competing approaches. It is plainly crucial, therefore, that an explicit account of how professional self-interests are to be conceived is given, together with a rationale for using the term in one way rather than another. To generate discussion here a number of distinct perspectives on the concept of interests will be analysed in turn, with the objective of developing a viable notion of professional self-interests to be employed in the research framework under consideration here. These perspectives fall into three main categories, each deriving from a distinct epistemological tradition, and have been termed by Saunders (1983) as the positivist, realist and conventionalist approaches.

The positivist approach

The positivist perspective rests on three main assumptions, which are conveniently outlined by Saunders as follows:

> First, an external world exists independently of our perceptions of it; secondly, . . . there are regular relationships between different elements of that world which may be expressed in the form of hypotheses and scientific laws; and thirdly, . . . such scientific explanations of real world events must be tested through observation or the collection of other direct sensory data.
>
> (Saunders 1983: 34–5)

As might be expected, positivist contributors to the analysis of interests are strongly opposed to claims that these might be unarticulated or unobservable; any attempt to delineate the interests of specific individuals or groups based exclusively on the assessment of outsiders is seen as being metaphysical, since it can have no valid empirical referent. For the positivist, therefore, interests can only be understood in terms of subjective policy preferences which may be articulated in a more or less overt manner. Dahl (1961; 1973) has provided one of the best-known expositions of this position, claiming that interests must be related to what people themselves perceive they want or prefer, as manifested by their political participation. Bachrach and Baratz (1962; 1963) regard interests as being defined by wants or preferences too – even if they stress, in contrast to Dahl, that interests can also be revealed in indirect and sub-political ways. In the field of health care the positivist approach is clearly exemplified by both Eckstein (1960) and Means (1963), who tend to equate the interests of the BMA and the AMA respectively with the explicit aspirations of the groups in question.

The application of such an approach to the determination of the interests of professional groups, however, is not particularly helpful, for the positivist standpoint is importantly flawed. More specifically, it runs into logical difficulties for it appears to rule out *a priori* the possibility of people mistaking their interests (Dunleavy and O'Leary 1987), even though it cannot necessarily be assumed that people know what is in their own interests (Plant 1991). The central problem here is highlighted by Runciman (1970b: 216) who argues that: 'Only when interest is so defined that it is possible for a man not to want his interests will the answer to the question whether his interests do influence his views be something to be demonstrated and not assumed.' This issue can be illustrated by the claim made by Means (1963), on the basis of his positivist definition of interests, that the consistent attempts by the AMA to obstruct large-scale state intervention in medicine in the United States have been in the interests of its membership. The deficiencies of associating the interests of the AMA with its actions in this case, though, are starkly revealed by Berlant (1975) who points to the fact that the monopolistic advantages of doctors can be augmented by greater state involvement in medicine, as happened in Britain where the interest position of the profession was improved with the advent of a national health care delivery system. Questions must, therefore, be asked about the extent to which a viable conception of interests can be based on empirically ascertainable subjective preferences.

Barry (1967a), however, has succeeded to some degree in reconciling interests and wants within the framework of positivism. He criticizes definitions which link interests to the common concerns of a given group, on the grounds that they conflict with a great many things that ordinarily might be said about this concept – including the notion of people misconceiving their interests. Barry (1967a: 113) suggests that this problem can be circumvented by adopting the position that 'a policy, law or institution is in someone's interest if it increases his opportunities to get what he wants – whatever that may be'. Clearly, this is compatible with the positivist perspective and represents an improvement on earlier accounts. Yet, as Saunders (1983: 36) points out, 'it remains a concept of interests which still rests ultimately on . . . subjective criteria since it takes wants as unproblematic'.

This being the case, Barry's account of interests continues to display, along with other positivistic analyses, a vulnerability to the charge of not adequately considering where wants actually come from. The dangers of equating interests and wants in this respect are accentuated by Hill and Bramley (1986) who note that stigma and ignorance can affect individual preferences and Mooney (1986) who suggests that much hinges on the supply situation because most people can only think about wanting things for which they possess a clear model. The positivist approach to interests also tends to play down the operation of power in both restricting and distorting the range of preferences open to any individual or group. Marxist critics in particular might assert that it is unwise to conflate objective interests and overtly expressed wants because of the problem of 'false consciousness' (Dunleavy and O'Leary 1987). The argument by Navarro (1986), for example, that the owners and controllers of the means of production stimulate artificial dependency and dissatisfaction in the sphere of consumption, and the belief of Marcuse (1991) that the repressive elites of advanced industrial societies have created, in commodity fetishism, false needs to divert attention from the real desire for liberty and thereby stifle dissent, both cast suspicion on the technique of using explicitly expressed preferences as a guide to true interests.

In addition to these weaknesses, a further criticism of the positivist approach to interests should finally be mentioned which rules out the adoption of this perspective in the research. If professional self-interests are to be defined in terms of the overtly manifested desires of professional groups, there is a danger that this strategy will simply tap the altruistic ideology characterizing the public pronouncements of the professions. As such, the question of the extent to which self-interests rather than the public interest shape professional decision-making may become a rather empty one, in which the interests of professions and those of the wider community merge one into the other. But if the positivist conception of interests will not do, what of that of the realists?

The realist approach

According to Saunders, the realist shares the positivist view that

> an external reality exists and that the task of science is to generate theories which can explain features of this reality, but argues against positivism that this reality is not necessarily observable. The realist is thus concerned to develop causal explanations of what we see through the generation of theories about underlying and unobservable structures and forces.
>
> (Saunders 1983: 35)

On this analysis, therefore, the positivist tenet that interests must be directly observable is rejected. Marcuse (1991), who argues that individuals are unable to recognize their true interests so long as they remain subject to the distorting effect of dominant ideologies, is one of the most prominent advocates of this school of thought. He believes that interests can only be determined in the last instance when people operate within a situation of ideological neutrality and political equality. Habermas (1976), another key figure in the Frankfurt tradition, concurs, claiming that the empirically existing world cannot provide the basis for discerning interests because of normative constraints. The structuralist Marxist strain within realism represented by Poulantzas (1973a), however, avoids the subjectivism and individualism of the accounts of Marcuse and Habermas by locating the concept of interests firmly within the framework of class struggles and asserting that the interests of a class are determined by what it can objectively attain as a social force in conflict with other classes. All of these explications, though, are underpinned by the assumption that interests are real, even if they are not usually manifested in overtly expressed preferences.

This is not the only factor which these realist conceptions have in common. Unfortunately, it must be said that they all seem singularly immune to operationalization and therefore cannot satisfactorily permit the identification of professional self-interests in the context of the research. Even if it is accepted that manifest wants are mere will-o'-the-wisps, products of a manipulative system – as Navarro (1976), for instance, claims is the case in Western capitalist societies where he sees the addictive behaviour of the population in the medical arena as a creation of the prevailing mode of production – it is not easy to see how real interests can be empirically determined. The 'false consciousness' debate appears to leave the issue open to theoretical anarchy, since problems arise in generating the counterfactual conditions by means of which it is possible to imagine a disconfirming instance in relation to any claims about the true interests of individuals and groups. As Saunders (1983: 37) says, the kind of analysis set out by Habermas is based on ascertaining interests through engagement in a hypothetical exercise akin to a mental experiment which 'under normal conditions, will not be capable of empirical confirmation or falsification'. Poulantzas also comes under attack for *a priori* theorizing, because his account rests upon a reflexive acceptance of certain central aspects of Marxist philosophy, especially the acknowledgement of the existence of two conflicting classes in capitalist societies. In the words of Saunders (1983: 41): 'The problem with Poulantzas's conception of interests as class interests specifically defined is that we need to believe it before we can accept it.' This problem, moreover, is accentuated in relation to the professions not only by the current sociological debate over where to draw the boundary line between the bourgeoisie and proletariat, but also by the contentious question of whether such a line is worth drawing at all – given claims that professional interests in areas like medicine cannot be systematically equated with a determinate set of class interests (Hart 1985).

Before leaving this field of analysis, though, it should be noted that Lukes (1974) has taken up the dilemmas posed by the work of contributors like Habermas and Marcuse, in an attempt to show that interests are open to empirical inquiry in situations where there is a false or manipulated consensus. He argues that the determination of such interests does not require absolute independence from prevailing ideologies but simply conditions of relative autonomy in which the influence exercised by the powerful over a particular actor's choices is comparatively weak. In these circumstances, Lukes (1974: 25) claims that the identification of real interests 'ultimately rests on empirically supportable and refutable hypotheses' in which evidence consists of observations of how people behave when the apparatus of power is removed or relaxed and when opportunities for escape are offered in 'normal' times. However, the work of Lukes – interesting as it is – fails to rescue the realist account of interests, for his strategy is far from watertight. Bradshaw (1976) has validly noted, for example, that the case is seriously weakened by the fact that the hypothesized independence of people from one source of power fails to rule out the likelihood of their subjection to other powerful groups in society. And since it is impossible to overcome this difficulty by manipulating society as a huge laboratory, there must be grave doubts about whether the basis Lukes provides for the empirical identification of real interests is operational. The deficiencies of his analysis in fact are even more clearly highlighted if his method is taken to extreme lengths. Then, as Bradshaw (1976: 122) points out, the purpose of the whole enterprise is thrown into question, for the result is a scenario in which the actor occupies 'a ridiculously barren, asocial arena'.

Although the work of Lukes has been considered here under the heading of realism, it is important to recognize that his position is actually closer to that of the conventionalist. Whilst his contribution shares several similarities with the accounts of writers like Marcuse and Habermas – not least because he adopts a subjectivist and individualist conception of interests – there is one crucial difference. This is expressed by Saunders (1983: 39) in the following terms: 'For Marcuse and Habermas, it seems that real interests exist, and the problem lies in illustrating what these interests are in a context of political and ideological repression . . . for Lukes, real interests need to be demonstrated, empirically if possible'. Herein lies the flaw of all realist analyses of interests; real interests exist merely to be recognized, not empirically established. But if Lukes has stepped outside this perspective and failed to produce a convincing basis for the identification of interests in general and professional self-interests in particular, can a conventionalist conception of interests contribute in any way towards the development of a research framework for investigating the degree to which altruism is manifested in the professions?

The conventionalist approach

The essence of conventionalism, according to Saunders (1983: 35), is that its proponents do not accept the distinction drawn in positivist and realist accounts between theory and external reality and believe that 'observation is itself determined by theory, that different theoretical frameworks cannot therefore be assessed through recourse to empirical evidence, and (in some versions at least) that there is no external reality outside of our perceptions of it'. In this vein, Lukes (1974: 34) clearly takes a conventionalist position in arguing that the concept of interests is irreducibly evaluative in so far as 'different conceptions of what interests *are* are associated with different moral and political positions'.

The extreme relativist version of this approach, though, which suggests that any conception of interests is as valid as any other and that the sociological enterprise simply consists of the acceptance or rejection of particular lines of argument depending on personal preference, must be considered untenable. As Saunders (1983: 42) says, this standpoint is beset by an important logical contradiction, for to assert that 'real interests do not exist independently of our concepts about them is to make an absolute statement which is clearly inadmissible in terms of a relativist epistemology'. In addition, he correctly argues that this variant of conventionalism leads inexorably to the absurd position in which mutually incompatible conceptions of interests – such as those of Dahl and Marcuse – must be accepted as equally valid. This problem seems to stem from a failure to appreciate that recognition of the influence of theoretical perspectives on conceptual constructs does not preclude the existence of theory-independent criteria for evaluating differing notions of interests. Indeed, it was only by assuming that there are such criteria that it was possible to dispose of the inadequate positivist and realist accounts of interests earlier in this chapter.

In this light, it is apparent that any viable definition of interests from a conventionalist perspective must side-step the trap of extreme relativism and reconcile the not unreasonable notion that interests are essentially contestable – resting as they do on personal moral and political values – with an avoidance of the primary weaknesses of the two other mainstream approaches considered. It is particularly crucial here that the naive positivist practice of reducing interests to subjective preferences is avoided given the way in which individual attitudes and beliefs may be limited and shaped by wider socio-political influences. Similarly, it is important not to replicate the failure of realist accounts to produce an operational concept of interests open to empirical investigation.

It is argued here that a conventionalist definition which meets these minimum requirements not only can be established, but can also be used as a basis for identifying professional self-interests in the context of the research. Such a concept is in fact set out – and fleetingly applied – by Saunders himself. He argues that real interests, whilst ultimately contestable, should be taken to 'refer to the achievement of benefits and the avoidance of costs in any particular situation' (Saunders 1983: 45) where the necessary utilitarian calculations are undertaken objectively by an external observer. But even though this basic definition escapes the pitfalls of subjectivism and opens up claims about interests to rigorous empirical scrutiny, the question remains of by what criteria the costs and benefits are to be assessed. Although it will be recalled that some writers on the sociology of professions – like Barber (1963) and Tawney (1921) – have tended to view calculations about interests in narrowly economic terms, the range of criteria employed to gauge the nature of professional self-interests in a given situation plainly needs broadening out to encompass issues of power and prestige. As Runciman observes, to assert

that something is in a man's interest is to say that it will result in an improvement in his position with respect to one or more of these three; and this is a matter which will be established quite independently of his wants and tastes and of how he may happen to choose to employ such wealth, power and social prestige as he has already.

(Runciman 1970b: 218)

Saunders, though, has argued that this still does not go far enough, because the indices of wealth, power and prestige do not cover every conceivable context in making assessments of the balance of gains and losses involved in calculating individual or group interests, especially as far as the allocation of scarce public resources is concerned. But whilst it is true that the costs and benefits resulting from, say, the distribution of state-provided hospital services cannot be fully evaluated in terms of these indices alone, Saunders exaggerates the extent to which other criteria will need to be employed in gauging interests. This is readily apparent in the case of the two examples that he himself cites to make his point about the costs and benefits associated with state allocative processes – namely, the quality of schooling available and the level of local taxation. Notwithstanding his comments, gains or losses in wealth, power and prestige are still likely to be the most significant indicators of the interests of individuals and groups in policy formation in these areas. It may reasonably be concluded, therefore, that these yardsticks will normally suffice as the main basis on which to make calculations of interests in this book.

It is worth noting, though, that such calculations may not always be as straightforward as Saunders indicates, for there are problems in implementing such cost-benefit criteria. Admittedly, he does rightly acknowledge that it may not be possible to express all, or even most, values in quantifiable form when engaging in the social accounting exercise – a difficulty which, as was seen in the discussion of the preponderance approach in Chapter 2, is particularly apparent in relation to issues like the relief of pain and the preservation of life in the health field. Nonetheless, Saunders does not draw attention to the problem of the uncertain consequences of action in identifying interests, nor, indeed, does he consider the ambiguous case in which the parties concerned may gain on one dimension of the cost-benefit scale, but lose on another following a given policy or decision. His insensitivity in the latter instance is clearly brought out by his criticism of Lukes for suggesting that, in some circumstances, poisoned air may be in the interests of town dwellers. The paradox is that even Saunders' own conceptualization of interests – based on an objective, rather than ultimately subjective, frame of reference – may not give rise to clear-cut conclusions, because of the conflicting pattern of gains and losses involved. This point is aptly illustrated by the discussion by Crenson (1971) of air pollution in Gary, a town in the United States, which could be seen to run against current lobbies for more emphasis to be placed on public health (Ashton and Seymour 1988). There is no doubt that the delay in dealing with air pollution in Gary was a cost to local residents because of its objective ill-effects on health. On the other hand, there were benefits in not taking up this issue, in that Gary was dominated by a single industrial corporation – which provided the basis for its prosperity – and there was a risk that the introduction of an expensive pollution-control ordinance could have led to a reduction or withdrawal of its investment in the town. This almost certainly would have had negative effects on the wealth, power and prestige of most residents in view of, amongst other things, the likely consequent increased rates of unemployment and decline of secondary industries.

Such objections, however, are not fatally damaging given, *inter alia*, the possibility of specifying the overall pattern of gains and losses without affixing standardized measures, the use of probability analysis to cope with the uncertain effects of actions and the rarity with which cases are liable to arise with a serious incongruity between the balance of costs and benefits on differing dimensions of the scale. It would seem, then, that a defensible and operational – if not uncontentious – concept of interests has been developed that enables the inquirer to assess empirically the extent to which any policy or decision is compatible with professional self-interests. Its utility can now be illustrated with reference to examples drawn from the field of health care.

OPERATIONALIZING THE CONCEPT OF PROFESSIONAL SELF-INTERESTS: THE CASE OF HEALTH CARE

The contributors so far considered who come closest to exemplifying the application of such a conception of interests to the medical profession are Jamous and Peloille who, as was seen in Chapter 1, implicitly employ the notion adopted here in their discussion of the resistance of the French University-Hospital Corps to the discoveries of Pasteur and Bernard in the nineteenth century. In these terms, they certainly do begin to adduce evidence for their claim that the interests of French clinicians at this time were unequivocally opposed to sharing in the new knowledge stock which was developing outside the elite circles of orthodox medicine. For instance, in noting that Bernard had failed the *agrégation* of medicine, which was the usual route to a Faculty chair, and that Pasteur was a chemist who did not work in either a hospital or a Faculty, they clearly indicate that the monopoly of the clinicians, and its associated privileges, was under threat. In the words of Jamous and Peloille:

> From the moment when profitable discoveries could also be made by people who were not treating the sick, or who had not followed the apprenticeship and training considered until then as the necessary way of obtaining such results, this monopoly was endangered. There appeared the need for a differentiation of functions, where the clinical doctors risked losing the monopoly over the production of medical knowledge. What is more, they were in danger of being gradually reduced over a longer period to the role of simple practitioners of this knowledge, and by the same token, of no longer being considered as those best-placed to transmit it.
>
> (Jamous and Peloille 1970: 139)

The benefits of spurning the advances in bacteriology and physiology, though, did not just involve the maintenance of power and prestige, but also perpetuated the lucrative financial position of a significant proportion of hospital doctors in private medicine. As Jamous and Peloille (1970: 132) relate: 'The expansion of the experimental sciences which transported the place of research from the hospital service to the laboratories, obliged doctors who wanted to devote themselves to research to give up an appreciable part of their income.'

But if this analysis indicates some of the relevant arguments that might be advanced to establish the nature of the interests of elements of the medical profession in nineteenth century France, the process involved in determining the interests of doctors in the central illustrative case of the United States in the twentieth century can be highlighted with reference to the growth of government intervention in health care. Earlier in this chapter it was made clear that professional self-interests in this context should be based on an objective assessment of the balance of gains or losses associated with particular pieces of legislation, not the subjective perceptions of bodies like the AMA, as the positivists would claim. In this sense, it must be stressed that whilst increased state involvement in health care could carry heavy costs for the medical profession, state intervention in the United States has not posed such a threat in practice to the medical profession in the contemporary period. This point is accentuated by the introduction of the Medicare programme which provided for health insurance for the elderly in the mid-1960s. As Stevens (1971) suggests in her account of the early stages of the implementation of this legislation, it is difficult to see that it brought anything but benefits for the medical profession; far from leading to intensified federal control of doctors, it actually increased the pool of funding for medical fees whilst giving doctors an extraordinary amount of freedom to prescribe, treat and charge for services, with all the resulting potential for significantly increasing their incomes. As such, the Medicare legislation manifestly appears to have been compatible with the furtherance of the interests of the American medical profession, even though stricter limits have now been imposed on payments under this scheme (Higgins 1988).

It is instructive to compare this conclusion with that to which a positivist conception of interests would lead in the period immediately preceding the introduction of the Medicare scheme. At this time there was bitter opposition to the programme from many quarters of the medical profession (Moran and Wood 1993) – with, for instance, only 38 per cent of private practitioners in New York State in favour of compulsory health insurance to cover hospitalization for those over the age of 65 (Colombotos 1969). This being the case, positivists would be likely to conclude that Medicare was not in the interests of doctors at this stage and to attribute the dramatic shift in support for the legislation amongst the American medical fraternity in the bonanza which followed its implementation (Starr 1982) not so much to physicians coming to a subjective realization of where their interests objectively lay, as to an actual change in their interests in this period. This perverse position underlines the limitations of the positivist approach to interests and the advantages of the type of conventionalist analysis proposed in this book.

The concept of professional self-interests advocated here, however, can be no less readily operationalized in the British context where, as has been seen, similar conclusions about the relative compatibility of state intervention with professional self-interests can be reached on the basis of an empirical consideration of the effects of such government action (Berlant 1975). Importantly too, this case highlights the merit of dividing professions into sub-groups for analytical purposes, since the objective interests of some segments of the medical profession seem to have been served more than others when the NHS was introduced. The interests of specialists and consultants in particular were advanced by their incorporation into the state medical service because of their advantageous bargaining position. As Gill says:

> Conditions of service, pay, permission to continue with private practice including access to National Health Service hospital beds, a high degree of control over appointments and promotion, and control over the merit awards system were all negotiated successfully by the representatives of the medical elite, the English and Scottish Royal Colleges.
>
> (Gill 1975: 168)

But if there is evidence that specialists and consultants improved their position in terms of wealth, power and prestige on joining the NHS, the gains for other medical groups were less substantial. Thus, Gill points out that general practitioners did not benefit as much from the continuation of private practice alongside the state system because it represented a smaller part of their work, whilst, according to Forsyth (1966), hospital doctors became less dependent on them because they no longer needed to rely on referrals for their income. Public health practitioners, though, probably fared worst of all; although there was no major deterioration in their position, this group not only failed to realize the objective of a fully integrated health service with strong links between prevention and cure, but also 'came under the control of the government almost as soon as its recognition as a medical specialty had been achieved' (Gill 1975: 168).

Notwithstanding these divisions, however, the advantages of the coming of the NHS to most medical groups definitely outweighed the disadvantages – not least because it consolidated the monopolistic privileges of the profession as a whole (Elston 1991). In contrast, governments in socialist societies have posed a far greater threat to the interests of doctors as here defined, which is clearly symbolized by the

abrogation of the collective power and autonomy of the medical profession following the Bolshevik takeover in Russia in 1917 (Field 1957).
This challenge is thrown into focus by state endeavours in the former
Soviet Union to compel doctors to practise in rural areas for a given
period on qualification. As Raffel (1984: 494) comments: 'The disadvantages of living in remote regions . . . and the decrease in opportunities
to advance have not been offset by any inducements yet offered.' The
position of doctors in Soviet society has been paralleled in China, where
the erosion of financial privilege, power and prestige was most marked
during the Cultural Revolution with its stress on reducing income
inequalities and breaking down the hierarchical division of labour (Sidel
and Sidel 1983). In these circumstances, it is not unreasonable to regard
efforts by doctors in China to evade manual labour and regain an elite
status in the period following the mid-1960s or more recent attempts by
their urban-born and city-trained counterparts in the former Soviet Union
to find ways of avoiding placement in the countryside as strategies
designed to protect their respective self-interests.

Yet if these illustrations point to the fact that the definition of
interests proposed can be readily operationalized, the concept is still
open to criticism – just as is the notion of the public interest – for its
inherent conservatism, especially in its application to the Anglo-
American milieu on which this book is primarily centred. The main
objection, as Saunders (1983: 47) observes, is that 'in taking . . . the
existing context as the basis for attributing interests . . ., it ignores what
could be achieved through the revolutionary rejection of that context'.
Marxist critics might therefore dispute the formulation outlined here,
on the grounds that the long-term interests of all groups in Britain and
the United States ultimately lie in the overthrow of capitalism, not in
the pursuit of parochial concerns within it. This applies no less to
professions in Western capitalist societies, which, as was seen in
Chapter 1, have frequently come under attack from Marxists for
supporting, rather than subverting, the existing system.

However, this attack is muted when it is recalled that Marxist
contributors themselves sometimes employ short-term definitions of
interests in their analyses to explain the compromised role of professions under capitalism, in so far as a self-serving attachment to
financial privilege, power and status is held to account for the continuing willingness of such occupational groups to act as agents of
capital in capitalist societies. There are difficulties too in empirically
grounding the notion of long-term interests at the heart of most Marxist
analyses. This is because the identification of policy decisions consistent with the interests of a given group necessarily involves making

comparisons with some other policy – in this case usually the perpetuation of the status quo. Yet, as Saunders relates:

> The problem with a conception of long-term interests is that there is no immediate comparative reference – the comparison is with something that has not yet occurred and which is not yet possible . . . . The identification of long-term interests would therefore seem to depend on ontological assumptions about human nature which can have no empirical reference.
>
> (Saunders 1983: 47)

The Marxist notion of long-term interests, moreover, cannot be accepted because it is incongruous with other elements of the research framework that have already been established for dealing with the debate about the altruistic orientation of the professions. In this respect, it should be re-emphasized that it is underpinned not only by a view of the public interest incompatible with that developed in Chapter 2 of this study, but also by a unitary conception of the relationship between group interests and the common good which rules out *a priori* empirical inquiry into possible conflicts between the two.

Potential objections from the Marxist camp, therefore, do not seem to represent a fundamental challenge to the employment in the research enterprise of the concept of interests articulated here. This concept both is operational and dovetails neatly in with the frame of reference within which the notion of the public interest favoured in this book is embedded. As such, it clearly assists the inquirer to assess empirically how far any policy or decision serves professional self-interests, the common good or a combination of the two. However, although criteria have now been established for gauging the direction of professional self-interests in any particular case, it must be remembered that an affinity between such interests and a given policy outcome is not sufficient in itself to demonstrate the causal efficacy of the former in decision-making – it is merely a minimal prerequisite for so doing. The important question of how to evaluate the role of the self-interests of professional groups in policy formation and implementation, therefore, now needs to be tackled in a more systematic manner.

ASSESSING THE CAUSAL ROLE OF PROFESSIONAL SELF-INTERESTS IN DECISION-MAKING

How, then, might an inquiry into the causal influence of professional self-interests on decision-making proceed? It should be stressed at the outset that the question of causality is much debated in sociology. Indeed, some schools of sociological thought – most notably those of interactionism and phenomenology – reject the very notion of causality itself, in the belief that it imposes an illegitimate structure which limits understanding of the way in which actors see and interpret the world (Cuff *et al.* 1990). Nor should it be imagined that the adoption of such a negative position is confined to the ranks of sociologists, for scepticism about causality is even more deep-rooted in philosophy. David Hume, for instance, classically denied that there was any valid ground for the attribution of cause and effect, challenging critics to discover anything more in the world than one object following another (Chalmers 1982). Still others, moreover, discount the possibility of establishing a specific causal nexus by taking the extreme view that the cause of a particular phenomenon can only be seen in terms of the total antecedent situation – resulting in the analytically sterile postulate that everything causes everything else (Blalock 1968). But these objections need not detain the inquirer here. As MacIver (1964) argues, whilst there is no way of decisively proving the universality of causation, this difficulty can be circumvented by transforming it into an axiomatic proposition. Similarly, the critique based on the problems raised by the infinite regress of causes can also be dismissed. In the words of MacIver (1964: 66), there is 'no reason why we should not seek the connection between an immediate phenomenon and its immediate antecedents. It is a curious logic that would allow us nothing because we cannot have everything.'

The most pressing issue in this area, therefore, concerns not so much the question of the fruitfulness of accepting the principle of causality as that of deciding the most useful way of inquiring into the causal influence of the interests of professional groups in a given case. Although there is not always a one-to-one relationship between research techniques and the theoretical perspectives on offer in sociology (Bechhofer 1981), Smelser (1976) has rightly pointed to the impossibility of discussing causal linkages in abstraction from the theoretical presuppositions of the inquirer which he claims will influence a range of aspects of the investigation, from the types of associational methods used to the choice of variables to be analysed. But whilst statements on the question of causality are destined to remain contested, it is clearly crucial to furnish at least some viable guidelines here for assessing the causal role of professional self-interests in decision-making, given the grave inadequacies of existing research in this field. These deficiencies, which were highlighted in Chapter 1, are interestingly not restricted to the work of sociologists alone. As MacIver found from his broad survey of publications offering causal explanations in the social sciences generally:

In the vast majority of instances either no grounds or quite inadequate ones were given in support of the causal imputations they presented. Sometimes there was displayed a meticulous care in the refinement of statistical indices or in the calculation of correlation coefficients, followed by a sweeping, unguarded, or wholly unwarranted conclusion regarding the causal nexus. Sometimes a selective description of conditions attendant on the phenomenon was the only basis for quite definite imputation. Sometimes cases or examples were offered showing the presence of the alleged cause, as though they were sufficient to establish its causal relation to the social phenomenon. Not infrequently an order of priority or importance was assigned to a number of 'causes', with little or no attempt to justify or even to elucidate this rating.

(MacIver 1964: 73–4)

A number of recommendations, though, can be made for overcoming such weaknesses which are largely replicated in the sociology of professions. An initial step which must be taken is to reject the cruder functionalist interpretations of causality that tend to explain social phenomena in terms of the positive effects of their existence (Hage and Meeker 1988). Although his own work was by no means free of functionalist fallacies, even Durkheim was aware of the dangers of reasoning about causality on this basis for:

To show how a fact is useful is not to explain how it originated or why it is what it is. The uses which it serves presuppose the specific properties characterising it, but do not create them. The need we have of things cannot give them existence, nor can it confer their specific nature upon them. It is to causes of another sort that they owe their existence.

(Durkheim 1938: 90)

The flaws of the functionalist approach as a whole, discussed in Chapter 2, need to be recalled at this juncture too. It is very difficult to see how a perspective which is based on the tenuous assumption that societies are goal-directed and purposive, and which disallows justifiable conflicts between the public and group interests, can be of any assistance in evaluating the influence of professional interests on decision-making.

Having dismissed the functionalist contribution in favour of a less tautological and teleological approach, claims about the causal role of professional self-interests can, of course, only be contemplated if it can be demonstrated that these interests have been consistent with the policy followed or decision reached in the area under scrutiny.

Assuming, however, that the self-interests of a profession, or of a segment of a profession are found to be compatible with a particular outcome, such groups also need to be shown to have possessed sufficient resources to have implemented their interests against the actual or potential resistance of others before the imputation of a causal relationship can be seriously considered. Such political resources are not equally distributed and it is worth underlining that the professions in general and the medical profession in particular possess more leverage than many other groups in the Anglo-American context in this respect (Child and Fulk 1982); it was not without reason that Eckstein (1960) reached his classic conclusion about the great influence of the BMA over medical policy in Britain, nor that the editors of the *Yale Law Journal* (1966) were similarly able to suggest that the AMA was the most powerful legislative lobby in Washington, such that the political authority of the state itself had in effect been delegated to organized medicine in the medical arena.

This situation makes the study of the influence of the self-interests of the medical profession over decision-making in Britain and the United States all the more compelling, but before progressing further, some words of caution are needed about the resource prerequisite for assigning a causal role to the operation of such interests. In the first place, notwithstanding a group's apparent command of political re-sources in a given decision-making context, it cannot be inferred that influence has been exerted on the basis of interests unless the actors under consideration were able to choose to act in alternative ways in relation to the issue being studied and were not the subjects of structural determinism. As Lukes says,

> to identify a given process as an 'exercise of power' rather than a case of structural determination, is to assume that it is in the exerciser's or exercisers' power to act differently. In the case of a collective exercise of power, on the part of a group or institution . . . this is to imply that the members of the group or institution could have combined or organised to act differently.
>
> (Lukes 1974: 55)

Following on from this point – which is brought very much to mind by the renowned critique by Poulantzas (1973b) of Miliband's analysis of the capitalist state for focusing on the values and social background of decision-makers rather than their role as bearers of structural relations – it is also crucial to note that the possession of a degree of autonomy and substantial political resources only constitutes a potential capacity for exercising power by professional and other groups. As Saunders

(1983: 23) relates, 'it is one thing to be in a position that affords the opportunity for effective political action, but quite another to use that position to engage in such action'. This distinction between having power and exercising it means, therefore, that if the causal role of professional self-interests in decision-making is to be established, further evidence will still need to be adduced.

In this respect, arguments about the influence of such interests will obviously be strengthened if other plausible alternative explanatory variables can be ruled out of consideration. This procedure was put forward *in extremis* by J. S. Mill whose 'method of residues' involved determining the cause of a phenomenon by excluding all known possible causes, with the remainder constituting the cause (Smelser 1976). However, Mill's position is untenable, a fact which was apparent even to early sociological contributors. Thus, Durkheim (1938) felt the method in its stated form to be inappropriate for sociology, as it assumed known laws to exist and was plainly impractical. It is difficult, too, to square Mill's method with the strong rebuttal by Weber (1949) of the notion of a 'presuppositionless' sociology and his related belief in the necessary selectivity of attempts to grapple with a complex reality. More recently, such criticisms have been echoed by Blalock (1968), who asserts that there are so many unknowns that the investigator is always forced to make assumptions about the behaviour of variables left out of any causal analysis according to his/her theoretical perspective. But this does not diminish the relevance of ruling out what seem to be the most reasonable competing explanations to that of professional self-interests in decision-making. Admittedly, even if this can be achieved, the strategy cannot logically ever firmly establish the causal significance of interests, since some hitherto unsuspected and unexamined factor may ultimately prove to have been of greater moment in accounting for the phenomenon in question. But this strategy can be effective as part of a battery of methods used to build a case, providing its limitations are appreciated. Indeed, Durkheim (1952) himself discovered this in his well-known study of suicide, where he cast empirical doubts on previously accepted theories based on, amongst other things, psychologistic reasoning and imitation, before developing his own claims about the importance of group integration to the phenomenon of suicide.

This raises the question of what type of evidence should be used in evaluating the part played by professional self-interests in decision-making both in this indirect sense – through the systematic attempt to exclude the most plausible alternative explanatory factors – and in a more direct manner. This is not the place to discuss comprehensively all the methods commonly used in sociology to assess the causal efficacy of a given variable. It is, however, worth making reference to perhaps the most basic ground rule in establishing causality – namely, that there must at least be an association, in the appropriate temporal sequence, between the dependent variable and the independent variable (Hage and Meeker 1988) which represent the decision under consideration and either professional self-interest or a competing explanatory factor respectively in this instance.

Special mention here should also be made of the utility of comparative studies in evaluating the causal efficacy of a particular variable – as illustrated by the work of Weber and Durkheim who, for all the differences in their epistemological assumptions, were both aware of the merits of comparative analysis in constructing explanations in the social world (Aron 1970). This type of analysis, though, is not without its difficulties. Given the ethical and political constraints on tightly controlled experimentation, the sociologist engaged in comparative work is usually faced with the task of dealing retrospectively with data that has already been created. Smelser (1976) has provided an extensive account of the comparative methods which can be employed to shed light on causal relationships in these circumstances. The methods which he describes that are of potential relevance to the problem at hand include systematic comparative illustration and, where the number of cases is smaller, deviant case analysis, the aim of which is to locate independent variables that set off exceptions to the general trend. Both involve the rigorous manipulation of what Smelser terms parameters and operative variables in order to develop sustainable explanations of given phenomena. Smelser also argues that even a case study of a single society can be used suggestively in making causal inferences – particularly if the prospect of investigating empirical co-variation is introduced by including the time perspective and/or a consideration of internal variations in the society in question. Irrespective, though, of the kind of comparative analysis that is undertaken – and much will depend on the information available – problems do exist, as with the study of cause and effect more generally, in ensuring the functional equivalence of cases, coping with the situation in which causal factors are not operating independently of each other and dealing with the recurring possibility that any associations found are simply a facet of a more global variable (Reid and Boore 1987). But these problems are far from intractable and should not mask the value of this method in causal analysis, not least in examining the role of professional self-interests in decision-making.

Rather than dwelling on the abstract methodological questions involved here, however, it is probably more useful in this context to highlight briefly some of the more specific procedures that might be followed in assessing the causal influence of the interests of professional groups, again with reference to concrete illustrative cases centred on the arena of health care.

THE ROLE OF PROFESSIONAL SELF-INTERESTS: HEALTH CARE ILLUSTRATIONS

The need to show that professional self-interests have been consistent with a given policy or decision before considering a causal imputation is no more clearly illustrated than by Strong (1979) in his review of the work of a range of sociological proponents of the thesis of medical imperialism, the notion that there has been an increasing and illegitimate medicalization of the social world as a result of self-interested professional expansionism. He suggests not only that there has been an exaggeration of the threat of medical imperialism, but also that advocates of the thesis have been all too ready to infer, rather than demonstrate, that the self-interests of groups like doctors are furthered by expansionist endeavours. This is exemplified in the British welfare state, where there are clear financial constraints on the drive to corral new categories of patient regardless of the clinical benefits of such action. Strong (1979: 208) argues that, in contrast to the United States where the structure of health care tends to provide greater pecuniary incentives for doctors to intrude into new areas of life, 'British hospital doctors who garner large numbers of fresh patients without first gaining extra resources from a higher level of authority, merely increase their workload'. This argument, of course, underplays the growing importance of private practice in British medicine and requires some reinterpretation in light of the recent establishment of the internal market in the NHS (Baggott 1994). But it does accentuate the flaws of the approach of many sociologists of the professions in this field – especially in relation to specialisms like geriatrics where there is sufficiently little prestige and opportunity to engage in private practice to temper the interests of doctors in casting more elderly people under the medical net (see, *inter alia*, Levitt and Wall 1992).

Yet if this example indicates that caution is needed in making inferences about the direction of professional self-interests, the theme of medical imperialism also provides a useful platform for highlighting other methodological issues involved in determining the causal role of such interests in decision-making. An interesting illustration in this respect is the claim by Shaw (1946) that the pecuniary interests of members of the medical profession led to a large amount of unnecessary surgery in Britain in the early twentieth century; he felt that surgeons in what was then a predominantly fee-for-service system had a financial interest in amputating limbs and that 'tonsils, vermiform appendices, uvulas, even ovaries are sacrificed . . . because the operations are highly profitable' (Shaw 1946: 68–9). Leaving aside the question of whether a great number of the operations carried out at this time could in fact be described as 'unnecessary', Shaw realized that if his claims were to be sustainable he had to establish not only that the performance of such surgery advanced medical interests, but also that members of the medical profession used their power to implement their interests. But whilst he made some inroads into these areas – albeit with an overly restricted financial definition of interests – he did not provide enough direct evidence on the centrality of self-interests in the explanatory process. In this respect, he particularly failed to expose his belief that unnecessary surgery was primarily a product of financial greed in private medical practice to comparative analysis by scrutinizing the relative rates of needless surgical intervention in the limited public medical sector of his day and in societies with more extensive provision of state-financed health care. Nor, indeed, did he satisfactorily rule out plausible competing accounts by examining the importance of such factors as the wishes of consumers which Parsons (1952: 467) has remarked cannot be ignored in this sphere because the bias in favour of active intervention in situations of uncertainty in surgical practice 'tends to be strongly shared by patients and their families'. More recent research showing the heightened influence of fee-paying clients over the nature of medical practice in private health care systems (Rothstein 1973) and exploring lay models of illness management (Calnan 1987) also underlines that the views of the client – along with other potential alternative explanations of unnecessary surgery – need to be carefully examined in any rigorous inquiry into the influence of professional self-interests in this area.

This critique of Shaw for downplaying the significance of factors other than the interests of professional groups in British medicine may seem unduly harsh given that he was writing as a playwright, not a sociologist. But it does help to illuminate the procedures which should be followed in analysing the effect of professional self-interests on decision-making. In fact the failure to scrutinize systematically plausible competing explanations is one of the most common faults in the sociological literature on this subject. Strong (1979: 205) highlights this point when he argues that critics of modern gynaecological practice have been prone to accuse doctors of self-interestedly invading the area of childbirth without considering the evidence that 'the plea of working women fifty years ago was for more proper medicine to save them from the horrors that childbirth then entailed'. He also draws attention to the frequency with which studies intent on establishing the causal primacy of professional self-interests exclude more convincing alternative explanations by erroneously attacking the medical profession with the benefit of hindsight. This problem, as will be recalled from Chapter 1, is especially apparent in the study by Jamous and Peloille (1970) of the defensive reaction of clinicians to the new systems of medical thought that were emerging in France in the nineteenth century. These authors preclude the possibility that ignorance, rather than self-interest, was the main reason for the development of this caste-like mentality because they do not explore the availability of medical knowledge at this time. They also fail to do justice to the historical context about which they write by following Shaw in overlooking the role of consumer demand in the web of causation, despite the existence of a predominantly fee-for-service system in this period which Williams (1983) suggests gave patients a disproportionate influence on the form of French medical practice.

It can be seen from the above examples how the basic requirements for an adequate analysis of the impact of professional self-interests on the decision-making process can be traced through the deficiencies of existing literature in the field. This is no more evident than when the claim by Means (1963) that the self-interests of the AMA have been responsible for blocking widespread government intervention in American medicine is considered. Although he does indicate that the AMA has possessed sufficient resources – including money for lobbying and propaganda activities – to impede the development of 'socialized' medicine in the United States, he fails to show that the AMA's capacity to influence decisions in this area has been consistently applied in policy formation. Indeed, Means, as has been seen, does not even satisfactorily demonstrate that the interests of this body run counter to extended government participation in health care, still less produce evidence on other superficially plausible explanations of the survival of a mainly private medical system. Yet in this latter regard it is plainly necessary to adduce comparative data to assess the claim by Doyal (1979: 37), amongst others, that the existence of a relatively non-militant labour movement in the United States has been a 'major reason for the failure to develop an American state health service' – especially since Navarro (1978) has argued that the inception of the NHS in Britain was precipitated by a high level of working-class pressure, channelled in large part through the Labour Party. Equally, Means does not examine the influence of elements of capital, such as private health insurance companies – which have the political resources to affect health legislation and a position to protect in face of increasing state encroachment in health care (Navarro 1986) – despite their centrality to assessing the causal role of professional self-interests in this context.

This consideration of the influence of capital is a reminder of the importance of taking into account the political milieu in which professional groups operate in any examination of the impact of their self-interests in capitalist societies, not least because it raises the crucial question about how far professions themselves have been subject to structural determinism under capitalism – an issue which McKinlay (1977) has usefully explored in relation to medicine in the United States. The question of structural determinism is, of course, just as relevant to the evaluation of the influence of the self-interests of groups like doctors in socialist societies where the methodology for making assessments of causality remains the same – even though the constraints on the autonomous expression of their interests are liable to be greater and based more heavily on party policies than capitalist relations of production. This is exemplified in the Soviet Union where, as Freidson (1970: 41) relates, doctors formally had 'no sociopolitically independent position from which to stand outside the state'. This situation, moreover, is officially paralleled in China in so far as the 'medical professional association, the Chinese Medical Association . . . follows medical policies set by the government' (Hu 1984: 136). But if these illustrations highlight the care that needs to be taken in investigating the causal role of professional interests in decision-making, some final points of clarification should be made on the subject of causality before drawing this chapter to a close.

CAUSALITY, INTENTION AND PROFESSIONAL SELF-INTERESTS

In the first place, it is important to emphasize that, in the research framework developed here, it is not necessary for the professional group under scrutiny to intend to bring about a particular effect before imputing a causal relationship between group interests and a given policy outcome. This issue is discussed in broad terms by Saunders (1983) in his analysis of the concept of power, of which he takes causality to be a central component. In brief, he argues that whilst many established definitions of power involve the deliberate and conscious intention to produce a given state of affairs, it is crucial to distinguish between causality and intention. Saunders holds that the demonstration of intention is only necessary if the concern is to attribute moral, and not causal, responsibility for actions. Since it is no part of the research enterprise to engage in debates about who is morally reprehensible for specific policies, this is a key distinction in this context. Indeed, the advantages of following the division made by Saunders are even more apparent when the difficulties of discerning the motives of individuals and groups are considered. Problems arise here because actors' testimonies about the reasons for their actions cannot be taken at face value since they may have incentives, amongst other things, to conceal their designs from outsiders to preserve credibility and status, or even to engage in self-delusion. As Papineau relates,

> agents' accounts of their intentions cannot always be regarded as authoritative, however thoroughly they might be negotiated. People will, if challenged, generally try to place their actions in a good light, emphasizing reputable motives and playing down unacceptable ones. Who does not obscure the less attractive aspects of their character from others and from themselves?
>
> (Papineau 1976: 9)

Yet whilst these dilemmas – which are especially accentuated with regard to the professions in view of the disputes by sociologists over the relationship between professional ideologies and professional practice – can be avoided by deeming the causal role of self-interests amenable to assessment irrespective of the subjective motivations of actors, the knowledge possessed by professional groups about the effects of their actions remains relevant to the evaluation of the role of self-interests in policy formulation. In this sense, Lukes (1974) differentiates situations in which the agent does not have certain factual and technical knowledge available to assess the consequences of a specific action and where the agent either possesses the pertinent information or lacks this data but could have found it out within culturally accepted limits. Although, as Saunders points out, Lukes himself uses this distinction to identify occasions when power has been exercised and thereby confuses moral and causal responsibility, the categories he delineates serve as a useful check on those who too readily implicate the causal role of professional self-interests in decision-making. As was seen in the evaluation of the work of Jamous and Peloille (1970), it is only in the latter instance – where there are no grounds for assuming ignorance – that it is possible to consider attributing the behaviour of professions, or segments thereof, to interests *per se*. The same principle also applies to the analysis of alternative explanations to those directly involving professional groups in the web of causation. Thus, drawing on an example related to health care that is cited by Lukes, a minimal requirement for assigning causal responsibility to the interests of a pharmaceutical company for the appearance of a dangerous drug on the market is to show that the company's scientists and managers either knew that the effects of the drug were dangerous or were in a position of remediable ignorance within existing cultural boundaries in this regard.

One final comment which should be made about the appraisal of the causal role of professional self-interests in decision-making using the battery of methods set out here is that, no matter how careful the investigation, the conclusions reached can never be more than tentative and probabilistic because of the unavoidable backdrop of untestable assumptions which shape and guide the analysis in every specific case. As MacIver (1964: xiii) says, the complexity of the causal network is such that 'our discovery of causation is . . . always incomplete and at best progressive, always leaving room for future investigation'. But although causality can never be definitely established, irrespective of how often an association is observed and how thoroughly competing explanations can be excluded by the manipulation and control of key variables, the inquirer can, as Smelser (1976) notes, be more or less confident of the existence of particular causal relationships on the basis of the logic and validity of the arguments leading to the conclusions reached. As such, the foregoing account should be regarded as providing grounds on which the researcher can be more, rather than less, confident in the outcome of analyses of the degree of influence of professional self-interests on policy-making at the formal and informal levels.

CONCLUSION

The assessment of the extent to which professional groups can be seen to pursue strategies serving their own interests at the expense of the public interest in the Anglo-American context is a far from easy task. The dichotomy frequently drawn between the public interest and self-interests may be misleading (Badhwar 1993) – in fact many possible permutations exist. As Watson (1987: 162) observes: 'Self-interests and altruism may often clash in the politics of work but this is by no means necessarily the case. The best way for a group to serve its self-interests may well be to do the best for others.' In addition to these possibilities, professional workers may refrain from following their own interests and thereby advance the public interest in the process of decision-making. On still other occasions, such restraints may result in policies which meet neither the interests of professional cliques nor those of the wider public.

However, a sufficiently sophisticated set of research tools has now been developed – culminating in this chapter in the identification of criteria for both defining the notion of professional self-interests and evaluating its role in policy formation – to lay bare the situation in any particular case and thus to assess the strength of professional altruism claims. Whilst this theoretical and methodological framework is by no means the only one possible for examining the relationship between professional self-interests and the public interest, it does have the merit of not simply being internally consistent, but also translating the questions arising here into a form whereby potential answers can be subjected to rigorous empirical scrutiny. Thus far, though, the application of the various elements of the framework outlined in Chapters 2 and 3 of this study has only been exemplified in a partial and heterogeneous manner – over a range of separate and largely un-connected cases drawn from the field of health care. The time has now come to illustrate the way in which the research framework can be operationalized all of a piece, in relation to a single case study. The case study which has been chosen, and which is set out in Part II of the book, retains the health theme emphasized throughout – taking the reader into the realm of alternative medicine through the analysis of the response of the medical profession to acupuncture in nineteenth- and twentieth-century Britain.

Part II

An empirical application: the response of the medical profession to acupuncture in Great Britain

4 Alternative medicine

The case of acupuncture

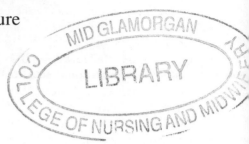

A prime justification for choosing acupuncture in Britain to explore the empirical applicability of the research tools forged in Part I of the book for assessing the altruism claims of professions is that sociologists have all too rarely studied alternative medicine in this country – especially as compared with the United States (Saks 1992a). The current chapter begins the foray into this still much neglected field by charting the response of the British medical profession to acupuncture and outlining its implications for the public availability of the technique. This provides the empirical basis on which to ground the central analytical tasks of evaluating the influence of professional self-interests on the position of acupuncture in nineteenth- and twentieth-century Britain and examining the extent to which the outcomes of such influence have been compatible with the public interest in the chapters which follow in Part II.

However, before the reception which acupuncture has received in British medical circles in the historical and contemporary context can be fully detailed, a certain amount of scene-setting is required. It is first necessary to elucidate the meaning of the concept of 'alternative medicine' and to deal with the distinctive problems involved in its study to inform the subsequent examination of the response of the British medical profession to acupuncture. The nature, origins and development of acupuncture in the international context then need to be considered to place the pattern of the medical reception of the procedure in this country into a wider perspective and pave the way for a comparative analysis of the British case at a later stage in the proceedings.

ALTERNATIVE MEDICINE: A FRAMEWORK FOR ANALYSIS

The label 'alternative medicine' applies to a wide span of therapies practised in Britain today including, amongst others, homoeopathy, chiropractic, osteopathy, spiritual healing, herbalism and, of course, acupuncture (see, for example, Stanway 1986; Olsen 1991; Grant 1993). Many of the practitioners of these therapies share a holistic emphasis on individualizing treatment and stimulating the life force to combat illness, in contrast to the dominant allopathic approach that treats disease as a breakdown to be repaired by direct biochemical and/ or surgical intervention (Stacey 1988). However, what is distinctive about alternative therapies is not so much their content – which can differ considerably, even as far as their epistemological base is concerned (Taylor 1985) – as their marginal position in the power relations surrounding health care. More specifically, alternative medicine consists of the range of therapeutic techniques that do not receive the backing of medical orthodoxy at an institutional level – as, for instance, through the systematic funding of research or by being routinely taught in officially designated medical schools (Saks 1992a). In this sense, the nature of alternative medicine will vary from period to period according to the social construction of the boundary between orthodox and unorthodox forms of health care, with the heterodox practices of one age becoming the conventional medicine of the next, and vice versa (Bynum and Porter 1987).

Wallis and Morley (1976) relate this definition to the division of labour, by linking marginal medicine with the clusters of occupational specialists who are concerned with the treatment of illness, yet practise outside the confines of organized medicine. Although this linkage obscures the growing number of practitioners in the orthodox fold who employ alternative medicine to treat their patients (see, for instance, Sharma 1992a), it does underline the mainstream interface between such therapies and the occupational structure in health care. Within this structure in contemporary Britain, organized medicine encompasses not only the medical profession – on which this study focuses – but also subordinated groups like nurses and the professions supplementary to medicine, and limited practitioners such as opticians and dentists who practise independently of medical supervision but limit their work to particular therapeutic methods or parts of the body (Turner 1987). These groups have exclusive rights over the title to their trade and enjoy a virtual monopoly over NHS practice – thereby sharing a position of legal privilege with their orthodox counterparts in other modern Western societies (Huggon and Trench 1992). In contrast, alternative therapists who operate outside mainstream medicine are usually heavily constrained by the law; whilst they are not formally prohibited from treating patients in Britain as in many other industrial societies, the strict limitations on their employment within the state health system are reinforced by the fact that it is illegal, amongst other things, for them to claim to possess remedies for certain diseases, including diabetes and cancer (Fulder 1988).

Having clarified the meaning of alternative medicine, of which acupuncture in Britain currently forms a significant part, some basic philosophical guidelines for studying this subject should now be provided before moving on to the substance of the case study. The most important general point to be made is that it is vital not to make the mistake of earlier commentators like Jameson (1961) and Roebuck and Quan (1976) in inferring that the marginal standing of alternative therapies is necessarily due to their intrinsic worthlessness. To take this line in the case of acupuncture would close off the opportunity of examining both the influence of professional self-interests on the position of this technique in British medicine and the possibility that its marginal status may not be in the public interest. There are clearly parallels between the difficulties associated with this one-sided approach to alternative medicine and those of the blinkered taxonomic view of professions considered in Part I of the book, not least because both tend to accept uncritically the ideologies of dominant professional groups in the health field in societies in which, as Esland (1980b: 216) remarks, 'professional legitimacy is often so strongly embedded and taken for granted that the cognitive frameworks through which we think through various social issues appear entirely self-evident and rational'.

The theoretical basis for dealing with this problem in the analysis of acupuncture as a form of alternative medicine is to be found in the debate over orthodox rationality in the sociology of science. Until recently, as Wallis (1979) points out, it was widely assumed that the acceptance and rejection of ideas in Western science – including medical science – was only of fleeting sociological concern because scientific knowledge represented the truth as it was based on open-minded, impartial and objective investigation. This was very much the trademark of the functionalist view of science as expounded by Merton (1968), who argued that the scientific enterprise in the Western world was characterized by universalism, communism, disinterestedness and organized scepticism – conjuring up an image of scientific activity in medical and other fields as impersonal and collaborative in which scientists were paragons of integrity. This reverence of institutional science, though, reflects the ethos underpinning the constraining and reflexively cynical view of alternative medicine referred to above. The adoption of a Mertonian perspective should therefore be avoided in any inquiry into the extent to which medical scientists respond altruistically to unorthodox ideas, especially since non-orthodox practitioners frequently employ different criteria to validate knowledge-claims to those of medical orthodoxy (Dolby 1979).

Fortunately, however, from the standpoint of analysing the position of alternative medicine in a more open-ended fashion, the functionalist conception of science has not passed without challenge in recent years. Merton's interpretation of Western science has in fact been heavily criticized for failing adequately to describe and explain activities in this sphere (Mulkay 1991; Webster 1991) as sociologists of science have increasingly subscribed to a more methodologically agnostic view of the truth claims of scientists. This shift has been fuelled in large part by the critique by Popper (1963) of the inductive method and verificationism and the stance taken by Kuhn (1970) that science normally takes place within paradigms embodying irrefutable sets of assumptions which lay down, amongst other things, the entities making up the conceptual universe, questions which can be legitimately asked and appropriate techniques of inquiry. This has led to the denial of a clear dividing line between science and non-science and the associated beliefs that the facts of science are not theoretically neutral; that bias, prejudice and emotional involvement cannot be removed from scientific observation; and that there are no common criteria and rules of evidence for assessing scientific knowledge-claims. On this basis, sociologists like Barnes (1974) and Mulkay (1979) have fully exposed orthodox scientific behaviour in medicine and elsewhere to sociological inquiry, opening up the possibility of treating the norms traditionally linked to science as the ideology of the scientific community and examining scientific activity in terms of both the interests of scientists and wider social factors. The importance of such work in this context is that it not only provides an appropriate theoretical backcloth to the study of alternative therapies like acupuncture and their relationship to medical orthodoxy, but also is highly compatible with the research framework set out in Part I of the book for evaluating the altruism of professions – primarily because of the common concern with professional self-interests as an explanatory variable and the recognition of the relativity of the criteria for assessing both scientific knowledge-claims and the direction of the public interest.

With the establishment of a sociological bridge between the research framework developed in this book and the analysis of the medical reception of alternative medicine in general and acupuncture in particular, attention can be turned to the task of outlining the nature, origins and development of acupuncture in the international context to complete the scene-setting exercise for the case study of the response of the medical profession to this procedure in nineteenth- and twentieth-century Britain.

ACUPUNCTURE: ITS NATURE AND VARIANT FORMS

A basic definition of the long-established and widespread practice of acupuncture is given by Rosenberg (1977: 3) as 'the insertion of one or more needles into various parts of the body for therapeutic purposes'. The strength of this definition is that it is sufficiently broad to encompass the range of different types of acupuncture employed throughout the world, without associating the method too closely with any one tradition. The most important distinction here is between acupuncture in the classical Oriental mould and that based on modern Western medical conceptions (Lever 1987) for it is around this axis that a number of other cleavages devolve. These include, *inter alia*, divisions over the optimal location of the acupuncture needles for particular disorders (Lewith 1982); the kinds of conditions which can be effectively treated using acupuncture (Macdonald 1982); the accept-ability of formula acupuncture involving the needling of set, rather than individually tailored, points for given maladies (Fisher 1973); and the value of electrically stimulating the needles to enhance their effect (Campbell 1987).

But if Rosenberg's definition has the merit of avoiding the limitations of classifications like that of Stanway (1986: 67), who views the method almost exclusively in modern Western terms as 'a therapy based on the principle that there is a nervous connection between the organs of the body and the body surface', and Lu Gwei-Djen and Needham (1980), who conversely tie acupuncture rather too closely to traditional Chinese medicine, its very breadth renders it problematic. Admittedly, the definition is not so broad as to incorporate either therapies that may indirectly have acupuncture effects without using needles or the medical employment of needles for diagnostic purposes. Difficulties arise, however, in relation to surgical techniques like suturing and probing and treatments based on the injection of substances into the body which fall within the basic definition, yet would not normally be regarded as acupuncture. The solution to this dilemma, though, lies in following Rosenberg (1977) in restricting the scope of the initial definition to what is conventionally labelled as acupuncture in the medical literature. This qualification keeps any analysis of acupuncture within reasonable bounds, whilst preserving a sense of eclecticism about the nature of this subject that dovetails neatly in with the research framework adopted in this study.

Attention should also be drawn here to therapeutic methods closely allied to acupuncture which, unlike such variants as ear acupuncture (Hsü 1992), do not strictly fall under the rubric of the foregoing classification. Prominent amongst such procedures are shiatsu in which direct finger pressure is applied to acupuncture loci (Rudolfi 1990), transcutaneous electrical nerve stimulation in which electrodes rather than needles are used to stimulate the acupuncture points (Lewith 1985) and the more recent development of laser acupuncture (Marcus 1992). Special mention in this context should be made of moxibustion which involves the burning of moxa on, or slightly above, acupuncture sites as either an alternative or complement to classical acupuncture therapy (Mole 1992). The significance of moxibustion is that more than any other therapy its fate has been linked historically with the fortunes of acupuncture (Lu Gwei-Djen and Needham 1980). Although such related procedures do not form the central focus of the case study, awareness of them is important to clarify the boundaries of interpretation of acupuncture in both Britain and the wider international setting.

Like many other alternative therapies, the particular form which acupuncture takes manifestly varies over time and between societies – as indeed does the response of medical orthodoxy to its practice in situations where a dominant group has established itself in the health care arena (Fulder 1988). The origins and development of acupuncture on the international scene will now be explored within this frame of reference, given the importance of understanding this setting for interpreting the medical reception of acupuncture in Britain.

THE DEVELOPMENT OF ACUPUNCTURE IN CHINA AND THE EAST

The origins of acupuncture can be traced back to ancient China, where its documented history runs from the oldest extant mentions of the therapy in 600BC to the present day (Lu Gwei-Djen and Needham 1980). The early years of this period saw the development of the classical system of acupuncture, based on the fundamental philosophical tenets of traditional Chinese medicine in which a homoeostatic universe was held to be governed by the dynamic interplay of the polar forces of yin and yang (Chow 1985). Since disease was seen as resulting from disequilibrium between these two types of energy flow, the role of classical acupuncture was clear. It was to restore the balance between yin and yang through the strategic insertion and manipulation of acupuncture needles at points along the meridians – surface channels connecting the twelve vital organs of the body through which the life force (Qi) was believed to circulate (Webster 1976). In this form, the traditional practice of acupuncture was extensively employed as a general therapy for a wide span of conditions from time immemorial in China (Pei 1983).

Traditional acupuncture – along with other aspects of classical Chinese medicine like moxibustion and herbalism – was very much part of the established medical orthodoxy at least until the nineteenth century when it was used by a whole network of practitioners up to the rank of royal physician and taught at the Imperial Medical College (Lu Gwei-Djen and Needham 1980). However, the status of acupuncture as a mainstream medical therapy in China, which contrasts so starkly with its classification as an alternative medicine in modern Britain, was jeopardized from the early nineteenth century onwards when the Ching government passed a decree eliminating acupuncture from the Imperial Medical College curriculum and then dropped it from the list of subjects to be taken in official medical examinations (Wei-kang 1975). Subsequently, the newly ascribed marginal standing of acupuncture was reinforced by the Kuomintang's attempt to modernize China in face of Western encroachment, which involved banning the practice of traditional Chinese medicine in 1929 (Hillier and Jewell 1983). Nonetheless, acupuncture has now re-established itself as part of the prevailing medical orthodoxy in the wake of the rise to power of the Chinese Communist Party, with its policy of integrating classical Chinese and modern Western medicine, particularly under the impetus of the Cultural Revolution in the late 1960s (Rosenthal 1981). In consequence, acupuncture is widely taught, practised and researched by doctors in China today in both its traditional and modern Western forms (Shao 1988), including its most well-known recent application as an analgesic in surgical operations (Stanway 1986).

In view of the fact that acupuncture originated in China and has long been established as an orthodox mode of treatment there, it is not surprising that it should have spread most rapidly to, and been most influential in, other countries in the Orient – especially in its classical mould. One of the first societies in the local culture area in which acupuncture became implanted was Korea, where clear evidence exists of the practice of this method and knowledge of the major Chinese classics as early as the beginning of the seventh century (Lu Gwei-Djen and Needham 1980). Another country in close geographical proximity to which acupuncture spread at an early stage was Japan, where it was incorporated into mainstream medicine by the eighth century (Lever 1987). The parallels between China and Japan are interesting here because there was also an attempt to legislate acupuncture out of existence in the Meiji drive to modernize Japan along Western lines towards the end of the nineteenth century. This, as in China, was followed by a period of resurgence, with acupuncture ultimately preserving its foothold in orthodox medicine (Hashimoto 1968) and retaining public respectability (Powell and Anesaki 1990). Indeed, with 6,000 doctors actively using the technique (Bannerman 1979) alongside 30,000 other qualified practitioners of acupuncture (Stanway 1986) and large-scale programmes of clinical and experimental research in this field (Huard and Wong 1968), Japan is probably the strongest traditional centre for acupuncture outside China.

Although acupuncture did not take strong root in every Eastern country (Lu Gwei-Djen and Needham 1980), many other examples of its influence on medical practice in this area of the world could be given – from Vietnam to Singapore and Malaysia (Kun 1983). But if China is not the only society in the Orient in which acupuncture has become part of orthodox medicine, the procedure has been much slower to diffuse and far less likely to have become even tangentially incorporated into mainstream practice outside this culture area – particularly in its traditional form. This is certainly true of the diffusion of acupuncture to the West, which will now be charted.

THE DIFFUSION OF ACUPUNCTURE TO THE WESTERN WORLD

The spread of acupuncture beyond the Oriental culture area to the Western world occurred earlier than is popularly believed. Marco Polo, for instance, mentioned the 'needles that cure' in a letter to the doge of Venice in the thirteenth century, although the main early disseminators of knowledge of acupuncture in Europe were undoubtedly the Jesuit missionaries who visited China in the fifteenth and sixteenth centuries (Roccia 1974). In the context of medical practice, the first books making substantial reference to acupuncture were texts published on Oriental medicine in the seventeenth century by authors such as de Bondt and Cleyer, surgeons from Denmark and Germany respectively who had come into contact with the procedure whilst practising in the East (Lu Gwei-Djen and Needham 1980). The most notable early medical works on this subject, however, were the doctoral dissertations completed at the end of the seventeenth century by Ten Rhijne and Kaempfer who both served with the Dutch East India Company and drew on their experience in Japan to describe the equipment used in acupuncture and the technique of needle insertion – albeit in fairly rudimentary and fragmentary fashion (see Carrubba and Bowers 1974; Bowers and Carrubba 1970). By the end of the eighteenth century, then, there was awareness of acupuncture in European medical circles, but details were sketchy and the interest displayed in the method was pitched mainly at a theoretical, as opposed to a practical, level (Lu Gwei-Djen and Needham 1980).

This picture changed dramatically in the early decades of the nineteenth century, when there was a vogue for acupuncture treatment in Europe which spread to the United States where the method had been newly introduced (Cassedy 1974). Even at this stage, though, the popularity that acupuncture enjoyed on both sides of the Atlantic did not wholly remove the procedure from its position as an alternative therapy and the use of acupuncture was still based on a less than full knowledge of the classical principles which underpinned it (Lu Gwei-Djen and Needham 1980). The practice of this method amongst both the medically and non-medically qualified, moreover, went into a marked decline in the West by the end of the nineteenth century (Chow 1985) and was not resurrected until after the mid-twentieth century (Bowers 1978).

The revival of acupuncture at this time – which was facilitated by the era of 'ping-pong' diplomacy between China and the West in the early 1970s – led to growing numbers of publications and research projects in the acupuncture field (Davis 1975), culminating in the claim by the British Acupuncture Association (BAA) (1982: 6) that: 'There are now over five thousand practitioners in Europe. Its use is spreading dynamically throughout the Western world, particularly in the United States, where it is finding ever-increasing acceptance.' Admittedly, this does not as yet approach the scale on which acupuncture is employed in countries like China and Japan. And the acupuncture which is practised – especially by the medical profession – does still tend to be based more on the allopathic than the classical tradition (Campbell 1987). But the fact that acupuncture has been brought to the fringes of orthodoxy today outside the Oriental setting signals a significant change in the response to this method as compared to the early half of this century.

Caution is clearly needed, however, in sketching out the overall pattern of reception of acupuncture in the West. This is highlighted by the account by Webster (1979) documenting the recent spread of acupuncture to the Western world, in which he tends to treat the response of the medical profession as monolithic, using the United States as a model for all countries. Such an approach conceals considerable societal variation in the reception of acupuncture – a variation that is crucial to some of the arguments pursued later in the case study. These differing Western medical responses to acupuncture will be briefly examined in the context of its diffusion to Europe and the United States.

VARYING PATTERNS OF MEDICAL RESPONSE TO ACUPUNCTURE: EUROPE AND THE UNITED STATES

In the European setting, acupuncture has been given a particularly icy reception in some countries. In Italy, for example, despite a flurry of interest among influential medical specialists in the first half of the nineteenth century and the more recent formation of a society for research into acupuncture, the orthodox response to the procedure has largely been one of rejection, epitomized by a reluctance to make official teaching appointments in this area (Roccia 1974). Acupuncture also still remains far from orthodoxy in Sweden, where doctors require special permission even to practise the method for research purposes (Macdonald 1982). In most other European societies, however, acupuncture has been more favourably received. In Finland, for instance, where the State Medical Board has recently approved acupuncture as a valid medical treatment, many local health centres now provide such treatment, which has also been increasingly incorporated into the medical curriculum (Vaskilampi 1991). Acupuncture has taken off in an even bigger way in Austria, where officially funded research into the technique has been conducted since the 1950s (Bischko 1973) and acupuncturists cooperate in ministering to patients in the hospital sector (Brelet *et al.* 1983). In Germany too, where acupuncture has a long history going back to Cleyer (Lu Gwei-Djen and Needham 1980), this procedure is also available from some hospitals, with expenditure by the patient being recouped through the national health insurance scheme (Stanway 1986).

The two countries in Europe where acupuncture has come closest to losing its label as an alternative medicine, though, must surely be Russia and France. In the former country, where links with acupuncture can be traced back three centuries (Bowers 1978), the medical establishment has never treated the method more seriously than over the last three or four decades. The new wave of interest began in the mid-1950s, when several doctors from the Soviet Union were sent to China to study traditional Chinese medicine (Stovickova 1961) and a number of research centres and clinics for acupuncture were set up (Veith 1962). Although there was a lull in this interest in the 1960s, the 1970s saw acupuncture emerge once again as a significant aspect of Russian medicine; more than a thousand doctors are now said to be engaged in acupuncture practice (Stanway 1986) and elements of the method which are felt to be scientifically sustainable are taught at institutes of postgraduate training as well as universities (Brelet *et al.* 1983).

France, however, has an even better claim to be the acupuncture centre of Europe. Linked in the eighteenth century with the famous physiological anatomist Vicq-d'Azyr (Lu Gwei-Djen and Needham 1980), acupuncture became extremely popular in the nineteenth century, when it was associated with names such as Berlioz, Sarlandière, Cloquet and Dantu (Baptiste 1962) and used to treat all manner of ailments from gout and pleurisy to ophthalmia (Quen 1975a). Although acupuncture was practised without a full understanding of classical theories and slipped into decline before the end of the nineteenth century (Lavier 1966), it reached a position bordering on medical orthodoxy in its time, with experimentation into the method taking place at Paris hospitals like La Pitié and La Charité (Haller 1973). Acupuncture, though, reached its zenith in France under the influence of Soulié de Morant who resurrected the procedure in its traditional Chinese form in the 1920s and 1930s (Campbell 1987). Under his sway, growing numbers of training courses for doctors were set up and acupuncture became increasingly available from qualified medical practitioners – with their patients receiving state reimbursements for treatment (Baptiste 1962). Today, official teaching facilities continue to exist for acupuncture (Brelet *et al.* 1983) which is extensively practised in many hospitals and clinics within the French health service (Fulder 1988). In this light, it is difficult not to concede that acupuncture has been more strongly accepted by the medical establishment in France – in both its classical and its Western forms – than anywhere else in Europe (Bowers 1978).

But if acupuncture has made a substantial impact on the medical profession in France – even though it cannot quite yet be said to be fully integrated into mainstream medicine (Bouchayer 1991) – the relatively favourable medical reception of this procedure has been rivalled to some degree by the United States. Here, the response of the medical profession to acupuncture merits slightly closer scrutiny than the previously mentioned societies given the focus on the comparative Anglo-American context that runs through this book.

The roots of acupuncture in the United States, as has been seen, go back almost two centuries. Physicians in America, however, were not directly influenced by countries like China and Japan traditionally associated with acupuncture in the same way as their European counterparts, but rather by books and articles published on the subject in Europe itself which found their way across the Atlantic (Cassedy 1974). These early nineteenth-century contacts resulted in an immediate flurry of indigenous medical publications on acupuncture by practitioners like Bache and Lee who employed the method on an experimental basis at this time – albeit for a narrower range of conditions than in most of Europe and with a similar degree of ignorance of its traditional underpinnings (Rosenberg 1977). As in many other Western countries, though, this did not provide a sufficiently firm platform to bring acupuncture squarely within the medical orthodoxy of the day (Quen 1975a). What was distinctive about the American experience, however, was that after the mid-nineteenth century acupuncture continued to be discussed in medical journal articles, textbooks, dictionaries, encyclopaedias and the like (Rosenberg 1977). It thus remained a fairly respectable procedure of the regular medical profession well into the nineteenth century and beyond – a point underlined by the involvement of the eminent physician Osler with the technique around the turn of the century (Wensel 1980). Although acupuncture did not entirely shake off its position of marginality in the United States in this period – in part because the association with the medically unqualified persisted even longer than in Europe (Haller 1973) – the method survived as a medical procedure until the late 1960s. It was around this time that the major American revival of the ancient Chinese medicine began.

After channels of communication with China were re-established in 1971, a number of American physicians visited the People's Republic to witness the much-publicized method of 'acupuncture anaesthesia', which sparked off a period of intense interest in acupuncture in the United States (Drake 1972). Whilst the initial response from some American doctors was disparaging (Duke 1972), the interest of those who were more receptive to acupuncture has been increasingly mirrored at the institutional level in American medicine. A number of courses were set up from the early 1970s onwards for doctors to learn about and/ or train in acupuncture (Rosenberg 1977). In addition, research funding was made available by official bodies like the National Institutes of Health, particularly for the study of the use of acupuncture in surgical analgesia and the treatment of pain (Webster 1979). In this light, it is easy to understand why the research output in this field in recent times in the United States should have been so prolific (Lewith 1982) – and, indeed, why some 2,000 American physicians are currently said to be involved with the procedure (Taylor 1985). But, although the medical profession has now also largely cornered the market for acupuncture by legally excluding unlicensed acupuncturists from practice in most states of America (Chow 1985), it would be dangerous to assume even at this stage that acupuncture has shed its label of alternative medicine, given that it has still to become an accepted and widely taught part of the medical curriculum in accredited medical schools (Wensel 1980). However, there is no doubt that acupuncture has made an impact in medical circles in the United States today, on a scale which rivals its reception in France – even if this interest has tended to be more heavily focused in the hands of medical practitioners on its specific application as an analgesic and modern Western scientific, rather than classical, theories of its *modus operandi* (Rosenberg 1977; Fulder 1988).

The pattern of response of the medical profession to acupuncture, therefore, has varied considerably between Western societies outside of the Oriental culture area. Whilst acupuncture has not gained unqualified acceptance as conventional medicine in any of the countries so far considered, in some of these it has come close to shedding its label as an alternative therapy and being accepted as part of medical orthodoxy. The central question of how far the response of the medical profession in Britain compares to this benchmark can now be pushed to its rightful place at the forefront of the analysis.

THE RESPONSE OF THE BRITISH MEDICAL PROFESSION TO ACUPUNCTURE

In this regard, the reception of acupuncture in Britain has not been as well documented as in many of the societies already reviewed. As a result, this case study draws heavily on the large amount of independent research undertaken by the author into this subject (see Appendix 1). The evidence that exists suggests that acupuncture not only has consistently failed to transcend its position as an alternative medicine in this country over the past two centuries, but has also been less favourably received historically by the medical profession than in the United States and many other parts of Europe. The fluctuating pattern of reception of acupuncture in Britain in the nineteenth and twentieth centuries will now be detailed – with rather greater emphasis being given to the modern period, from the mid-twentieth century onwards, about which most information exists and in which most developments have taken place in the field.

It is first necessary to note that acupuncture reached Britain much earlier than the start of the nineteenth century. The origins of acupuncture in this country can in fact be traced back to the late seventeenth century when Ten Rhijne's classic dissertation on this theme was published in London and Sydenham – an eminent clinician of the day – made reference in his work to the technique being a 'famous cure' for dropsy (Lu Gwei-Djen and Needham 1980). Information about acupuncture continued to reach Britain from abroad in the eighteenth century – not least through the reports of surgeons employed by groups like the London Missionary Society and the Edinburgh Medical Missionary Society (Haller 1973). The significance of such links with other countries is illustrated by the publication of an abridged and paraphrased version of Cleyer's important text on Oriental medicine in Sir John Floyer's *Physician's Pulse-watch*, which appeared in two volumes in 1707 and 1710, and the demonstration given by a Chinese merchant in London in 1775 of a medical figure with the acu-tracts and loci marked upon it (Lu Gwei-Djen and Needham 1980). However, whilst acupuncture did receive occasional exposure in the medical literature and elsewhere at this time, its clinical employment seems to have waned in the eighteenth century – only to resume in the first half of the nineteenth century, which was to become a central period for the diffusion of knowledge, and medical take-up, of acupuncture in these early days in Britain.

Early to mid-nineteenth century

This surge of medical interest in acupuncture was scarcely evident in the first two decades of the century when Coley (1802a; 1802b), a country general practitioner, appears to have been one of the only medical men to have published in this field. However, from the early 1820s onwards there was a wave of enthusiasm for the technique in medical circles – paralleling that occurring in America and several other European countries (Lu Gwei-Djen and Needham 1980) – which was reflected in the sharp growth in the numbers of items on the subject appearing in the leading British medical journals (Saks 1985). At this time the greatest protagonist of acupuncture was undoubtedly Churchill, a Fellow of the Royal College of Surgeons (RCS) who practised in London and produced two major texts in this area, *A Treatise on Acupuncturation* (1822) and *Cases Illustrative of the Immediate Effects of Acupuncturation* (1828). The aim of these works, which gave an account of Churchill's encouraging clinical experiences with acupuncture, was to kindle the interests of doctors in Britain in the subject. This they certainly seemed to do, for whilst Churchill himself was mainly concerned to apply the procedure in cases of rheumatism and injuries of the muscular and fibrous structures of the body, several publications by British medical practitioners appeared in the 1820s and 1830s favourably recounting their use of acupuncture in an even wider span of conditions, ranging from anasarca, hydrocele and ascites to ganglions on the tendon (Tweedale 1823; Lewis 1836; Furnivall 1837; Vowell 1838).

Admittedly, acupuncture in this period was still not generally employed by doctors in such a broad range of cases as, say, in France and was mainly practised pragmatically, following the pattern adopted in many other societies outside the Orient, doubtless because of the lack of understanding of the classical theories associated with acupuncture and the failure of its proponents to produce fully convincing alternative explanations of its *modus operandi* (Elliotson 1850). But it had become reasonably popular in at least some medical quarters by the 1820s and 1830s, and those using the method seem to have regarded it as a helpful therapy in the limited band of maladies to which it was usually applied. Thus Churchill not only claimed that he himself had found acupuncture to be 'a valuable curative measure' (1822: 12), but also that he was 'continually hearing of successful cases from respectable members of the profession' (1823: 372). Wansbrough, a practitioner in Fulham, spoke even more glowingly of acupuncture when he observed that in cases of local rheumatism it was 'a more expeditious and efficacious mode than any other remedy' (1826: 846). And the popularity of acupuncture amongst doctors can have been done no harm – in the initial stages at least – by Elliotson who, after taking up the procedure in 1824 whilst at St Thomas' Hospital, acted as one of its most forceful advocates throughout a career in which he held the prestigious posts of both Professor of Medicine at the University of London and President of the Royal Medical and Chirurgical Society (Haller 1973).

For all this, acupuncture did not become anything more than a marginal therapy in terms of the emerging medical orthodoxy of the time, particularly since members of the two most powerful medical bodies of the day – the RCP and RCS – took a none too positive view of the procedure. Indeed, in the early 1820s Churchill had publicly rebuked the RCS for ignoring his work on acupuncture (Haller 1973) and expressed his annoyance at the incredulity with which his establishment colleagues viewed the technique (Churchill 1823). Given that the *Lancet* (1827) later reported that Dr Yates of the RCP had called acupuncture – along with the stethoscope – an 'ephemeral folly', it is small wonder that one medical commentator noted that acupuncture had received the sneers of 'certain learned sages' (Wansbrough 1827). The marginal position of acupuncture was reinforced, moreover, by the fact that even amongst individual medical practitioners at the grass-roots level its popularity seemed to ebb and flow (Ward 1858) and those practising the method tended to use it only very sporadically (see, amongst others, Hacket 1837; Furnivall 1837). This should not be surprising because acupuncture was not routinely taught at medical schools in this period, with most of its practitioners learning the technique themselves on an individual basis (as, for example, Lewis 1836; Hacket 1837). Thus, although it is questionable how far a distinct system of medical orthodoxy could be identified in the first half of the nineteenth century in light of the wide variations in educational standards and the large number of medical licensing bodies in existence (Parry and Parry 1976), acupuncture does seem to have at best been tangential to the concerns of the developing medical establishment at this time.

Additional testimony to the marginality of acupuncture, even at the height of its popularity in the 1820s and 1830s, is provided by its association with unlicensed practitioners (see Churchill 1822), over whom there was no effective medical control and who substantially outnumbered those with more orthodox qualifications in medicine (Holloway 1964). But if the take-up of this method by fringe operators on a fairly small scale alongside such therapies as mesmerism and hydropathy (Inglis 1980) underlined the status of acupuncture as an alternative medicine in the early nineteenth century, its marginality became even more apparent from the 1840s onwards when the non-orthodox practice of acupuncture expanded with the spread of the Baunscheidt device to many parts of Europe, including Britain – for this device, which was based on the principle of driving a series of spring-attached needles into the body to create artificial eruptions on the skin and so cure all kinds of internal maladies, consolidated the earlier panacea claims of unlicensed practitioners of acupuncture and increased the public demand for treatment from them in this country (Haller 1973).

The arrival of Baunscheidtism in Britain in fact coincided with a distinctly more hostile shift in the response of the medically qualified to acupuncture. The reception given to unlicensed acupuncture practitioners and other medical outsiders from the late 1830s onwards made the fairly ambivalent response of medical orthodoxy in the two previous decades appear restrained. The Council of the Provincial Medical and Surgical Association (PMSA), which saw quackery as a central problem facing qualified doctors, agreed in 1839, for example, to stage popular lectures and circulate tracts to highlight the dangers of 'quack' remedies (Vaughan 1959). Wakley, one of the leading campaigners for the reform of the medical profession also used his position as editor of the *Lancet* in an attempt 'to expose, to discredit, and if possible, to prosecute quacks' (Parssinen 1992: 70). The leading medical journals had not given much credence to the work of fringe practitioners even in earlier periods of the nineteenth century, a point accentuated in the case of acupuncture by the failure of the major medical journals to publish a single item on the use of this method as a panacea in Britain at a time when reporting on acupuncture was most prolific – despite evidence of its growing employment in this manner by the majority of unlicensed practitioners and a small minority of qualified doctors (Elliotson 1850). But by the end of the 1830s this implicit check on fringe acupuncture by the mainstream medical journals was transformed into a more direct assault on quackery in all its guises. The overtly negative response of the emerging medical establishment to unlicensed practitioners of acupuncture and other fringe methods, however, was not just restricted to outsiders – insiders practising such therapies also came under increasing pressure.

In this respect, a growing number of attacks on licensed practitioners of deviant systems of medicine like homoeopathy, hydropathy, mesmerism and, by extension, acupuncture appeared in the medical journals with the express purpose of discrediting those involved (Parssinen 1992). Indeed, Elliotson even lost his chair at the University of London as a direct result of his involvement with the fringe – albeit in this case as a consequence not of his association with acupuncture, but with mesmerism, a cause which he increasingly championed towards the end of his career (Inglis 1980). In the specific case of acupuncture, however, the ever-expanding climate of medical rejection was no more clearly manifested than by the steep decline in items appearing in the leading medical journals on the subject in the 1840s (Saks 1985), which was clearly reflected in the reporting of acupuncture in the *Provincial Medical and Surgical Journal* (*PMSJ*) and the *Lancet* (see Appendix 2). Only one item in fact seems to have been published in such journals in this period – a short and somewhat implausible report from Italy on the use of acupuncture of the heart as a means of reviving 'drowned' cats which it was felt should be tried in cases of human asphyxia (Carraro 1841). In this light, it is not surprising that by the middle of the nineteenth century in orthodox medical circles, as Lu Gwei-Djen and Needham (1980: 299) observe, 'very little acupuncture was being done, though it could still find an entry in surgical treatises'. And when acupuncture did appear in such treatises – as it did in the case of those of both Fergusson (1842) and Hooper (1848) – the comments of the authors only served to emphasize that the procedure had increasingly slipped into disuse within the orthodox profession in Britain.

Mid-nineteenth to mid-twentieth century

But if a predominant climate of rejection of acupuncture as practised both inside and outside the ranks of medical orthodoxy had been established by the mid-nineteenth century in Britain, the response of medical practitioners in general and the emerging medical elite in particular scarcely became any more favourable in subsequent years. Indeed, the overall pattern of response in the period leading up to the mid-twentieth century was, if anything, even more negative than that which had begun to develop in the 1840s. This is again well illustrated by the number of publications in the major British medical journals of the day; only about two-thirds of the number of items on acupuncture appeared in these leading journals in the period from 1850 to 1949, as compared with that spanning from 1800 to 1849 alone (Saks 1985). Since these figures are inevitably only fairly crude indicators of the response of the medical profession to acupuncture in the years between the mid-nineteenth and mid-twentieth centuries – which do not take into account the possibility of selective editorial bias, amongst other things – a more detailed exploration of the situation is obviously required. The second half of the nineteenth century will first be examined as part of this exercise.

In this period acupuncture clearly continued to be of little interest to the vast majority of doctors. This is borne out in articles by Ward (1858), Teale (1871) and Lorimer (1885) which affirm at regular intervals in the latter part of the Victorian era that acupuncture had largely passed out of fashion. As such, Britain contrasts starkly with countries like the United States where, as has been seen, the method remained a significant part of the orthodox medical repertoire after the mid-nineteenth century. This is not, however, to claim that acupuncture had been entirely abandoned by British medical practitioners as an experimental procedure. A few isolated pockets of practice persisted. At Leeds Infirmary and Birmingham General Hospital, for instance, acupuncture was employed as a traditional therapy for such conditions as chronic rheumatism and sciatica (Teale 1871). Evidence also exists of medical interest in the method being displayed at Sheffield Eye Hospital (Snell 1880) and University Hospital in London, where Ringer is said to have taught Osler the procedure (Rosenberg 1977), as well as by general practitioners such as Ward (1858) in England and Munro (1874) in Scotland, who both continued to treat patients using this type of therapy.

The overall medical climate, however, remained one of rejection. This is even to some degree apparent in the work of the small number of medical practitioners who persisted with the use of acupuncture. They continued to follow their early nineteenth-century counterparts in restricting its application to a limited range of conditions, which mainly included the pain experienced in sciatica (Belcombe 1852), rheumatism (Banks 1856), cancer (Craig 1869), chronic pelvic inflammations (Aust-Lawrence 1889) and acute tympanies of the abdomen (Oliver 1889), together with the occasional treatment of dropsy (Munro 1874). For all their apparent success in such cases, though, the adoption of acupuncture on this partial basis – legitimated by a variety of tentatively espoused Western 'scientific' theories ranging from counter-irritation (Ward 1858) to fluidism (Druitt 1859) – only reinforced the earlier implicit rejection of the method as a wider therapy in its classical Oriental mould. The ensuing position of marginality of acupuncture in the latter part of the nineteenth century in Britain, moreover, was accentuated further by the fact that the doctors who employed the method usually did so only on a very occasional basis (see, for instance, Teale 1871 and Munro 1874) and – with the notable exception of Gibson (1893) who assessed the efficacy of acupuncture in the treatment of one hundred consecutive cases of sciatica – conducted relatively little larger-scale research into this area at a time when the value of more systematic inquiry was being increasingly recognized within the medical profession (Vaughan 1959).

The main evidence for the continuing climate of rejection of acupuncture after the mid-nineteenth century, though, lies not so much in the stance adopted by its medical advocates, as that of the leadership of the medical profession, around which doctors had become increasingly unified following the passing of the 1858 Medical Registration Act (Parry and Parry 1976). It is noteworthy that no funding appears to have been forthcoming for research into acupuncture from such key bodies within the profession as the BMA, although money had gradually started to become available for conducting medical research at the tail end of the century (Thomson 1973). Nor, indeed, did acupuncture seem to have been any more strongly incorporated into the orthodox medical curriculum than it had been in earlier times, despite the efforts of the General Medical Council (GMC) to impose a greater degree of educational homogeneity on the profession (Stacey 1992). But if acupuncture had no more of a stake in the formal undergraduate curriculum at this time than homoeopathy (Nicholls 1988) or bonesetting (Cooter 1987), its treatment by the mainstream medical journals confirmed its position as an alternative therapy; whilst the relatively small quantity of items published on acupuncture by journals like the *British Medical Journal (BMJ)* and the *Lancet* from 1850 to 1899 (see Appendix 2) was probably not too disproportionate to the extent of its employment by doctors, its medical standing was not enhanced by editorial decisions to include reports referring to the irrational and stigmatized nature of the practice – particularly when applied as a broad-ranging remedy (see, for instance, Dudgeon 1872).

This point highlights the fact that the medical establishment in the second half of the nineteenth century – following the style of the 1840s – responded negatively not just to those with an interest in acupuncture within the profession, but also to acupuncturists drawn from the large cohorts of practitioners outside its ranks who were still permitted to practise under the common law and were far more likely to be linked with therapeutic panaceas (Vaughan 1959). The specific employment of acupuncture as a cure-all by practitioners not on the medical register seems to have grown at this time under the impetus of both Baunscheidtism and the obsessive sexual fears of Victorian males, to whom medically unqualified acupuncturists offered remedies for such complaints as spermatorrhoea, impotence and urethral irritation (Lu Gwei-Djen and Needham 1980). The leaders of the medical profession reacted by becoming involved in a propaganda war with outsiders who engaged in the treatment of patients using acupuncture and other medical heresies. The *BMJ* in particular launched an attack on everything from homoeopathy to the patent medicine business (Vaughan 1959). But the assault on alternative practices like acupuncture, homoeopathy and herbalism did not end simply with sharp words in medical journals and tracts; the GMC also actively inhibited the practice of those without legitimate medical qualifications by deeming it unethical for doctors to refer their patients to be treated by them (Inglis 1980).

The judgement by Haller (1973), therefore, that the British medical profession maintained 'a generally skeptical posture' towards acupuncture in the latter half of the nineteenth century seems accurate on a number of counts. The climate of rejection which existed at the turn of the century, however, was further stiffened thereafter; whilst acupuncture, as has been seen, continued to be used on a limited scale in orthodox medicine in the United States in the twentieth century and was resurrected as a medical procedure in France in the 1920s and 1930s, it had reached the brink of extinction in Britain by the mid-twentieth century.

This is again well illustrated by the fact that seven times fewer items on the procedure were published in the leading medical journals in the first half of the twentieth century as compared to the last fifty years of the nineteenth century (Saks 1985) – which had itself represented a lean period for acupuncture. The three publications that appeared in this period, moreover, were hardly likely to have inspired members of the profession to take up acupuncture, in so far as they consisted of no more than a short report on the experimental use of the method in France in the early 1930s (Monod 1932) and two items from the 1940s suggesting that acupuncture had little value outside the treatment of sciatica (*BMJ* 1945; Stacey-Wilson 1945). Judging from other sources – such as the occasional entry in contemporary medical cyclopaedias and dictionaries (see, for example, Ballantyne 1906) – this highly restricted range of orthodox publications on acupuncture seems to have reflected the dearth of interest in the field in medical circles of the day. This is not to say that there was no bias against acupuncture on the part of the editors of the major medical journals in the first half of the twentieth century in Britain. Moss, for instance, who was to become one of the leading medical proponents of the method in the modern era, certainly claims that his own work on a technique closely related to acupuncture was subjected to medical censorship by the *BMJ* and the *Lancet* in the 1940s (Ewart 1972). Either way, however, the pattern of appearance of items in the leading medical journals bears witness to the developing climate of rejection of acupuncture in the profession at this time – a negative climate that is also confirmed by the fact that acupuncture does not seem to have been actively promoted by any of the Royal Colleges in existence by the mid-twentieth century (Stevens 1966), nor indeed to have received any funding from the growing numbers of private and state-financed institutes for medical research in Britain (see, amongst others, Thomson 1973).

Against this backcloth, it does seem anomalous that the profession should have devoted so little time to attacking the practice of acupuncture by the medically unqualified in the first half of the twentieth century as compared to earlier times. Admittedly, restrictions on referrals persisted and the medical establishment continued to fight its general battle against encroachment on a number of fronts (Inglis 1980), albeit usually in more muted form. But acupuncture itself was rarely explicitly mentioned in this process, not even meriting a direct reference in the GMC-inspired *Report as to the Practice of Medicine and Surgery by Unqualified Persons in the United Kingdom* (1910). The most obvious explanation is simply that the practice of acupuncture by those not on the medical register had more or less sunk without trace by the end of the nineteenth century (Lu Gwei-Djen and Needham 1980). Dolby (1979: 13) says that scientists 'often ignore work with which they disagree, rather than openly challenge it'. The near ex-tinction of the practice of acupuncture by unregistered outsiders in Britain would probably have made this an attractive strategy for the medical establishment in the first fifty years of this century.

In this light, the British medical profession clearly appears to have perpetuated and extended the climate of rejection which acupuncture faced at this time. The strength of this negative climate is indicated by the fact that unlike most alternative practices of the day – such as homoeopathy and manipulation – acupuncture seemed to lack even a tenuous foothold in orthodox medicine, not to mention unorthodox practice itself (Inglis 1980). This being the case, the reception of acupuncture in British medicine from 1850 to 1949 was surely one of the least favourable in the European and American context. What, though, of the modern era in Britain?

Mid-twentieth century to the present day

In general terms, interest in acupuncture amongst both medical and non-medical practitioners increased after the mid-twentieth century, and particularly from the early 1970s onwards. However, as will be seen, the position of acupuncture in contemporary Britain has still not come to rival that attained by the method in the United States and some parts of Europe, and even today has not yet fully entered the portals of medical orthodoxy. This trend is once again mirrored in the pattern of publication on this subject in mainstream British medical journals, where the number of items on acupuncture has expanded from a mere trickle in the two decades following the mid-twentieth century to a steadier stream in the 1970s and beyond as it has gradually begun to outgrow its status as a medical curiosity (Saks 1985). The section begins, though, by documenting the medical response to acupuncture in Britain in the period from 1950 to 1969 before this therapy started to re-establish itself in this country in a more substantial way.

That the profession made only a limited response to acupuncture in the 1950s and 1960s is borne out by the content of the two most well-known British medical journals of the day, the *Lancet* and the *BMJ*; in this period no items were published on the procedure in the former and only three short entries appeared in the latter, all of which stressed the lack of a rational basis for its use (*BMJ* 1953; 1966; 1968). The tentative nature of the reception given to acupuncture at this time is also apparent from the restricted take-up of the method by doctors. Despite the early work of pioneers like Moss, who began using acupuncture after making contact with French practitioners around the middle of the century (Ewart 1972), there were literally only a handful of medical acupuncturists in Britain by the late 1950s (Inglis 1964). One of these was Felix Mann, who founded the Medical Acupuncture Society (MAS) in the early 1960s which played a central role in the survival and propagation of the procedure in medical circles before it became more fashionable from the 1970s onwards (Eagle 1978).

An intriguing aspect of the practice of the few early modern proponents of acupuncture which contrasted with that of their nine-teenth-century counterparts was their overall commitment to using the technique as a broad-ranging therapy in the classical Oriental mould – even if they too were wary of accepting *in toto* the traditional theories of its *modus operandi*, which were increasingly becoming known in detail in the West at the time (see, for example, Mann 1962a; Moss 1964). For all this apparent liberality, however, the position of acupuncture as an alternative medicine in the 1950s and 1960s is not in dispute. Aside from the fact that there were even fewer medical practitioners of acupuncture than of most other marginal therapies in this period (Inglis 1964), acupuncture also paralleled such techniques as radiesthesia and osteopathy in not being taught as part of the basic medical curriculum (Ewart 1972). Nor indeed did it even become incorporated into the fringes of orthodox postgraduate training programmes, as homoeopathy had been (Inglis 1964). Up until the late 1950s doctors wishing to study acupuncture after qualification, therefore, had little option but to teach themselves. Privately-run training courses were, however, gradually set up in this country thereafter – such as that offered by Mann for medical practitioners from 1963 onwards and the less exclusive and more lengthy programmes of the College of Traditional Chinese Acupuncture and the British College of Acupuncture from 1963 and 1964 respectively – thus following the pattern established by several other alternative therapies (Fulder 1988). But, like deviant medical practitioners more generally, doctors wishing to take such courses were placed at a considerable disadvantage as they did not receive the subsidies available for more orthodox elements of the postgraduate curriculum (Inglis 1980).

Further testimony to the marginality of acupuncture within the profession in the 1950s and 1960s is provided by the fact that there is no evidence of any systematic orthodox funding of research into acupuncture in this period through either the BMA, the Medical Research Council (MRC), the medical trusts or universities and hospitals themselves. In this light, it is not surprising that the few research papers produced by doctors on acupuncture at the time should have relied so heavily on independent endeavour (as, for example, in the case of Mann and Halfhide 1963) – often in face of the scorn and disbelief of the medical profession (Ewart 1972). As such, the position of this therapy did not differ substantially from that of other unorthodox techniques which – leaving aside the investigation by the BMA of spiritual healing and hypnosis in the 1950s (Inglis 1964) – also tended to be starved of official research interest and support, given the stigma and hostility that existed in the ranks of orthodox medicine (Bradbury 1969).

The climate of professional rejection, moreover, extended to the

small, but growing, numbers of non-medical practitioners of acupuncture too. The GMC, supported by the BMA, continued to prohibit
links between doctors and medically unqualified acupuncturists and
other such alternative practitioners who retained the right to practise
under the common law (Inglis 1980). Although a few individual doctors
informally directed patients to the fringe, despite the risk of being
disciplined (Inglis 1964), the stance of the medical establishment makes
it easy to understand why unregistered outsiders practising methods like
acupuncture and chiropractic were so often subjected to bitter opposition and ridicule by rank-and-file members of the profession (Bradbury
1969). It is somewhat ironic that this denigratory line was supported by
most medical acupuncturists of the time (see, for instance, Moss 1964;
Inglis 1964), even though they themselves were not exempt from the
negative backwash of its influence. The position of both medically
qualified and unqualified acupuncturists in this sense is appropriately
summed up by Ewart at the beginning of the 1970s as follows:

> Officially . . . [acupuncture] is beyond the pale, although interest in
> it is growing and the day may not be far away when the medical
> establishment will be forced to bow to public pressure. But British
> acupuncturists, and there are an increasing number of them, have so
> far been unable to break down the prejudice against this well-tried
> system of treatment.
>
> (Ewart 1972: 37)

This prejudice began to crumble in the period from the 1970s to the
early 1990s, as is suggested by the rise in the number of items that
appeared on acupuncture in mainstream medical journals, which now
quantitatively outstrips several times over all of the publications on the
subject in the preceding 170 years in Britain (Saks 1985). Just as in the
United States following the reopening of diplomatic relations with
China, several doctors – including representatives of official bodies like
the MRC – visited the Chinese mainland in the early 1970s to witness
the much-publicized method of 'acupuncture anaesthesia' (see, amongst
others, Capperauld *et al.* 1972; Brown 1972). Such visits clearly played
a part in inspiring the growth that has occurred in the use of acupuncture
by medical practitioners and, to a lesser degree, auxiliary personnel like
physiotherapists operating under their supervision (Lewith 1985). An
increasing amount of research into the mechanism and effects of
acupuncture has also begun to be undertaken in a range of medical
institutions from the Royal Edinburgh Hospital (Stewart *et al.* 1977)
and St Bartholomews Hospital (Clement-Jones *et al.* 1979) to the
National Hospital for Nervous Diseases (Loh *et al.* 1984) and the Royal

London Hospital (Ho and Bradley 1992). At the same time, the number of training courses in acupuncture for doctors and other orthodox health personnel has expanded (Campbell 1987) as interest in alternative medicine in general and acupuncture in particular has risen amongst medical practitioners (as shown, for instance, by the surveys of West and Inglis 1985; Nicholls and Luton 1986; Stephens 1989). This rising interest has been reflected in the growth of the newly formed British Medical Acupuncture Society (BMAS), which was set up to promote the use and scientific understanding of acupuncture as part of the practice of medicine; the exclusively medical membership of this organization, which superseded the MAS in 1980, has escalated from around fifty at its inception (Grant 1986) to close to 1,000 today (Marcus 1992).

However, whilst increasing credence is being given to acupuncture and other unorthodox techniques by the medical profession in this country, it would be a mistake to infer that acupuncture has yet transcended its position as an alternative medicine. Notwithstanding the above trends, the standing of acupuncture in Britain still lags behind its position in such societies as Russia, France and the United States, for the limited degree of acceptance of the method at the grass-roots level has not been matched by the official response of the medical establishment to acupuncture in the years from the 1970s to the early 1990s.

The marginality of acupuncture in Britain even today is highlighted by its persisting exclusion from the orthodox medical curriculum. The GMC has made no recommendation that acupuncture be taught at undergraduate level (see, for example, GMC 1980) and such instruction does not seem to have been systematically provided in practice in medical schools in this country at any stage over the last twenty years. Indeed, a recent approach by the BMAS to all Deans of medical faculties in the United Kingdom produced little interest in even providing brief instruction in acupuncture as part of the core undergraduate syllabus (Marcus 1992). As in the 1950s and 1960s, moreover, the method has not formed a part of the required teaching in the post-registration education of doctors overseen by the Royal Colleges. Doctors interested in practising acupuncture, like those in areas of alternative medicine such as herbalism and chiropractic, have therefore once more been forced to look outside the orthodox medical curriculum for training (Fulder 1988) – and if they enrol on one of the mushrooming span of courses on this subject, there is still no guarantee of receiving financial subsidies for attendance, especially if the programme is not exclusively run for practitioners on the medical register (Stephens 1989). Financial barriers, though, are not the only obstacle to medical practitioners wishing to take up acupuncture and other forms of alternative medicine today; although the stigma associated with the fringe is declining (Eagle 1978), insiders who employ unorthodox methods like acupuncture continue to face the disdain of many of their colleagues (Macdonald 1982). This position has hardly been ameliorated by the publication of the distinctly hostile BMA Report (1986) on alternative medicine, even though the latest BMA Report on this subject (1993) is considerably less negative in tone.

Whilst there has been no shortage of demand for courses in acupuncture from doctors in recent years despite such constraints (as indicated by the surveys of Reilly 1983; Wharton and Lewith 1986), acupuncture cannot be said even today to have a firm foothold in orthodox medicine. Although it is difficult to know exactly how many doctors actually practise the method in Britain, it was estimated in the mid-1980s that the number was probably around 550 (Camp 1986), of whom some 300 were members of the BMAS (Fulder 1988). Even allowing for some subsequent growth in this figure, however, it still only represents fewer than one in every 100 doctors in this country. It is also numerically lower than that for medical acupuncturists in several other Western societies (see, for instance, Stanway 1986) and is not too dissimilar to that for other more popular alternative therapies in this country (Fulder 1988). As such, it is hard to accept that the procedure is anything more than tangential to mainstream medicine in contemporary Britain.

This point is reinforced by the generally limited use to which the small band of medical acupuncturists have put the method in the contemporary era. Although most of the early pioneers and some doctors with a newly developed interest in acupuncture do apply this technique to conditions as far-flung as ulcerative colitis, allergies, asthma and addictions, amongst others (as witnessed, for example, by Mann 1973; Macdonald 1982; Campbell 1987), the medical practice of acupuncture has largely focused on its application in cases of severe pain – including its modern employment in surgical analgesia (Saks 1992b). This pattern of adoption follows the characteristically narrow span of employment of acupuncture in orthodox medicine in the nineteenth century. The limited medical focus today, though, is perhaps best illustrated by the reporting of this subject in the *BMJ* and the *Lancet*, where far more items on the use of acupuncture as an alternative to surgical anaesthesia and as a means of alleviating painful conditions have been published over the past two decades than on the employment of acupuncture as a wider therapy, and these narrower applications have generally been evaluated more positively (Saks 1991b).

Yet if acupuncture is seen by doctors primarily as 'a potentially cheap and safe form of treatment for relieving some types of pain' (*BMJ* 1981: 746) – an emphasis which is reflected in its widespread availability in pain clinics in this country (Camp 1986) – it is important to note that this limited form of practice has been justified as in earlier times with reference to theories drawn from contemporary medical science. Such theories, as the BMA Report (1986) on alternative medicine demonstrates, serve as a basis on which the policy of limiting acupuncture to a narrow sphere of operation can be rationalized whilst traditional explanations of its use as a panacea are rejected for being unscientific and irrational. Initially the orthodox theories advanced to sustain the case for making only restricted use of acupuncture were mainly psychological in nature (Capperauld 1972; MacIntosh 1973). But these theories soon came under attack and have now been largely supplanted by a range of legitimating neurophysiological explanations – spanning from the once much-vaunted 'gate control' theory (Mann *et al.* 1973) and 'busy cortex' hypothesis (Bull 1973) to more fashionable beliefs about the role of endorphins and other neuroactive substances in producing states of analgesia (see, for instance, Chung and Dickenson 1980). Paradoxically, however, although such accounts seem to place acupuncture at the forefront of modern medicine, they ultimately shore up the position of the method on the fringes of the British health care system, since they continue to be so heavily centred on explaining its efficacy in the relief of pain alone.

The continuing marginality of acupuncture also appears to be manifested again in the response of the major medical journals to this therapy. Whilst the volume of publications on acupuncture in the mainstream medical journals has certainly grown sharply in recent times, not least in the *BMJ* and the *Lancet* (see Appendix 2), the number of articles and leaders, as distinct from letters and short reports, in these latter publications has still only averaged around two each year since 1970. This has led to some medical acupuncturists becoming suspicious that the editors of the leading medical journals may be biased against publishing material from doctors on acupuncture – even when cast in Western scientific form. Questions have also been raised about the adequacy of the representation of the minority form of traditional acupuncture in this mould because – despite the recent publication of such work as that by Jobst *et al.* (1986) on breathlessness and Dundee *et al.* (1986) on perioperative nausea and vomiting – classical acupuncture has tended to be covered all too rarely even in proportion to the extent of its medical practice, and in an excessively disparaging manner. It is, of course, difficult to assess suggestions of bias without more information about the number and content of submissions to the journals in question. Understandably too, the editorial staff of the *BMJ* and the *Lancet* are adamant that all contributions submitted to them are considered on their scientific merits. But this view perhaps needs to be tempered by the claims of Mulkay (1972) about the negotiability of the criteria employed for assessing 'good quality' work in the gatekeeping function performed by the editors and referees of professional journals in the scientific world.

The climate of rejection of acupuncture which is still maintained within the medical profession, albeit in diluted form, however, is even more clearly evident in relation to orthodox funding of medical research into the procedure. Whilst more research into acupuncture has been supported by the medical establishment in Britain in the past two decades than in the 1950s and 1960s, the work on acupuncture that has been financed – in common with other alternative therapies – can hardly be described as extensive (Fulder 1988). The MRC and the Department of Health (DoH) and its predecessors have done little more than award small occasional grants for doctors to learn about the subject, mainly through training fellowships and scholarships (see, for example, Stewart *et al.* 1977; Clement-Jones *et al.* 1980). Acupuncture projects financed through the universities and the largely non-commital Royal Colleges have also been few and far between. And notwithstanding contributions from such bodies as the Laing Foundation, the King's Fund and the Mental Health Foundation, most major privately-funded organizations involved in financing medical research have given negligible backing to doctors working in this field. Members of the medical establishment who play such a crucial role in decisions about the direction of research in both the public and private sectors, therefore, have not strongly promoted the investigation of acupuncture – still less in its application as a wider therapy as compared to its employment in analgesia. As a result, medical researchers interested in studying the procedure have all too often been left to look for funds from the relatively meagre pool of resources available to bodies lying outside the direct control of medical orthodoxy, such as the Institute for Complementary Medicine (Davies 1984). Whilst this picture is beginning to change following the formation of the Research Council for Complementary Medicine, which has started to attract official funding for research in unorthodox areas – including a £60,000 grant from the government to finance its work (Saks 1991a) – the stance of the medical establishment on research expenditure has placed therapies like acupuncture in a double-bind situation; the essence of this double bind for medical acupuncturists is that they are generally unable to attract the kind of funding necessary to produce the results to justify the method breaking out of the vicious circle in which it currently finds itself (Fulder 1988).

The generally negative attitude adopted towards alternative therapies like acupuncture by significant elements of medical orthodoxy since 1970 has also caused practical as well as financial difficulties to medical researchers in this field, in an age in which research activity has become a vital part of the process of establishing scientific credibility (Thomson 1973). Substantial barriers seem, for example, to have been put in the way of doctors wishing to conduct clinical trials of acupuncture in some British hospitals because their colleagues, assuming that the method does not work, have demanded that only patients whose problems are entirely psychological are referred for acupuncture therapy, or have insisted on orthodox treatment being continued alongside acupuncture – both of which could seriously prejudice the outcome of the trials (Macdonald 1982). Such cases of institutional scepticism and non-cooperation only reinforce the view that acupuncture still occupies a marginal position in contemporary medicine.

Further confirmation of the negative regard in which this therapy has continued to be held in orthodox circles is provided, as in previous eras, by the reception given to the considerable numbers of acupuncturists in this country whose qualifications and mode of practice lie outside organized medicine (Fulder 1988). This is exemplified in the sphere of research, where non-medical acupuncturists, who tend to subscribe to a wider and more traditionally rooted view of acupuncture (Mole 1992), have been not only shunned by most medical practitioners with interests in this field, but also deprived of orthodox funding for their investigative work. However, this situation – which has parallels in other fringe areas (Eagle 1978) despite long-standing in-principle government support for the idea of involving non-orthodox practitioners in trials of therapies like osteopathy, chiropractic and acupuncture (Inglis 1980; Sharma 1992b) – is really only the tip of the iceberg as far as non-medical acupuncturists are concerned. This is highlighted by the fact that, although the GMC has now relaxed its stringent ruling on referrals by doctors to the medically unqualified in face of stiff opposition from the BMA, such practitioners are still hedged in by professionally inspired legal restrictions on, amongst other things, the possibility of working in the NHS and the types of illnesses that they can claim to treat (Huggon and Trench 1992).

Non-orthodox practitioners of acupuncture, moreover, have also received an even more hostile response from the leading medical journals than their medical counterparts, as reporting in the *BMJ* over the past twenty years particularly illustrates. Although coverage of alternative medicine is now slightly less one-sided than once it was, most references to non-medical acupuncturists in this period strongly associate the treatment given by such practitioners with untoward side-effects. This trend is epitomized by the reports on the non-medical acupuncture therapy held responsible for the spread of hepatitis B infection (*BMJ* 1977) and cases of pneumothorax (*BMJ* 1978). The negative stance that is still generally taken towards non-orthodox practitioners of acupuncture and other marginal therapies, though, is even more overtly expressed in a number of recent editorials in the *BMJ* which variously suggest that the wider application of fringe methods 'ought to be as extinct as divination of the future by examination of a bird's entrails' (1980: 1); that alternative practitioners, in contrast to orthodox doctors, are long on caring and short on curing (1983); and that the therapies that they practise 'make no scientific sense' (1985: 1745). But if these items resurrect claims of continuing editorial bias against such alternative methods as acupuncture, so too does the assertion by the President of the BAA that the *BMJ* 'will not publish research reports submitted by traditional acupuncturists' (Webster 1979: 137) – indicating that there may be still other grounds on which the orthodox medical response to acupuncturists without medical qualifications can be considered unfavourable.

As in the 1950s and 1960s, though, non-orthodox practitioners of acupuncture have come under attack not just from the medical establishment, but also from medical acupuncturists themselves. This is evident from the published accounts of several doctors in this field which warn against both patients consulting acupuncturists who are not on the medical register and medical practitioners referring patients to them (see, for example, Mann 1973; Macdonald 1982; Marcus 1992). This follows the official line of the BMAS (*Lancet* 1987) and supports the view expressed by the BMA that 'doctors can only remain responsible clinically if they recommend patients to a medically qualified acupuncturist' (Fulder and Monro 1981: 13). Despite this additional obstacle, however, the numbers of lay acupuncture practitioners have been steadily increasing in recent years, following the general pattern for alternative therapists as a whole (Fulder 1988). This growth culminated in the major non-medical acupuncture organizations – the BAA, the Traditional Acupuncture Society (TAS), the International Register of Oriental Medicine (IROM) and the Register of Traditional Chinese Medicine (RTCM) – with a membership of around 800 practitioners, joining forces in the 1980s under the mantle of the Council for Acupuncture (CFA) to press, amongst other things, for state registration (Silverlight 1983). This search for legitimacy, though, has served more to affirm the marginality of acupuncture in contemporary Britain than to bring it within the orthodox fold, because such acupuncturists have failed to gain incorporation into mainstream medicine in face of successful opposition to date from establishment bodies like the Royal Colleges and the BMA. Their resistance has ironically been stiffened by official representations made by medical acupuncturists (see, *inter alia, Hansard* 1977) who have themselves only gradually been able to begin to break down the antagonism towards the practice of acupuncture within the profession.

It is difficult to avoid the conclusion, therefore, that acupuncture has faced a persisting climate of orthodox medical rejection in postwar Britain – albeit one which has begun to be slowly eroded, especially since the mid-1970s as far as the limited use of acupuncture by medical practitioners is concerned. Nevertheless, the general response of the British medical profession to acupuncture has scarcely been one of the more encouraging outside of the Oriental culture area in the modern era, with the result that the method has been left in a similarly disadvantaged position to other forms of alternative therapy in this country. As such, the reception given to acupuncture by orthodox medicine in more recent times has broadly mirrored that of the preceding 150 years; for all the variations in the medical response to the procedure in the nineteenth and twentieth centuries, it has not at any stage passed beyond the status of an alternative medicine in Britain. This brings back into focus the central issue to be addressed in this illustrative case study – namely, that of how far the medical response to acupuncture over the past 200 years can be seen to be altruistically oriented. This question, however, cannot be fully answered without a basic understanding of the effects of the marginal standing of acupuncture on its availability to the wider public in the historical and contemporary context – a task to which this chapter now finally turns.

ACUPUNCTURE AS AN ALTERNATIVE MEDICINE: THE SOCIAL IMPLICATIONS

The most striking aspect of the fluctuating response of the medical profession to acupuncture in nineteenth- and twentieth-century Britain is the negative repercussions that this seems to have had on the availability of the method to the public in general and groups in society disadvantaged by their class and/or regional location in particular. These negative social implications associated with the status of acupuncture as an alternative medicine began to become apparent in the first half of the nineteenth century. Although the availability of medical acupuncture increased in the 1820s and 1830s as growing numbers of doctors adopted acupuncture in their practice – albeit sporadically and for a limited range of conditions – the bulk of medical acupuncture still appears to have been undertaken in the private sector on a fee-for-service basis in patients' own homes (see, for example, Tweedale 1823; Wansbrough 1826), thus largely restricting its use to the middle and upper classes (Stacey 1988). That regional as well as class inequalities of access also prevailed in this era is indicated by the fact that the numbers of medical practitioners of acupuncture were never very substantial, even in the heyday of the procedure in the first half of the nineteenth century, especially in comparison with the 11,000 qualified doctors listed in the first Medical Directory of 1845 (Levitt and Wall 1992). These differentials were reinforced in the 1840s as an ever-stronger professional climate of rejection emerged, reducing still further the general level of availability of the medical variant of the method.

But if the at best equivocal response of the developing medical establishment to the practice of acupuncture by doctors in the period up to 1850 must surely have had a highly restrictive effect on its accessibility to the public from within the ranks of the medically qualified, the increasing practice of acupuncture on the fringe from the 1840s onwards with the arrival of Baunscheidtism in Great Britain clearly offset some of the limitations imposed by medical orthodoxy. This is underlined by the use of this method as a general therapy by unlicensed outsiders at a time when 'quack' practitioners were relatively popular with the working classes, who widely distrusted the official medical services (MacLaren 1976). However, even here the growing number of attacks made on external competitors by leading members of a medical establishment that was fast gaining public credibility (Parry and Parry 1976) probably acted as a restraining influence on patients turning to non-medical acupuncturists.

This restraining influence was all the greater as far as the alternative practice of acupuncture in the latter half of the nineteenth century was concerned as the medical profession, in the wake of the 1858 Medical Registration Act, used its growing powers against the 'evils' of quackery. That acupuncture practice amongst the medically unqualified dwindled so dramatically by the turn of the century seems to bear witness to the very real checks that the profession was able to impose on the public availability of non-medical acupuncture in its struggle for dominance at this time. The introduction of a more intensive system of internal control within the profession following the 1858 Act, moreover, cannot be dissociated from the further decline in the general availability of acupuncture from medical practitioners themselves. Paradoxically, class inequalities in access to doctors practising acupuncture may have been reduced as the method found a more secure niche in the hospital sector (see, for instance, Teale 1871; Aust-Lawrence 1889) where the poor formed by far the largest part of the clientele (Stacey 1988) and private medicine became more accessible to working-class wage-earners with the growth of schemes organized by friendly societies, trade unions and similar associations (Levitt and Wall 1992). But, against this, geographical inequalities in the provision of medical acupuncture doubtless widened as such practice became confined to a limited number of centres unevenly distributed throughout the country. The overriding trend in the period to the turn of the century, then, was the ever-decreasing availability of acupuncture from both medical and non-medical sources, linked to the climate of rejection established by the medical profession – a response that was to culminate in the situation in the first half of the twentieth century, in which it was virtually impossible for a patient to find an acupuncturist of any kind to consult.

Yet if considerations of class and regional inequalities of access to acupuncture paled into insignificance under such circumstances, these are of greater moment in assessing the availability of acupuncture to the public in Britain in the 1950s and 1960s when the method was resurrected by a small group of doctors in face of strong opposition within the profession. Whilst the generally wide scope of practice of these pioneers increased opportunities for patients to be treated by acupuncture for a broad range of conditions, their low numbers and London residential focus (see Mann 1971; Ewart 1972) inevitably meant that some sections of the public were disadvantaged in terms of geographical location. The fact, moreover, that medical acupuncturists at this time primarily worked in the private sector, as opposed to the newly founded NHS, would also have had similar implications for the differential class take-up of the method as in other areas of private practice in health care in this period (Higgins 1988).

Although the unfavourable reception of acupuncture by the medical establishment could only have retrogressively influenced the amount of acupuncture practised by doctors and the form of availability of the therapy from the few practitioners involved in this field, the negative effects of its stance were counterbalanced to some degree in the period from 1950 onwards – as in the nineteenth century – by the growth of a more numerous body of acupuncturists without orthodox training (Gould 1972). The existence of this group of acupuncturists certainly helped to compensate for the shortfall of medical exponents of the method in a comparable manner to earlier times, especially since they were even more committed to the traditional, broader-based variant of acupuncture. However, the numbers and use of such alternative therapists were scarcely encouraged by the animosity displayed towards them by the medical profession at both the institutional and individual level – so much so that even at the beginning of the 1970s only about one in four general practitioners approved of their patients turning to non-medical acupuncturists for treatment (Consumers Association 1972). Nor were class inequalities surrounding client access to lay acupuncture substantially diminished in the 1950s and 1960s; the procedure continued to be excluded from coverage within the professionally-dominated NHS (Inglis 1964), although the cost of a course of treatment from a non-medical acupuncturist was by no means negligible at this time (Consumers Association 1972).

Public access to acupuncture, though, has improved since the early 1970s, not least because of the gradual moderation of the line adopted by the British medical establishment. The availability of acupuncture from doctors in particular has grown in this period, reducing earlier regional imbalances in provision (Camp 1986). Class inequalities in the take-up of medical acupuncture have been mitigated too by the increasing use of the procedure in the NHS (Consumers Association 1981), even if the provision of alternative therapies in the state sector generally tends to be patchy and localized (Sharma 1992a). Having said this, the medical response to acupuncture over the past two decades has continued to restrict its availability to the public. Medical acupuncture is still heavily employed in private practice (Camp 1986), which tends to perpetuate class differentials in access based on persisting inequalities both in income and wealth and membership of private health insurance schemes (Griffith *et al.* 1987; Blane 1991) – although private medical practitioners of acupuncture and other unorthodox therapies do occasionally treat socially disadvantaged patients for reduced fees (see, for example, Moore *et al.* 1985). Geographical variations in the supply of medical acupuncture, moreover, have yet to be fully eliminated, particularly as between the well-provided South-East and the more poorly served areas of Wales and Scotland (Camp 1986). It is also worth recalling that the range and type of acupuncture available within the profession is inevitably limited by the fact that it is now most frequently employed by doctors for analgesic purposes within a Western scientific framework – and, indeed, that the profession has still to provide the stimulus for more than a small proportion of doctors to take up the method in any of its various forms. Furthermore, despite the more liberal climate of medical opinion prevailing today, only a minority of

general practitioners actually make referrals to doctors who are operating in this field (as highlighted by the surveys of Nicholls and Luton
1986; Wharton and Lewith 1986), thus restricting the availability of
acupuncture within the profession by making it more difficult for
prospective patients to find a medical acupuncturist who will treat them.

The even less favourable stance of the medical profession towards
non-medical acupuncture practice in recent years seems to have again
played a part in limiting access by the public to such provision.
Admittedly, there are now more non-medical acupuncturists in this
country than ever before, with a wider conception of the applicability,
and a deeper understanding of the classical basis, of the technique than
many doctors who practise the procedure – as in the case of several
other alternative therapies (Sharma 1992a). Nonetheless, the general
efforts of the medical establishment to keep lay acupuncturists outside
the NHS have meant that their fees are still not usually covered by the
state (Consumers Association 1986) which has obvious implications for
access by socially disadvantaged groups despite the charitable treatment of some patients of limited means (see, for instance, BAA 1985).
That non-medical acupuncturists have been compelled by the medical
profession to operate more or less exclusively on the private market –
in which payment is typically not even met by private health insurance
schemes (Davies 1984) – has also helped to generate substantial
regional variations in both the provision (Fulder and Monro 1981)
and the use (Halpern 1985) of non-medical acupuncture. Patient consultations with such practitioners of acupuncture can hardly have failed
to have been affected, too, by the negative stance which continues to
be taken towards them at the grass-roots level in some sections of the
profession. This is accentuated by the fact that doctors still tend to be
more reluctant to refer patients to lay acupuncturists than medical
exponents of the procedure (see, amongst others, the surveys by Reilly
1983; Nicholls and Luton 1986), notwithstanding both the recent
abandonment of ethical prohibitions on cooperation with the fringe by
the GMC and evidence from some areas of the country that medical
attitudes towards alternative therapists outside the profession are
changing (Franklin 1992).

This brief outline of the social implications of the medical reception
of acupuncture in Britain appears to confirm that the response of the
profession to this therapy throughout the past two centuries has greatly
restricted its availability – both to the public as a whole and especially
to certain disadvantaged groups in society. These restrictions on access
to acupuncture, which have varied in degree, scope and intensity over
time, are symptomatic of the long-standing status of acupuncture as an

alternative medicine. As such, there are many parallels with other alternative therapies in this country. In the nineteenth and early twentieth centuries, for example, the exclusion of herbalism and homoeopathy from the basic undergraduate medical curriculum also seems to have restricted the availability of medical practitioners of these techniques – particularly with increasing professional unification after the 1850s (Brown 1985; Nicholls 1988). Equally, from the mid-twentieth century onwards, the opposition of the medical establishment to the incorporation of alternative practitioners such as chiropractors into the NHS not only has implications for class inequalities, but also again partially accounts for geographical disparities in the provision of such marginal therapies (Fulder and Monro 1981).

But if there are obvious similarities between the restrictive implications of the medical response to acupuncture and other alternative therapies in Britain, this should not mask the distinctive limitations on the availability of acupuncture in this country as compared to many other societies in the international arena. These limitations were evident as early as the mid-nineteenth century when the medical availability of acupuncture in Britain began to diminish – and at a far greater rate than in countries like the United States (Rosenberg 1977) and imperial China where the more traditional practice of acupuncture also came under forceful attack (Wei-kang 1975). The strength of the restrictions surrounding the technique in Britain, though, is most plainly highlighted with reference to modern China where acupuncture, having now been restored to a position closer to medical orthodoxy, is much more freely available to the public as a wide-ranging procedure and little affected by inequalities in access (Rosenthal 1981). The contrast with societies outside the Orient today is not quite so striking. In America, for instance, where regional and class inequalities in health care are already pronounced, non-medical acupuncturists are banned from practising independently in some states and in most cases the treatment they administer cannot be reimbursed through third party payment, private insurance schemes or public funds (Chow 1985). However, even here – and particularly too in countries like France and Russia – acupuncture seems to be more generally available than in Britain, especially from within the ranks of the medical profession (see, *inter alia*, Wensel 1980; Stanway 1986).

CONCLUSION

It is clear that the British medical profession has established one of the stronger climates of rejection of acupuncture worldwide over the past two hundred years and that this has had distinctly adverse consequences for public access to the procedure. The empirical applicability of the analytical framework developed in Part I of the book for assessing the altruism of professional groups can now be examined in this context. The crucial questions that need to be tackled here are twofold. First, how far can the persisting standing of acupuncture as an alternative therapy in Britain be seen to be a product of the self-interests of the medical profession, as opposed to other factors? Second, to what extent can the generally unfavourable response of the medical profession to acupuncture in the nineteenth and twentieth centuries, with all its negative implications for the availability of the method, be considered to be compatible with the public good? In answering these questions the study will again focus most heavily on the modern era for the reasons given earlier in this chapter, although the historical dimension will by no means be neglected. Within this frame of reference, Chapters 5 and 6 will explore the role of professional self-interests in the reception given to acupuncture in British medicine, whilst Chapter 7 will focus more pointedly on the extent to which the predominant climate of rejection established over the last two centuries has been in the public interest.

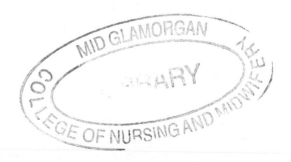

5 Potential explanations for the rejection of acupuncture in Britain

This chapter aims to heighten understanding of how far the response of the British medical profession to acupuncture has come about as a result of professional self-interests in the nineteenth and twentieth centuries. This is an important task in its own right given the continuing paucity of scholarly analyses of the influence of social factors on the medical reception of acupuncture in the West, as initially highlighted by Quen (1975a). However, the main rationale for studying the marginal practice of acupuncture in the British context is to illustrate the application of the research framework for examining the altruism claims of the professions. In this sense, it will be recalled that a central part of the strategy proposed for evaluating the role of professional self-interests in decision-making was to consider the most plausible alternative explanations of the phenomenon under discussion. It was argued that if these competing explanations could be dismissed this would considerably strengthen, if not conclusively demonstrate, the case for attributing decisive causal responsibility to professional self-interests. Accordingly, this chapter endeavours to assess systematically the superficially most plausible alternative explanations to that of the interests of the medical profession, or segments thereof, in accounting for the generally unfavourable medical climate of reception of acupuncture which has existed, to varying degrees, since the early nineteenth century in Britain – as a prelude to a more direct consideration of the evidence bearing on the self-interest hypothesis in Chapter 6.

It is worth, however, remembering that a major pitfall of this approach is that it is impossible to assess every possible explanation of any specific situation, since the causal web is infinite. In face of this difficulty and given that the inadvertent omission of a crucial variable from the analysis of competing accounts could have important consequences for the conclusions reached, as many potentially significant explanations as possible need to be examined in the case under consideration; although the outcome of the inquiry can never be more than probabilistic, the adoption of this procedure will at least lend more credibility to its findings. In this chapter, therefore, a wide range of what appear to be the most plausible factors, aside from professional self-interests, in explaining the largely negative medical reaction to acupuncture over the past two hundred years will be discussed. The explanations considered here have been drawn from work directly dealing with the reasons for the differential medical responses to acupuncture and other alternative therapies (see, for instance, Wallis and Morley 1976; Taylor 1985); the literature on the diffusion of innovations as a whole (of which classic examples are Linton 1936; Rogers 1962) and scientific innovation in particular (epitomized by Dolby 1979; Webster 1991); and studies of the history of medicine focusing on factors that have retarded or advanced knowledge and practice in this field (as represented by Stern 1927; Youngson 1979). The assessment begins with a discussion of the view that the form of the medical response to acupuncture in Britain has been a function of the diffusion of knowledge about this procedure.

THE DIFFUSION OF KNOWLEDGE OF ACUPUNCTURE

The notion that acupuncture has not been strongly taken up by the British medical profession in the period under consideration because knowledge of the method – and its allegedly beneficial effects – has been slow to diffuse to this country is consistent with the belief that scientific resistance to new ideas often derives from a lack of knowledge of the discovery in question (Duncan 1974), a claim which has also been put forward in relation to the form of the Western medical response to acupuncture (see, amongst others, Camp 1973). This explanation is given added plausibility by the lack of long-standing economic and cultural ties between Britain and China of the kind that facilitated the incorporation of acupuncture in particular and Chinese medicine in general into the orthodox health care system of societies like Japan (Powell and Anesaki 1990).

This reason for professional resistance to acupuncture in nineteenth-century Britain, however, is not very convincing. As has been seen, knowledge of the method had begun to filter through to this country from the East as early as the seventeenth century and it was practised in rudimentary form by at least some doctors from the beginning of the nineteenth century. Nor was this early practice in any way surreptitious; acupuncture not only was sporadically mentioned in mainstream medical journals at this time, but also had started to attract prominent advocates in the higher echelons of the British medical profession – including Elliotson, who was 'one of the most formidable medical men of his age' (Parssinen 1992: 62) and Ringer from University Hospital, a physiologist of some renown (Rosenberg 1977). It could scarcely be said therefore that the icy reception given to acupuncture after the 1830s resulted from the failure of leading intellectuals to endorse the method, particularly as the method was also supported by such significant international medical figures as Dunglison and Osler from the United States (Cassedy 1974; Fernandez-Herlihy 1972). Even more importantly, claims regarding the slow diffusion of knowledge about acupuncture leading to the professional climate of rejection of the method in the nineteenth century are further weakened by the Western penetration of China – especially following the Opium Wars – which provided ample opportunity for British doctors to learn about acupuncture, had they so wished (Bowers 1974).

However, although available indigenous and exogenous sources of knowledge about acupuncture belie this potential explanation as far as the nineteenth century is concerned, it is true, as will be recalled, that both the practice of, and publicity given to, acupuncture had petered out by the first half of the twentieth century in Britain. It therefore seems possible that the failure of the British medical profession to respond more rapidly and positively to acupuncture in the period after 1970 as international interest in the method spiralled is explicable in terms of a general lack of awareness of acupuncture, the principles on which it is based and the favourable results claimed by its practitioners.

This view, though, also fails to hold water for it flies in face of the impact of such pressure groups as the BAA, which has consistently aimed to promote acupuncture since its foundation in 1960 (Saks 1985), most recently in harness with other major acupuncture organizations under the umbrella of the CFA (Saks 1991a). This lobby has been paralleled within the medical profession by the work of pioneers like Moss and Mann who were amongst the first to draw public attention to the therapy in the postwar period, as well as the subsequent activity of the MAS and then the BMAS in propagating acupuncture in this country (Saks 1992b). At a wider level, moreover, acupuncture has gained further publicity from such overarching organizations as the Scientific and Medical Network (SMN), the Institute for Complementary Medicine (ICM) and the Council for Complementary and Alternative Medicine (CCAM) which have spread knowledge about a wide span of alternative therapies inside and outside of the profession (see Inglis 1980; Fulder 1988).

Claims about the lack of sufficient knowledge of the method and its application by doctors in the contemporary era seem all the more tenuous when the exposure that acupuncture has received in the mass media in modern Britain is considered. The surge of generally favourable media publicity for acupuncture – which has often been built around its growing number of famous patrons, including royalty and sporting personalities – began in the early 1960s and has since extended to include a burgeoning range of newspaper and magazine articles, television and radio programmes and popular books on this subject (Saks 1985). At the simple level of medical awareness it is therefore difficult to conclude that the availability of knowledge about acupuncture has had a significant bearing on the relatively small number of doctors practising the method, the virtual exclusion of this subject from the undergraduate medical curriculum and the very low research spending on this area in recent years.

This point is accentuated by the fact that the publicity given to acupuncture from the 1960s onwards also featured in the medical press. In this respect, Mann (1962a; 1962b; 1963; 1964; 1966) fulfilled an important role at the outset of this period in producing a pivotal series of academic texts on acupuncture. As was seen in Chapter 4, these books complemented the increasing number of items on acupuncture that were beginning to be published in mainstream medical journals in Britain in the 1960s – the content of which reveals that acupuncture and other forms of Chinese medicine were being brought to the attention of the medical community at this time, not least through an exhibition for doctors in London (*BMJ* 1966) and an address by Mann himself to a clinical meeting of the BMA on this subject (*BMJ* 1968). In addition, by the early 1970s the British medical literature on this subject was becoming larger and more positively disposed towards acupuncture as practised in its limited analgesic form – as well as being bolstered by a readily accessible and expanding American literature base in this field (see, for instance, Veith 1972; Tai 1973). This, coupled with the visits of British doctors to China to study acupuncture and regular questions in Parliament on its use in the NHS (Saks 1985), together with the continuing growth of British medical publications on the method up to the early 1990s (Saks 1992b), clearly indicates that the inquirer must look elsewhere for a plausible alternative explanation to that of professional self-interests for the predominantly negative medical response to acupuncture in contemporary Britain.

As was highlighted in Chapter 3, Lukes (1974) has noted that it is necessary in relation to explanations based on ignorance to differentiate situations where the agent does not have certain factual and technical knowledge available to assess the consequences of a particular action and where the agent claims to lack this data, but could have found it out within culturally accepted limits. The foregoing analysis leaves no doubt that where knowledge of acupuncture in the ranks of the medical profession has been absent at crucial stages over the last two hundred years, it has largely been remediable ignorance on this criteria. But if explanations based on the slow diffusion of knowledge about acupuncture to this country are implausible, what of the apparently more straightforward claim that acupuncture has not been favourably received simply because it has consistently been an ineffective therapy?

THE EFFECTIVENESS OF ACUPUNCTURE

This explanation is certainly worth considering because the effectiveness of a therapy has been identified in the literature as a factor influencing the acceptance or rejection of medical innovations (Stern 1927) and the value of acupuncture in this respect has been challenged by some commentators in both the nineteenth and twentieth centuries (see, for example, Ward 1858; Wall 1972). But before the impact or otherwise of the effectiveness of acupuncture on its fate in Britain in the past and present can be evaluated, some cautionary comments are needed on how the 'effectiveness' of this technique can best be gauged.

In this vein, it should be stressed that its effectiveness cannot be simply inferred from the long history of its use in China, as some authors have come close to suggesting (Lu Gwei-Djen and Needham 1980) for many therapies have been discredited after being practised for centuries – as, for example, bloodletting and other heroic therapies in the last century in Britain (Porter 1987). There are also alternative reasons why acupuncture and other forms of traditional medicine could have persisted for so long in China, including the dearth of modern medical facilities and Western-trained health personnel (Hillier 1988).

Having said this, the task is not made easier, as was seen in Chapter 4, by the argument of contributors like Mulkay (1991) that the cognitive criteria used to evaluate knowledge claims is negotiable, which in effect denies the existence of transcendentally objective standards of assessment in science in general and medicine in particular. The difficulties which this poses for evaluating the effectiveness of acupuncture are thrown into focus by the different bases on which alternative practitioners tend to make diagnostic judgements as compared to orthodox practitioners (Coward 1989) and the debate between such practitioners and the medical establishment about the importance of clinical trials as distinct from the case study approach to the assessment of treatment outcomes (MacEoin 1990). However, these controversies – which are mirrored in the acupuncture world where holistically-oriented traditional practitioners make diagnoses based on the balance between yin and yang and are not usually enamoured with trials centred on the principle of needling set points (Mole 1992) – can be circumvented by judging effectiveness with reference to the criteria which are most strongly supported by medical orthodoxy at any given point in time. This is not intended to imply a medical monopoly over scientific truth, but does enable the effectiveness of acupuncture to be considered as a reason why the medical profession has maintained a predominant climate of rejection of the technique in this country in terms which the medical profession itself could be expected to apply.

The net result of employing this yardstick to assess the effectiveness of acupuncture in the twentieth century, and particularly over the critical last twenty-five years, is to increase the weight given to the findings of controlled trials – the use of which has become increasingly accepted in the profession, notwithstanding the value which continues to be placed on the case study approach at the level of the individual practitioner (Cochrane 1972). It should first be emphasized, however, that many questions can be raised about the much-vaunted technique of 'acupuncture anaesthesia' – in terms of the necessary preselection of the patients involved and the levels of analgesia induced by this method alone (Saks 1985) – although it does appear to be cheaper and safer and to have fewer side-effects than chemical anaesthesia for the small proportion of people on whom it is effective (Lu Gwei-Djen and Needham 1980). This contrasts with the use of acupuncture as a treatment for chronic pain, for which there is now much extensive controlled and uncontrolled trial evidence in relation to back problems, headaches and other conditions, even if there are ongoing debates about such issues as the extent of long-term as opposed to short-term relief that it provides (Richardson and Vincent 1986). This evidence complements the less extensive body of work supporting the utility of acupuncture in related areas, such as its employment as an antiemetic in the postoperative, obstetric and cancer chemotherapy context (see, for instance, Dundee and McMillan 1991).

The disparity between the apparent effectiveness of acupuncture on orthodox criteria and the take-up of the method by the medical profession is also evident in its application as a general therapy. As will be recalled, this is an area in which the medical establishment has been most hostile in recent times. But, whilst there have been few controlled trials in this field – the small-scale study of Jobst *et al.* (1986) on acupuncture and breathlessness along these lines is the exception which proves the rule – acupuncture does seem to have been successfully applied in the modern era as a wider therapy in Britain and abroad. This is well illustrated by Mann (1973) who outlines the high proportion of patients reported as either completely cured or significantly helped by acupuncture in a large span of maladies, ranging from hay fever to peptic ulceration and glaucoma, in a number of international studies of consecutive patients whose condition had previously proved resistant to conventional therapies. This should not be too surprising given that the World Health Organization (WHO) has drawn up an extensive list of diseases which lend themselves to treatment by this method (Bannerman 1979) and the use of acupuncture as a general therapy in China is considered more important than its analgesic application (Lu Gwei-Djen and Needham 1980).

Yet if the results of contemporary studies of acupuncture cast doubt on attempts to account for the largely unfavourable medical response to acupuncture in the latter half of the twentieth century in terms of its lack of effectiveness, this form of explanation is no more applicable to earlier times. As has been seen, medical documentation of the beneficial effects of acupuncture in cases of pain – particularly those associated with conditions like rheumatism – can be traced back to the early nineteenth century and beyond (see, *inter alia*, Elliotson 1850). Much the same is also true for the broader application of acupuncture – although its range of uses were not as widely recognized as today, with attention mainly focusing on its employment in such ailments as dropsy (Tweedale 1823) and lockjaw (Finch 1824). The case study approach was typically used on varying scales to support the employment of acupuncture in such circumstances (see, for example, Banks 1831; Belcombe 1852; Gibson 1893), in an age in which the significance of carefully controlled trials had yet to be acknowledged. The conclusions reached about the efficacy of acupuncture in nineteenth-century Britain, moreover, were supported, as in more recent times, by international studies in countries like the United States and France (Quen 1975a).

Although acupuncture was not always seen to be successful in the nineteenth century in the rudimentary form in which it was practised (*Lancet* 1833), there are clearly strong contemporary parallels between this method and Perkins' patent metallic tractors and mesmerism, in so far as each of these seemed to be efficacious, but faced a strong climate of medical rejection (Quen 1975b). This mirrors the situation in the twentieth century in which acupuncture has tended to receive a similarly negative reception from the medical profession to that of other marginal practices like homoeopathy and chiropractic, despite growing evidence of their utility (Fulder 1988). It does not seem therefore that the increasing abandonment of acupuncture by the medical profession from the 1840s onwards, its almost total non-employment in the first half of the twentieth century and the generally less than enthusiastic medical response even after the 1960s can be attributed to the lack of effectiveness of acupuncture on orthodox criteria or an absence of knowledge of the studies suggesting its likely efficacy. Could it be, though, that the predominant climate of rejection surrounding acupuncture in this country is due more to its lack of safety than its lack of therapeutic promise?

CONSIDERATIONS OF SAFETY

This view receives support from Lloyd (1971) who suggests that considerations of safety impeded the adoption of such procedures as the utilization of chloroform as an anaesthetic in Britain in the last century. Cassedy (1974: 896), moreover, has argued that only a moderate amount of attention was given to acupuncture by the American medical profession in this period because of 'infections arising out of this pre-Listerian operation'. Safety therefore needs to be examined as a possible factor shaping the medical response to acupuncture in the British context, not least because of more recent claims about the dangers of the method being practised by the medically unqualified (see, for instance, Marcus 1992).

Having said this, as an explanation of the pattern of medical reception of acupuncture in nineteenth century, it remains singularly unconvincing. The claim by Cassedy about the inhibiting effect of infections on its medical take-up, for example, does not seem plausible in this country, as infections were not a prominent feature of any of the Western medical reports of the time (Quen 1975a). Knowledge of infection, indeed, was not generally available until the 1860s (Youngson 1979). This hardly squares with the strong climate of rejection of acupuncture that was established by the 1840s in Britain. And, as Rosenberg (1977: 91) points out, even if infection was perceived to be a problem later in the nineteenth century, doctors could simply have 'begun to prepare their needles, as they did other instruments, to avoid this complication', as aseptic and antiseptic procedures were increasingly incorporated into medical practice (Porter 1987).

The overriding emphasis of accounts of acupuncture in the nineteenth century in fact was not so much on its dangers as on its safety. Difficulties with the technique were only fleetingly touched upon in the international medical literature – with notable exeptions ranging from very sporadic reports in France about needles being lost inside the bodies of patients (Baptiste 1962) to an extreme case in England of infanticide caused by acupuncture of the brain (Elliotson 1850). From documentary sources of the day, practitioners in Britain generally appear to have been aware of the dangers of introducing needles into such places as the nerves, tendons, blood vessels and the spinal chord. This was certainly true of Churchill (1822: 9), one of the pioneer practitioners of acupuncture in this country, who expressed his amazement that the method had not been more favourably received by doctors, given his belief that the safety of acupuncture had been 'so fully demonstrated'.

In some ways, however, this early medical literature understated the risks from the procedure. There is now growing recognition in the modern era of the need to avoid the so-called 'forbidden points' of traditional Chinese acupuncture – not all of which correspond with those based on Western anatomic beliefs – lest dangerous consequences ensue (Lu Gwei-Djen and Needham 1980). A number of accidents involving acupuncture, moreover, have been documented in the international literature, such as fatalities due to the insertion of needles into the heart and bacterial infection as a result of failing to follow routine sterilization techniques (Peacher 1975), some of which are beginning to be reported in Britain too (Lonsdale 1991). Recent British cases range from bacterial endocarditis (Jefferys *et al.* 1983) to death arising from the accidental puncturing of a lung during acupuncture therapy (Gee 1984). Hepatitis B has also been contracted as a result of such treatment, the largest British outbreak of which occurred in Birmingham in 1977 and led to by-laws being introduced requiring the premises of non-medical acupuncturists to be regularly inspected by the Medical Officer of Health (Macdonald 1982).

This said, it is still difficult to believe that the dangers of acupuncture have played an important role in the at best equivocal response of the British medical establishment to the method as popular interest grew from the 1970s onwards. The incidence of accidents in Britain linked to acupuncture appears to be very low, as in China where the method is practised more extensively than anywhere else in the world (Sidel and Sidel 1974). In addition, the chances of acupuncturists who are not medically qualified causing damage have been reduced by the fact that most are now trained in organizations which ensure that students not only have a sound basis in anatomy and physiology, but also understand the need to sterilize needles to protect against the spread of infection (Saks 1992b). This, together with the introduction of a stringent code of practice by the CFA (1987), makes it even harder for the medical establishment to justify its attacks on the bulk of non-medically qualified acupuncturists who belong to one or other of the major acupuncture bodies in Britain (Fulder 1988). It is also pertinent to note that the contemporary safety of acupuncture has been much improved by the abandonment of the nineteenth-century practice of leaving needles *in situ* for a number of days, which occasionally led to their disappearance below the body surface (Baptiste 1962). Since acupuncture – like many other alternative therapies – appears to be relatively safe when used with care by those with appropriate training (Inglis 1980), other possible reasons need to be explored for the climate of orthodox rejection of acupuncture which has predominated in Britain over the last two hundred years if a viable alternative explanation is to be found to that of professional self-interests.

PROBLEMS OF RESEARCH

Although the existence of acceptable evidence for innovations in health care does not necessarily lead to their rapid absorption into orthodox medicine (Stern 1927), another potential reason why the British medical establishment might have shunned acupuncture for much of the period since the beginning of the nineteenth century is that there are intractable technical difficulties involved in researching this field. One form of this argument is that there has been insufficient information available on the classical practice of acupuncture for research purposes. This view certainly appears superficially credible for, whilst knowledge of acupuncture has been accessible from quite early times, doctors in Britain do not seem to have begun to understand the basis of the classical employment of the method until relatively recently. This is well illustrated by medical acupuncturists in the Victorian era, who deviated from traditional Chinese procedures by routinely treating their patients by inserting needles directly into the site where pain was experienced (Quen 1975b) and by the naive statement in the *BMJ* (1945: 34) that acupuncture is generally performed by needling 'a point situated a few centimetres above the internal malledus and just behind the posterior border of the tibia'.

For all this, however, such an explanation is again tenuous. If the lack of such information was so critical in the 1840s in Britain, why should the method have remained a significant part of medical practice in the United States in the second half of the nineteenth century when knowledge of classical acupuncture was no less limited? The generally good results obtained by the early pioneers on both sides of the Atlantic in cases of pain (Saks 1991b; Rosenberg 1977), coupled with current informed testimony on the helpful effects of needling sites of local pain

(Lewith 1982) sharpen the question as to why an understanding of traditional acupuncture should have been necessary before systematic research into the method could be conducted in the nineteenth century. In fact British doctors at this time had even less reason than their American counterparts to abandon the technique on such grounds, given the close Western European link with France where important accounts of classical acupuncture were published by Dabray de Thiersant in the 1860s (Baptiste 1962) and Soulié de Morant and his collaborator Ferreyrolles in the first half of the twentieth century (Lu Gwei-Djen and Needham 1980) – the work of the latter of which was even publicized at the time in the *BMJ* (Monod 1932).

The notion that a lack of in-depth knowledge of classical acupuncture delayed the full adoption of the method by medical orthodoxy after the mid-twentieth century is even more unconvincing. Although the degree of sophistication of the available literature on traditional acupuncture could be greater (Lu Gwei-Djen and Needham 1980), this is progressively being improved with the development of an international nomenclature (*BMJ* 1989) and the increasing translation of Chinese texts in this area (Mole 1992). It should also be stressed that many key publications on traditional acupuncture practice have been available since the late 1950s – and not only those previously referred to by Mann, but also texts by such respected authors as Lavier (1965), Lawson-Wood and Lawson-Wood (1959; 1964; 1974) and Austin (1972). Nor can the lack of classical practitioners of acupuncture be invoked as an explanation of the medical reception of the technique in view of the growing numbers of traditional acupuncturists that have been trained in this country in recent years (Fulder 1988). Such difficulties, moreover, certainly do not seem to have retarded developments in the modern era in other non-Oriental societies like France, Russia and the United States.

It has, nonetheless, been suggested that the greatest difficulty relating to research lies not so much in the availability of detailed knowledge of acupuncture, as in the fact that acupuncture is not amenable to scientific assessment in general or being subjected to tightly conducted controlled trials in particular (see, for example, Greene 1972). However, the former claim is clouded by the fact that, as has been seen, there is no universal agreement on the principles which demarcate science from non-science. At best it can be said that the idea of science in nineteenth- and twentieth-century Britain is associated with 'open knowledge-seeking systems, rather than with . . . closed knowledge-conserving systems' (Dolby 1979: 28). Since acupuncturists have generally sought over the years to consider critically evidence on the method and have not taken the self-sustaining position of the religiously based alternative health care systems of Christian Science and Pentecostalism (Saks 1985), medical disbelief in acupuncture does not seem to have stemmed from its unscientific approach – particularly since the openness of orthodox medicine itself to contrary evidence has not always been beyond reproach (see, *inter alia*, Inglis 1980; Collier 1989). What needs to be explored more fully, though, is how far the predominant climate of rejection of acupuncture has been sustained by the impossibility of carrying out rigorous controlled trials in this area – at a time when it is felt in some medical circles that 'it is essential that clearly controlled, randomized clinical trials become available . . . before this technique is accepted' (Lewith and Machin 1983: 111) and that the concepts and procedures of acupuncture 'do not always lend themselves readily to testing in double-blind studies or with other research tools' (Riscalla 1979: 221).

In this respect, it should be acknowledged that, as a result of imponderables such as the length of time for which a trial should continue (Hemminki 1982), there are difficulties in assessing any therapy using trials that compare outcomes associated with random allocations of subjects to a standard treatment and control group (Reid and Boore 1987). These difficulties are accentuated in the study of pain, for which the greatest claims have been made for acupuncture in this country, in part because of the problems of measuring 'subjective' reactions as opposed to 'objective' events (see, for instance, Richardson 1992). Although this is not an objection in principle to trials in this area, a number of more significant methodological issues do arise specifically in relation to acupuncture. These include problems in undertaking a double-blind study of this technique, where the acupuncturist will need to be sufficiently skilled to recognize when real – as distinct from sham – acupuncture is being administered and nonstandard points for sham acupuncture may have specific effects (Vincent 1989). Just as important is the claim that such trials are impossible because of the 'techi' sensation experienced by the subject when the needle is correctly inserted (*BMJ* 1981). These are not, however, fatal objections. The researcher may need to be content with a single-blind study to ensure the appropriate treatment expertise in administering treatment and could use minimally inserted needles to limit the difficulties posed by sham acupuncture (Vincent and Richardson 1986). Equally, the 'techi' effect linked to real acupuncture is not liable to be recognized by British patients who are unlikely to be familiar with the sensation associated with an appropriately needled point (Macdonald

1982) – and could in any case be mimicked if necessary by using an electrical stimulator (*Doctor* 1974).

Such resolutions are inevitably not perfect, but do at least highlight the ways in which some key objections might be countered in an assumption-laden field. Whilst there is still scope for improvement in the trials conducted to date in this area (Richardson and Vincent 1986), the difficulties associated with them can scarcely have been a significant factor in the ambivalent medical reception given to acupuncture in modern Britain. This point is reinforced by the fact that randomized trials are far from universally applied today, even in orthodox medical research itself; whilst drug therapy is routinely subject to this method of assessment, as Hemminki (1982: 711) notes, a mixture of technical and ethical problems has entailed that clinical trials 'are less well established in other therapies, such as surgical procedures, physiotherapy, and psychotherapy'. A further argument against this explanation of the contemporary British medical response to acupuncture is that such trials have not by any means always vindicated established medical practice (Cochrane 1972), still less been consistently rigorously conducted (Hemminki 1982). In many other countries in the modern context too, concern about the rigour of clinical trials in acupuncture, far from stemming the flow of medical interest, has if anything acted as a spur to further research – as, for example, in the United States, where the comparative absence of trials in the 1960s seemed to motivate the medical establishment to increase levels of funding for research into acupuncture (Davis 1975).

On this note, however, it should finally be emphasized that – as for many other alternative therapies – the randomized controlled trial runs counter to the holistic philosophy underpinning the traditional variant of acupuncture, in which treatment is tailored to the individual (Mac-Eoin 1990). Its importance may therefore be limited in relation to the assessment of acupuncture as a therapy in modern Britain. This comment applies with even greater force to the past, given that the randomized controlled trial did not receive its first medical application until 1952 (Strong 1979). The difficulties associated with trials of acupuncture could not therefore have been a stumbling block to its incorporation into orthodox medicine from the early nineteenth to the mid-twentieth century in Britain. Nor does it seem that any other technical problems concerned with evaluation could have resulted in its progressive rejection in this period, when the use of medical journals for research communications only began in the first half of the nineteenth century and statistics were first employed on a wider basis in assessing the value of specific remedies around the turn of the century

(Jewson 1976). Given the methodological flaws of even the more illustrious medical inquiries of the day (Youngson 1979), queries can scarcely be raised about the lack of scientific credibility of medical studies of acupuncture prior to the modern era – which, whilst usually small-scale in nature, followed the prevailing standards by basing their conclusions primarily on a range of individual cases (Saks 1985). But if claims about the problems of research in this area do not stand up, does the real key to the predominantly negative response of the British medical profession to acupuncture over the last two hundred years lie in the philosophical clashes between Western and Eastern medicine?

CONFLICTING PHILOSOPHIES OF MEDICINE

At first glance, this seems an appealing explanation. Cultural dissonance and lack of paradigm conformity are commonly cited as reasons for the rejection of innovations in scientific and other fields (see, for instance, Rogers 1962; Duncan 1974). The distinction between the ancient Chinese system of medicine on which acupuncture is based and that established in Britain from the early nineteenth century onwards is also apparent (Mole 1992). At its most general level this is represented in the holistic principles of classical acupuncture as compared to the mechanistic materialist approach of British medical orthodoxy, a distinction which is also accentuated by the absence of any known connection between the meridians along which acupuncture points are located and the conventional Western physiological structure (Lu Gwei-Djen and Needham 1980). Claims about the disjuncture between the philosophical underpinnings of classical acupuncture and orthodox medicine leading to the medical marginality of acupuncture in Britain, moreover, are supported by the influential work of Kuhn (1970) who argues that there are substantial advantages to be gained from scientists operating within a single paradigm which lays the basis for 'normal science' and provides 'the source of the methods, problem-field and standards of solution accepted by a mature scientific community' (Kuhn 1970: 103). These advantages include the opportunity for scientists to focus on narrow technical issues and rapidly accumulate precise knowledge, rather than engage in unending debates about the basic assumptions guiding their work; to progress to higher logical states through successive periods of normal science; and to minimize potential problems of communication and mutual understanding.

But if Kuhn seemingly provides strong theoretical grounds for paradigm-entrenchment in orthodox medical science, it is important to note that his work has been significantly challenged by other sociologists of science. Mulkay (1991), for example, has claimed that there are usually a number of candidates for paradigm status in science at any one time, centred on a myriad of problem networks with common sets of intellectual preconceptions. Dolby (1979) believes that it is vital for such a range of alternative approaches to coexist since it is impossible to prove conclusively the truth of any part of what is conventionally regarded as science. The best-known advocate of this position, though, is Feyerabend (1975: 10) who opposes one approach to theory and method dominating all others, asserting that the 'only principle that does not inhibit progress is: anything goes'. This anarchistic view of knowledge – which gains further support from Barnes and Mackenzie (1979) who argue that technical problems associated with the parallel existence of two or more incommensurable paradigms can readily be overcome by scientists in practice – clearly favours the full toleration of deviant science in general and alternative medicine in particular. As such, it offers a condemnation, rather than justification, of the hostility which the medical establishment has tended to display towards acupuncture both inside and outside the profession in nineteenth- and twentieth-century Britain.

Attempts to explain the rejection of acupuncture in Britain in terms of the conflicts between Western and Eastern systems of medicine are also weakened by the fact that they underplay the very real similarities between Western medicine and the ancient Chinese medical philosophy underlying acupuncture (Unschuld 1987). This is especially apparent in relation to the systems theory of disease inherent in the concepts of humoral and tension pathology widely applied in Britain and other Western societies until the early nineteenth century. In this respect, Quen observes:

> Asclepiades and his doctrine of strictum et laxum; Friedrich Hoffman's tonic and atonic states; and the Brunonian sthenic and asthenic conditions, as medical systems stressing a healthy balance between polar elements, are not so different as to make traditional Oriental concepts intellectually alien to the West. By the same token, the five elements of the Chinese system bear a marked resemblance to the four elements and the four humours of the Hippocratic school.
>
> (Quen 1975a: 198)

Even after the progressive demise of the systems explanation of disease with the rise of first hospital and then laboratory medicine (Jewson 1976), some similarities continue to exist – not least through the parallels between the Western notion of referred pain and the classical acupuncture principle of needling at a distance and the links between the circulation of energy in the traditional Chinese medical system and the theory of the circulation of the blood and circadian rhythms in modern Western medicine (Lu Gwei-Djen and Needham 1980).

The undeniable differences between the systems that still exist today, moreover, have not prevented both Western and Eastern philosophies from being integrated within modern Chinese health care provision (Shao 1988) or Western doctors from linking acupuncture to orthodox medical practice (see, for example, Marcus 1992). This has been facilitated by the development of theories relating this technique to contemporary Western medicine. Indeed, its medical use as an analgesic based on such recently generated theories as those focused on gate control and the release of endorphins (Lewith 1985) means that reservations about the ancient Chinese philosophy on which acupuncture is traditionally rooted can hardly be said to account for the failure of orthodox doctors to take up acupuncture in Britain in the modern era.

But if the problem of conflicting philosophies of medicine fails to account for the predominantly negative medical response to acupuncture in contemporary Britain, it is an even less convincing explanation of the climate of rejection in earlier times. In the first place, it is not consistent with the fact that acupuncture was spurned in the nineteenth century before there was any real medical awareness of the traditional Chinese roots of the method (Quen 1975b). It also seems to fly in the face of the efforts of some earlier practitioners to wed acupuncture to popular science and relevant medical conceptions of the day – such as through the fluidist notion of acupuncture with its links to the much in vogue theory of electrical conduction (Druitt 1859; Craig 1869) and the even more orthodox medical notions of counter-irritation and tension pathology (Ward 1858; Teale 1871). Finally, this explanation ignores the part that acupuncture played in the subsequent development of orthodox medicine through the role of the needle as a surgical device. As Quen says, as a result of acupuncture practice in the early nineteenth century:

> The needle needed to be looked at anew, and surgeons started experimenting with it as a surgical instrument. James Young Simpson, in the mid-nineteenth century, introduced, or re-introduced, the use of acupressure, using the shaft of the needle to apply localized occluding pressure on a vessel. Arterial aneurysms treated by acupuncture would develop occlusive thromboses that would canalize. Sir William Macewen, dissatisfied with the incidence of emboli occurring with this method, studied the process and, in 1890, reported that the use of an acupuncture needle to scratch and damage the

endothelium of an aneurysm would result in a mural thrombus less likely to embolize. This kind of interest in the use of the needle, and the early Western acupuncturists' work on electrical stimulation of discrete muscle groups, led to the development of modern techniques for electromyography and electroneurophysiologic research with implanted micro-electrodes.

(Quen 1975a: 200)

In this light, it is genuinely difficult to believe that the ties between acupuncture and Oriental philosophies of medicine held back the development of this method in either the nineteenth or the twentieth century.

This view is reinforced by the fact that cognitive dissonance as an explanation does not square with the greater degree of acceptance of acupuncture by medical orthodoxy in other Western societies with similar scientific traditions – and especially France where, as has been seen, the method was resurrected in its classical form in the 1920s and 1930s. Attempts to explain the unfavourable medical climate of reception of acupuncture in Britain over the last two hundred years in terms of the failure of the traditional Chinese account of its *modus operandi* to mesh with the philosophical underpinnings of Western science in general and British medicine in particular, then, simply will not do.

THE *MODUS OPERANDI* OF ACUPUNCTURE

Having said this, it might be claimed that the reason for the predominant climate of medical rejection of acupuncture is that doctors in this country have failed to provide a satisfactory orthodox explanation of the *modus operandi* of this method. Certainly, Dolby (1979) has emphasized how important it is for any deviant form of medicine to possess an adequate justificatory theory if it is to compete successfully with medical orthodoxy. Both Haller (1973) and Stanway (1986), moreover, hold that the reluctance of the medical profession to accept acupuncture in contemporary Britain is centrally related to the unsatisfactory nature of accounts of its *modus operandi*. Quen (1975b) and Inglis (1980) also argue that the method fell into disuse in the nineteenth century because of a lack of a convincing explanation of the results it produced.

The view that the rationale of acupuncture was 'not evident' from the standpoint of medical orthodoxy as far as Victorian Britain was concerned (*BMJ* 1973b: 687) is not too far off the mark. As has been seen, a range of medical explanations of the method were put forward in the nineteenth century in this country, including those based on tension pathology, counter-irritation and the conduction of electrical energy. Other theories were also advanced – not least being those explaining the success of acupuncture in terms of the escape of morbific vapours (Churchill 1822) and bloodletting (Hooper 1848). Although accounts based on electricity were only loosely bound to conventional medicine because of their links to mysticism and fringe practice (Haller 1973), theories rooted in the systems view of disease were close to mainstream medical philosophies, especially in the first half of the nineteenth century before the emergence of modern allopathic medicine. Yet despite their compatibility with medical orthodoxy, such indigenous theories of acupuncture could be discounted for their implausibility. Churchill (1822), for example, distinguished acupuncture from blood-letting because it was rare for blood to be drawn in treatment, whilst Wansbrough (1826: 848) was sceptical about theories involving the release of vapours because the 'very form of the instrument is a barrier to the escape of air, and . . . the cure is often performed before the needles are withdrawn'. Elliotson (1850) too dismissed counter-irritation as an explanation because similar results were obtained irrespective of the pain experienced in treatment and equally opposed galvanism because needles of gold and silver were as efficacious as those made of steel. Even accounts based on tension pathology had their detractors, who raised questions about how far the nerves were the main agency in acupuncture therapy (see, for instance, Lorimer 1885).

But if an adequate Western medico-scientific theory of how acu-puncture worked was lacking in the nineteenth century, by the early 1960s the action of acupuncture was 'still poorly understood' within a Western medical framework (Huard and Wong 1962: 336), with none of the arguments advanced proving very satisfactory. This was, how-ever, the start of the period when more powerful attempts were made to account for acupuncture in terms of the neurophysiological mechan-isms on which so much of orthodox medicine is now based. Two mainstream explanations stand out in this respect. The first is the gate control theory put forward by Melzack and Wall (1965), and sub-sequently modified (Melzack 1975), which is centred on the notion that a gate mechanism in the substantia gelatinosa in the dorsal horn of the spinal chord blocks pain impulses to the brain when the large pain fibres in the skin are stimulated by acupuncture. The second is the theory advanced by a growing number of acupuncturists since the mid-1970s that endorphins and other neuroactive substances are released into the nervous system following acupuncture treatment and have a similar effect to the injection of a narcotic – hence accounting for the often dramatic impact of acupuncture in cases of pain (see, *inter alia*, Pomeranz 1977; Chung and Dickenson 1980).

Despite the interest that these medical theories have generated, though, they are still not entirely convincing. The gate control theory cannot explain, for example, why acupuncture should work at a distance as there is typically no anatomical correlation between the site at which analgesia occurs and the points at which the acupuncture needles are inserted (Bowers 1978). Equally, this theory does not fully account for the prolonged effects of acupuncture, nor its apparent efficacy in a range of non-painful conditions (Lewith 1982). These pitfalls also apply to medical explanations based on the release of endorphin-like substances. Lever (1987) additionally notes that the endorphin theory does not explain why the stimulation of particular points seems to produce specific effects. A further query about the viability of this account of the mechanism of acupuncture is raised by the lack of consistent evidence that naxolone, the opoid antagonist, reverses analgesia induced by the technique (Filshie and Abbot 1991). Lewith (1982: 45–6) reinforces such doubts in suggesting that, whilst the effects of acupuncture can be instantaneous, 'the release of chemicals might possibly be too slow a process to have such a swift action'. All this indicates that acupuncture may have been largely disregarded in twentieth-, as well as nineteenth-, century Britain because its *modus operandi* has yet to be fully explained by orthodox medicine.

This, however, would be a premature conclusion – and not just because of confidence in a more plausible orthodox rationale for acupuncture being developed in the near future, or the defensibility of the traditional Chinese explanation of the technique in its own terms. A more important reason for rejecting this proposed explanation of the limited medical interest in acupuncture in recent times is that therapies are often introduced into orthodox medicine and widely utilized before a satisfactory account of their operation is developed. As Ewart observes:

The major problem with acupuncture in the Western world, and in Britain in particular, is that it defies any scientific explanation. But who can explain how aspirin works? Digitalis, the heart drug made from fox-gloves, slows the heart beat and increases its force, but nobody knows how it achieves this effect. Adrenalin constricts the blood vessels in normal doses and acts as a dilator in minimal doses – for no explained reason. They are all empirical, used as a result of observation and experiment, but with no irrefutable scientific explanation.

(Ewart 1972: 10)

Other mainstream examples could be given of treatments which are extensively employed without a convincing orthodox theoretical basis, including the use of electroconvulsive therapy in psychiatry which is far more controversial than acupuncture in terms of health outcomes (Gould 1985). Such examples highlight the emphasis that Mulkay (1991) places on the negotiability of the criteria by which scientific knowledge-claims are judged. The reasons why acupuncture occupies a marginal standing in modern Britain must, then, be sought elsewhere. This is confirmed by an editorial in the *BMJ* (1981: 747) which stated that if acupuncture is effective and safe 'then its mechanism of action is of secondary importance'.

An explanation based on the absence of a satisfactory *modus operandi* of acupuncture is even less convincing in relation to the strong climate of rejection of the technique that emerged from the 1840s onwards in the nineteenth century. At this time the British medical tradition still bore the mark of the eighteenth-century patronage system, in which medical careers were advanced by prescribing cures for ailments, rather than developing theories about disease and its treatment (Jewson 1974) – in a similar way to the United States where physicians were perhaps even more pragmatically oriented as a result of the anti-intellectualism of the Jacksonian era (Rosenberg 1977). In this light, it is understandable that Flood should write that he and other doctors were

> bound in many cases, to believe that which we can neither explain nor understand. Take, for instance, the action of many medicines; we know that some substances act almost specifically in curing certain forms of disease, and yet we know no more than the man in the moon how they do so; it would be an act of insanity on our part to refuse calling in their aid, simply because we are unable to understand their modus operandi, or the law which patterns their action.
>
> (Flood 1845a: 181)

The absence of a satisfactory orthodox theory of how acupuncture works does not therefore seem to be the main reason for the negative response by the British medical profession to this method in either the nineteenth or twentieth centuries – a point which is accentuated by the fact that this explanation does not adequately account for the less favourable medical response to acupuncture in Britain as compared to countries such as the United States. This is a problem which also besets the next potential explanation to be considered – namely, that acupuncture has tended to be rejected in Britain because its efficacy is a chimera, related to the power of the mind rather than the autonomous influence of the method itself.

ACUPUNCTURE AND THE POWER OF THE MIND

Claims about the power of the mind paradoxically suggest that acupuncture has been largely rejected by the British medical establishment not because its achievements cannot be adequately explained on orthodox criteria, but precisely because they can – albeit in terms of factors like hypnotism, cultural stoicism and the placebo effect which deny the independent efficacy of the technique. This thesis was particularly strongly asserted in the 1970s in Britain by Wall (1972; 1974) – mirroring a wider body of international opinion on this subject (Webster 1979).

Arguments advanced to sustain the view that acupuncture has been marginalized because of the influence of the mind – paralleling certain other alternative therapies like spiritual healing (Inglis 1980) – are not without foundation. The belief that cultural stoicism may affect the amount of pain relief experienced in acupuncture treatment, for instance, is supported by research highlighting the influence of culture in the social interpretation of pain (Helman 1990). Equally, the link between hypnosis and 'acupuncture anaesthesia' is not inconceivable, given that operations have been carried out using hypnotic techniques (Lu Gwei-Djen and Needham 1980). Suggestion in a broader sense than that of hypnosis may also be partially responsible for the success of acupuncture, given the emphasis which acupuncturists and other alternative therapists normally place on the need to build up a sympathetic relationship with clients (see, for instance, Sharma 1992a). Nor can the possible placebo effect of acupuncture be ignored in view of the classic finding of Beecher (1955) that some 35 per cent of Euro-American patients suffering from pain derive relief from drugs with no known pharmacological effect – and even greater placebo reactions are associated with medical procedures involving injections (Shapiro 1971). In addition to recovery from illness due to spontaneous remission, further evidence for supposing that the independent effects of acupuncture may be limited is provided by the fact that acupuncture seems to be most effective in functional disorders based on easily reversible physiological processes, readily influenced by the mind (Mann 1962a).

However, whilst it would be foolish to deny the psychological influences on the results achieved by acupuncture – or any other therapy for that matter – there are a number of strong arguments which contradict the view that the effects of acupuncture are wholly subjective and that the minimal autonomous efficacy of acupuncture has led to a less than enthusiastic medical reception of the method in Britain. In the first place, professional hypnotists have universally rejected the links between hypnotism and 'acupuncture anaesthesia', not least because those on whom acupuncture is employed display 'none of the trance-like or somnambulistic states characteristic of hypnosis' (Lu Gwei-Djen and Needham 1980: 226). The claim that suggestion is more broadly responsible for producing the effects of acupuncture is also weakened by the lack of a correlation between responses to acupuncture and individual suggestibility (Lewith 1985) – a point which is underlined by the positive outcomes achieved in its long-standing application to animals and children, who are less susceptible to suggestion (Mole 1992). Beliefs about the impact of cultural stoicism are similarly subverted by the successful employment of acupuncture in a wide range of conditions and socio-cultural settings, in both the East and the West (Macdonald 1982). And whilst the placebo effect cannot be entirely discounted, the controlled trials that have been conducted to date certainly indicate that this is far from being the only factor involved in its utility, particularly in cases of pain (Richardson and Vincent 1986). This position is reinforced, as Lu Gwei-Djen and Needham (1980) observe, by the identification of many of the classical acupuncture points through the measurement of electrical skin resistance and other methods – even if the meridians have still to be established as a separate physiological system. In this light, it is not surprising that they conclude that acupuncturists today

> have nothing to do with parapsychology, occult influences or 'psychic powers' . . . They do not depend entirely on suggestion, nor on hypnotic phenomenon at all . . . consequently they do not deserve the odium theologicum of the medical profession in the West.
>
> (Lu Gwei-Djen and Needham 1980: 318)

Much the same might also be said of the situation in the nineteenth century, although it is not quite as clear-cut in so far as early British acupuncturists did not, as has been seen, have a clear understanding of such aspects of classical acupuncture as the traditional point locations – – with the result that the form of acupuncture practised may have been more dependent on factors like the placebo effect and suggestion for success. Renton certainly noted that one reason why acupuncture may not always have been favourably received by doctors was that

> its boasted recoveries have been imputed more to mental reaction – that is to impressions acting upon the patient's mind from a fancied and mystical confidence in the use of the means employed – than to any real good effects resulting from the operation itself.
>
> (Renton 1830: 101)

However, his was a lone voice in the published literature of the day in this area. Elliotson seems to have been more representative in his view that the positive results of acupuncture were due to

> neither fear nor confidence; since those who care nothing about being acupunctured, and those who laugh at their medical attendant for proposing such a remedy, derive the same benefit, if their case is suitable, as those who are alarmed and who submit to it with faith.
>
> (Elliotson 1850: 34)

It is also true that while randomized controlled trials were not carried out on acupuncture at this time, the results of studies of the method reported in the medical journals suggested a higher rate of success than would be expected from the placebo effect alone (see, for example, Gibson 1893). Indeed, even if acupuncture was to have worked purely on the basis of placebo reactions, this would not have been an adequate reason for rejecting this technique so forcefully in the last century, especially as much of the medicine practised in this period was ineffective in its own right and hence more dependent than today on the placebo factor for any positive outcomes achieved (Porter 1987).

The reliance of orthodox medicine on the placebo effect is worthy of elaboration since there is a strong argument that doctors generally should make far more systematic and conscious use of the potent therapeutic force of the mind. In this vein, Quen (1975b) argues that mesmerism, perkinism and acupuncture were all shunned in the nineteenth century because the striking therapeutic responses induced were due to the 'imagination'. He thus asks why, given the long-standing medical awareness that 'passions' could cause disease states, there was 'no room in the contemporary medical or scientific conception of reality for an "imagination" that could treat or heal' (1975b: 156). Although Quen's view of the basis on which acupuncture worked in this early period is contentious, he does provide a further reason for rejecting the claim that the medical reception of acupuncture in Britain was heavily conditioned by the fact that the *modus operandi* of this method rested on the power of the mind. This rebuttal applies with equal force to the twentieth as well as the nineteenth century, in so far as the placebo effect is still a vital component of modern medicine and there is a growing body of opinion that doctors should be striving to build on its influence, rather than dismissing it as unscientific (see Pietroni 1991). Yet if accounts based on the power of the mind do not stand up as potential alternatives to that of professional self-interests in the explanation of the largely negative medical response to acupuncture over the last two hundred years, what of the claim that this method has been marginalized because of the practical difficulties of integrating acupuncture into orthodox medicine?

PRACTICAL PROBLEMS OF INTEGRATING ACUPUNCTURE INTO ORTHODOX MEDICINE

Such a claim does not seem too compelling when there are arguments that acupuncture falls into a common mould with many other forms of alternative medicine in that its very simplicity has led to opposition in medical circles in an age of increasing scientific sophistication. In this respect, Haller (1973: 1217) certainly notes that in nineteenth-century Britain – when the rudimentary type of acupuncture practised was indeed straightforward to learn and easy to apply – 'medical men and their suffering patients found it hard to believe that disease could be cured or pain alleviated with so trifling a procedure'. However, the notion that acupuncture was rejected on these grounds hardly squares with the fact that orthodox medicine itself continued to rely predominantly on the use of simple procedures like heroic purges and venesection (Porter 1987). In the modern era too, the plausibility of this argument diminishes because simplicity is actually widely sought in the formulation of orthodox scientific generalizations (Mulkay 1979) and it is increasingly appreciated that acupuncture may be even more effectively practised in its more complicated and highly skilled classical form (Mole 1992).

These comments lead to the conclusion that it may in fact be the complexity, rather than the simplicity, of the technique which has posed the greatest obstacle to its incorporation into orthodox medicine in contemporary Britain. This explanation is supported by the assertion in an editorial in the *BMJ* (1973b) at the start of the modern period of resurgence of acupuncture that this factor has weighed heavily against trials of the method in Britain and the observation by Lewith (1982: 37) that many doctors currently 'find the philosophical concepts of traditional Chinese medicine indigestible'. That this claim warrants serious attention is further endorsed by writers on the diffusion of innovations in general and medical innovations in particular who argue that the rate of adoption of new ideas is often adversely affected by the degree of difficulty involved in understanding and using the innovation in question (see, for example, Rogers 1962; Youngson 1979). The specific problems associated with acupuncture are the alleged difficulties of developing short courses on this method as a basis for research and practice and of introducing such a seemingly lengthy and labour intensive procedure into the financially hard-pressed NHS – not least given the time which is said to be needed in traditional acupuncture for pulse diagnosis (Macdonald 1982), individual consultations (Fulder 1988), repeat treatment sessions (Mole 1992) and preparing clients for 'acupuncture anaesthesia' (Inglis 1980).

Ultimately, though, arguments about the complexity of acupuncture seem no more persuasive than those concerning its simplicity as an explanation of the none too favourable medical reception of the method in recent times. Many authorities in this field believe that basic training in acupuncture can be adequately undertaken in weeks or months rather than years – especially for practitioners with a medical training who wish to use the method simply as an analgesic, without reference to classical theories (Lever 1987). Indeed, several weekend courses have already been established for doctors interested in practising the technique in this manner in Britain (Campbell 1987). Even an accelerated training in traditional acupuncture, moreover, may be feasible given that barefoot doctors during the Cultural Revolution in China appear to have been successfully prepared in this method in a very brief period (Sidel and Sidel 1974) – which helps to support the WHO view that a Western-trained physician may require 'no more than three months' training' to learn acupuncture in its classical mould (Bannerman 1979: 28). This prospect has been further enhanced by the introduction of electronic aids such as acupuncture point detectors and the Voll Dermatron, a diagnostic and therapeutic device centred on the classical principles of Chinese medicine (Lewith 1982). Notwithstanding the objections of some traditional acupuncturists to the reduction of the length of training programmes in this area (Webster 1979), therefore, it does seem as if it is possible for both doctors and non-doctors to gain a basic knowledge of the theory and practice of acupuncture in a short time.

The difficulties of introducing acupuncture into the British health service also appear to be overplayed. The New York State Commission on Acupuncture concluded that the method could be practised almost as effectively without the complexities of pulse diagnosis (Riddle 1974). And although there is little that can be done about the length of consultations and the typical need for repeat treatments, the involvement of doctors employing this method can be dramatically reduced by using electrical, as opposed to manual, stimulation of the needles (Lu Gwei-Djen and Needham 1980) and delegating the task of administering acupuncture to personnel such as nurses and physiotherapists (Downey 1988). It should also be noted that, in terms of time, 'acupuncture anaesthesia' represents a minority use of the technique and that protracted preparation is not normally needed for other applications of the method (Inglis 1980). Neither should cost be seen as a major obstacle to its incorporation into the NHS; notwithstanding the staffing requirements involved, the financial outlay for training and equipment in the acupuncture field is comparatively low (see, for instance, Selly 1991) and is more than offset by the considerable savings that can be made on drugs and expensive high-technology equipment (see, for example, Myers 1991). Indeed, even the labour intensive use of 'acupuncture anaesthesia' could entail significant savings on life-sign monitoring equipment and earlier patient discharge in the absence of the side-effects of more conventional forms of anaesthesia (Macdonald 1982).

But if claims relating the at best equivocal medical response to acupuncture in modern Britain to the complexity of incorporating this method into the health service seem tenuous, this explanation of the marginal position of acupuncture is even more implausible with regard to earlier times. As has been seen, detailed knowledge of classical acupuncture was lacking in the crucial period leading up to the mid-nineteenth century when the method faced an increasingly strong climate of medical rejection. Problems of providing systematic training in acupuncture, therefore, did not arise at this stage. As Churchill (1822: 13) said, the technique was 'simple and easy, requiring neither practice to give dexterity, nor adroitness that it may be done with propriety'. Nor, indeed, did practitioners see the need to repeat treatments as often as today; whilst Elliotson (1850), for example, had to administer acupuncture nine times to one patient before his lumbago would yield, he stressed that the operation was usually only required a second time. The cost of acupuncture in Elliotson's day, moreover, must have been minimal, given that none of the modern electronic acupuncture devices was available and that ordinary household needles with wax deposited on one end were generally used in treatment instead of specifically designed acupuncture needles (Churchill 1822). In this light, the practical problems of integrating acupuncture into mainstream medicine were even less likely to have acted as a deterrent to the medical adoption of the method in the nineteenth, as compared to the twentieth, century.

PRIORITIES IN MEDICINE

Another possible reason for the apparently blinkered medical response to acupuncture in Britain is that, notwithstanding the generally positive results claimed from studies of the method to date, competing priorities in medicine have been more pressing. Certainly Linton (1936) has argued that any innovation must significantly improve on existing techniques if it is to be widely accepted, and many writers have been prepared to testify to the effectiveness of modern medical orthodoxy – with some suggesting that its effectiveness was a major factor in the general decline of alternative medicine in early twentieth-century Britain (Wallis and Morley 1976). Indeed, in respect of acupuncture, the *BMJ* (1973b: 688) explicitly stated that the comparative lack of medical acceptance of acupuncture in this country is related to 'competing claims of seemingly greater priority'.

Again, however, this is not a very satisfactory rival explanation to that of professional self-interests in the modern era. The effectiveness of modern medical orthodoxy has been so powerfully challenged in recent years by the well-supported work of contributors like Dubos (1968), Powles (1973), McKeown (1979), Ashton and Seymour (1988) and Pietroni (1991) that its present value and future therapeutic potential seem much more limited than is commonly assumed. The key criticisms of modern medicine that such work contains are most forcefully expounded by Illich (1976) who suggests, with extensive documentation, that the medical establishment in the twentieth century has now become a major threat to health – which is manifested in a three-fold system of iatrogenesis. The main features of the clinical dimension of this are that the decline in death rates and the spread of mass killer disease is not centrally related to the progress of interventionist medicine; environmental factors such as the quantity and quality of the food supply and the use of soap are the primary determinants of health; most of the sky-rocketing medical expenditure in the industrial world is destined for diagnosis and treatment of doubtful effectiveness; and the most rapidly expanding epidemic today is illness caused by doctors through the application of standard medical procedures. Although Illich's account is itself open to criticism for being overly sweeping, providing one-sided interpretations of ambiguous data and failing to emphasize sufficiently the positive features of modern medicine (Horrobin 1978), the evidence that he and his fellow critics adduce leaves no doubt that even on its own terms the benefits of orthodox medicine in industrial societies like Britain are overrated. As such, the extent to which conventional medical procedures supersede acupuncture in the system of priorities today is questionable.

The competitiveness of a number of current aspects of orthodox medicine can be even more directly questioned since the most fruitful areas of application of acupuncture tend to correspond with those of greatest weakness in mainstream medicine – following trends in the relationship between the alternatives to medicine and orthodox medicine more generally (Taylor 1985). Thus, acupuncture appears to have much to offer sufferers from chronic degenerative disorders like arthritis and rheumatism which are now a major scourge of the middle- and old-aged population in the West (Lewith 1985), as compared to orthodox drug therapies which can have serious complications (Gould 1985). Acupuncture also seems to have advantages over orthodox biomedicine in cases of backache (Campbell 1987) through which millions of costly working days are lost every year in Britain (DHSS 1979; Humphrey 1989) and for which conventional measures tend to produce relatively poor results (see, for instance, Meade *et al.* 1990). Substantial benefits may exist too in using acupuncture rather than conventional medicine in the treatment of such conditions as strokes and Bell's palsy (Lewith 1982). The successful application of acupuncture to gallstones and acute appendicitis, moreover, has the added merit of avoiding the surgery often prescribed by orthodox doctors (Macdonald 1982). These and other advantages of acupuncture over more conventional treatments are reinforced by the numerous instances where patients have benefited from acupuncture after mainstream medicine has failed (see, for example, Mann 1973). This is not, of course, intended to indicate that acupuncture is always superior to medical orthodoxy; as has been seen, general anaesthesia, for instance, is preferable to 'acupuncture anaesthesia' for most patients during major surgery and even the Institut du Centre d'Acupuncture in France has acknowledged that antibiotics are a more effective treatment for infectious diseases than acupuncture (Locke 1972). But when the relative efficacy of this method in a number of areas of health care is taken together with its comparative safety at a time when orthodox treatments are increasingly coming under fire for their dangerous side-effects (see Fulder 1991), claims about the unfavourable medical reception of acupuncture in the modern era being due to competing priorities in medicine do not seem very convincing.

There may be a stronger case, though, for considering the competing priorities argument in nineteenth-century Britain, when the limitations of the new medical ideas being laid in bacteriology by key figures like Bassi, Schoenlein and Pasteur were not so evident. This explanation of the early negative medical response to acupuncture, however, does not adequately mesh with the temporal sequence of events as the medical profession intensified the climate of rejection surrounding this method in the 1840s before professional unity had begun to develop around the new medical perspectives (Youngson 1979). A further difficulty with this explanation is that the therapeutic benefits of the biological materialist approach to health care only began to become apparent towards the end of the nineteenth century, through the contributions of Lister and others (Lee 1976). Indeed, most of the crucial innovations translating the theories of early medical researchers into workable preventative and curative measures – including mass vaccination against tuberculosis and diptheria and the prescription of penicillin – were not introduced until the twentieth century (McKeown 1984). Since the medical rejection of acupuncture occurred before doctors had shaken off their dubious dependence on heroic therapies (Porter 1987), it is difficult to believe that acupuncture – which in these early days seems to have been a relatively effective and safe remedy for pain and more narrowly defined conditions such as dropsy – could have been increasingly abandoned in the period leading up to the mid-nineteenth century as a result of competing medical priorities. Admittedly, its range of application was not as widely acknowledged as today. However, set against a newly developing medical system which appeared to have no practical application and the fatalities caused by bleeding and purging and surgery without sterilization or anaesthesia (MacLaren 1976), acupuncture must have appeared promising even as a limited therapeutic technique at this stage.

It could, of course, be argued that the unfavourable medical response to the method arose because more effective specific remedies gradually became known as the nineteenth century wore on in those areas in which acupuncture had hitherto made a significant contribution. Certainly, Lorimer (1885: 956) suggested that acupuncture may have passed into neglect in Britain because 'in some conditions for which it had been used, it has been superseded by other and better means'. In this regard, Cassedy (1974: 896) believes a critical factor in its decline in the first half of the nineteenth century was 'the emergence during the 1840s of ether and the various other anaesthetics as effective means for the relief of pain in surgery'. But, as Quen (1975a) observes, this is unconvincing for it has only recently been discovered that acupuncture can be used as an alternative to chemical anaesthesia in major operations. The claim by Rosenberg (1977) that some of the problems that had previously been treated by acupuncture came to be cured through surgical procedures made possible by early anaesthetic techniques, moreover, is also flawed as an explanation; ether only began to be employed in Britain several years after the medical climate of rejection of acupuncture had been established (Parssinen 1992) and surgery under ether and subsequently chloroform was not only dangerous (Youngson 1979), but also no alternative to acupuncture in cases such as rheumatism and sciatica. Nor could the introduction of either morphine or aspirin account for the marginalized position of acupuncture. Morphine was increasingly given for pain in general practice from the 1840s onwards, but was not a strong competitor to acupuncture because of its addictive properties and the fact that it only offered short-term relief (Rosenberg 1977). And the development of aspirin could scarcely have jeopardized the position of acupuncture for, like morphine, it presented no real challenge in the treatment of persistent pain or of conditions such as hydrocele, ascites and lockjaw. Aspirin was also not launched until close to the turn of the century (Gould 1985), at which time acupuncture had already been pushed to the brink of extinction by the orthodox rejection of the technique.

The deficiencies of the competing priorities argument are accentuated in this early period – as in the modern era – by the fact that many contemporary acupuncturists discovered that, over a range of conditions, acupuncture regularly succeeded where more orthodox therapies had foundered. This is illustrated by the experiences of Churchill (1823), whose case of rheumatism quickly cleared up following acupuncture treatment when cupping and blistering had failed to subdue the disease, and Belcombe (1852), who managed to cure a patient of vexatious sciatica with acupuncture after several other measures had been unsuccessfully tried. As such, acupuncture in the nineteenth century paralleled methods such as astrology and mesmerism which were also rejected in earlier times, despite countering significant weaknesses in the mainstream medicine of the day (Wright 1979; Parssinen 1992).

CLIENT DEMAND AND THE DANGERS OF QUACKERY

But if the competing priorities explanation of the fate of acupuncture is inadequate in both nineteenth- and twentieth-century Britain, what of the role of consumerism? One obvious interpretation of the situation is that acupuncture has been predominantly rejected by the medical profession simply because the thought of being turned into a 'human pin-cushion' has consistently lacked appeal amongst the British public. This view is certainly worth considering in light of cultural influences on the demand for health care (see, for example, Currer and Stacey 1986) – even if there are difficulties in studying its independent impact, given the power of the medical profession itself in shaping such demand (Turner 1987).

As far as the nineteenth century is concerned, however, client demand is another explanation which fails to impress as an alternative to that of professional self-interests. To be sure, Ward (1858: 728) hinted that the lack of demand for acupuncture may have resulted in its early demise when he said that it was 'not unlikely that its disuse may be occasioned partly by fear of the pain, and partly by the difficulty the patient finds to believe so trifling an operation can produce such powerful effects'. But such an explanation is not consistent with the seeming popularity of acupuncture in Britain in the 1820s and 1830s, before the profession began to establish a strong climate of rejection. Public demand for acupuncture, moreover, appears to have continued beyond this point, particularly under the impetus of Baunscheidtism – following the pattern for alternative medicine generally in the latter half of the nineteenth century, albeit in more muted form (Saks 1992a). That there was a continuing demand for acupuncture at this time should not be surprising because, contrary to Ward's beliefs, the procedure was usually quite painless (Elliotson 1850) – and its apparent safety and efficacy may well have appealed to a public seeking cures and remedies more than theoretical explanations in medicine (MacLaren 1976).

Public demand for acupuncture, though, did seem to have fallen by the end of the century. Yet whether this contributed significantly to the perpetuation of the climate of orthodox medical rejection of the method in the first half of the twentieth century is a moot point. There are grounds for arguing that the reduction in demand for acupuncture by the first half of the twentieth century was mainly the self-fulfilling result of the medical profession's own hostility towards the method – particularly with the shift in the relationship between practitioner and patient in Britain from a patronage system in which wealthy clients were able to control the form and content of medical theories and therapies in the late eighteenth and early nineteenth century (Jewson 1974) to a system in which the consumer came to occupy a more passive and uncritical role, as the power of doctors grew in the broadening market for professional services – with the rise of first hospital and then laboratory-based medicine (Jewson 1976). In this situation, with their position reinforced by the passing of the 1858 Medical Registration Act, doctors were increasingly able to inhibit demand for deviant remedies and in the case of alternative therapies like acupuncture actively seem to have done so from the mid-nineteenth century onwards (Saks 1992a).

Yet if there must be reservations about the influence of consumer demand on the medical rejection of acupuncture in earlier times in Britain, these are strengthened in more recent years by the huge upsurge of interest in the method. As early as 1960, for instance, a leading women's magazine received over 10,000 inquiries from readers after printing a short article on acupuncture – most of which were from people who wanted to know where they could receive treatment (Inglis

1980). The expanding demand for acupuncture in Britain is also confirmed by the heavy pressure under which most practitioners in the field seem to be working; even by the early 1980s acupuncturists were dealing with some two million annual consultations (Fulder 1988). In this respect, acupuncture has now become one of the most popular alternative therapies, at a time when as many as one in seven of the population visit alternative practitioners for treatment (Saks 1991a). It is not difficult to explain why there are comparatively high and increasing levels of popular interest in acupuncture and many other forms of marginal medicine in contemporary Britain despite the power of the medical profession, in an age where, amongst other things, beliefs about the relative safety and efficacy of such methods have been sharpened by the growing critique of orthodox medicine and there is increased striving for self-determination and holistic engagement in health care (Bakx 1991). Explanations, however, are of less concern here than the fact that even the more equivocal, albeit still mainly negative, response of the medical profession to acupuncture in Britain today cannot be accounted for by low levels of public demand.

This does not mean that client demand has been irrelevant to the medical reception of acupuncture in this country over the past two hundred years. In fact, there is a more powerful case for arguing that it has been the growth, rather than the limitations, of demand for the method which has led to the predominant climate of rejection – in so far as this has heightened the profession's fears of encouraging the practice of acupuncture by the medically unqualified, which could endanger the public's health. Certainly, Stern (1927) claimed in his classic work that the medical profession is generally wary about accepting medical innovations, lest its support for any specific procedure be widely publicized and enables quacks, faddists and patent medicine manufacturers to exploit the lay public in their ignorance and desire for relief. And in the case of acupuncture, there has been a long-term concern by the medical establishment to clamp down on the activities of the non-medically qualified even more than doctors using the technique – in line with its characteristic pattern of response to other alternative medical practices (Inglis 1980). Moreover, claims about the rejection of acupuncture in Britain being due to its association with quackery in the nineteenth century have not only been explicitly advanced in commentaries on this period (as, for instance, Haller 1973), but also sometimes appeared in the medical literature of the day (see, *inter alia*, Lorimer 1885).

However, it is important to refrain from making blinkered judgements about the viability of such an interpretation, despite common preconceptions – which figure heavily in professional ideologies – about the dangers of quackery to the public (Johnson 1972). It is crucial to emphasize the difficulties in distinguishing the quack and the doctor historically (Cooter 1988) and to note that the quackery of one age often becomes the orthodoxy of the next (Saks 1992a). These difficulties are no more evident than in the first half of the nineteenth century in Britain, in which Vaughan contrasts the qualified doctor who may simply have trained at an older university 'where it was possible to collect a medical degree by merely remaining in residence for the required time and attending two dissections' with the non-orthodox practitioner who

> may have been a charlatan and a humbug, but not necessarily: though theoretically unqualified he was often widely experienced and able to cope as well as anyone with a wide variety of medical emergencies. Many unlicensed practitioners had received some medical training by the system of apprenticeship, or by walking the wards after an established surgeon or physician as he went his rounds in hospital.
>
> (Vaughan 1959: 36–7)

Of course, some quack practices may have been harmful in the nineteenth century – especially those associated with the patent medicine business which Vaughan (1959: 93) describes as frequently offering 'remedies of hopeless inadequacy for diseases of every imaginable kind'. But the fact that there was so little to choose between the medically qualified and unqualified by the 1840s when the medical war against acupuncturists and other marginal groups was stepped up weakens the force of the argument about protecting the consumer from quackery.

This explanation of the medical response to acupuncture is further attenuated by the fact that non-medically qualified practitioners of acupuncture in the nineteenth century could hardly have received any less formal training in the technique than qualified doctors who, it will be recalled, were primarily self-taught. There is no evidence either that the method at this stage was any more hazardous or ineffective in the hands of so-called quacks than orthodox practitioners. Admittedly, Haller (1973: 1219) has criticized the Baunscheidt device, on which much fringe acupuncture practice was based, for having 'all the properties of a medieval torture instrument' and for being used as a panacea and as a vehicle for the exploitation of sexual problems. Yet the Baunscheidt device was not introduced in this country until after the medical profession had stiffened its negative response to acupuncture (Quen 1975a). Its application, moreover, seems to have been no less horrendous or broad-ranging than such orthodox procedures as cupping and bleeding which were still prevalent in the mid-nineteenth century (Porter 1987). The claim about the sexual exploitation of the public by early quack acupuncturists too cannot seriously explain orthodox medical attacks on fringe practitioners of the method when the profession itself was recommending operations like clitorodectomy for female sexual over-indulgence in the Victorian era (Doyal 1979). In these circumstances, the view that acupuncture was rejected both inside and outside the profession in the nineteenth century because of the dangers posed to the public by quacks – at a stage when the relative safety and efficacy of acupuncture in a number of disorders was not seriously in dispute – does not seem very credible.

There may be stronger grounds, though, for accepting this interpretation in the twentieth century given that the standards of medical education have now improved immeasurably (Levitt and Wall 1992). Certainly too, non-medical acupuncture today has come under attack for postponing the take-up of effective orthodox treatment and masking the symptoms of underlying conditions and can still have ill effects 'when performed by amateurs, cranks or under-educated practitioners' (Lu Gwei-Djen and Needham 1980: xx). These arguments are thrown further into relief by the widespread concern about ensuring proper standards of hygiene and safety for the ever-expanding numbers of lay acupuncturists that followed a significant outbreak of hepatitis in this country in the late 1970s which was traced back to an unqualified practitioner (Macdonald 1982).

In the last analysis, however, the case is still not convincing because it again exaggerates the dangers to patients from the medically unqualified. Whilst the safety of the public may occasionally be put at risk by untrained practitioners, most lay acupuncturists in Britain now have both a grounding in the basic elements of classical acupuncture and at least a rudimentary understanding of the principles of orthodox medicine – including those of physiology and anatomy – because of the standards set by the acupuncture organizations to which they belong (Saks 1992b). But if the amount and level of training undertaken by non-medically qualified acupuncturists in this and other fields is generally increasing (Sharma 1992a), the possibility of delaying effective conventional treatment and engaging in long-term symptomatic treatment is also minimized by the fact that the majority of the clients of acupuncturists, like those of other marginal practitioners, have already received unsuccessful conventional treatment from doctors before seeking help outside the orthodox medical fold (Thomas *et al.* 1991). Lay acupuncturists in Britain today, moreover, have every incentive to treat patients as effectively and safely as possible given the statutory controls that now exist on their premises (Fulder 1988), the risk that they will be expelled from the acupuncture bodies to which they belong if they do not come up to standard (CFA 1987) and, most importantly, the fact that if they fail to satisfy their customers in a predominantly fee-for-service market situation, their very economic survival could be threatened (Cant and Calnan 1991).

When it is also considered that recent claims about the medical profession protecting the public from quackery in this field understate by implication the considerable hazards of orthodox medicine – as well as those of contemporary medical acupuncturists whose training is often sufficiently brief to warrant the charge of engaging in symptomatic treatment in terms of traditional theories of this technique (see Campbell 1987) – it is clear that the dangers of quackery do not provide an adequate explanation of the predominant climate of professional rejection of acupuncture established in either nineteenth- or twentieth-century Britain. But although such arguments are no more convincing than those related to client demand, might a viable alternative explanation of this situation lie in the divisions which have existed over the past two centuries within acupuncture itself?

SPLITS IN THE ACUPUNCTURE MOVEMENT

There have indeed been a number of splits in the acupuncture world in recent years, mirroring those in alternative medicine more generally in this country (Saks 1991a). As has been seen, these have centred on the debate over how far acupuncturists should follow Oriental precepts rather than Western-style medical theories, which have in turn created further divisions – including those concerning its therapeutic scope and the level of qualification necessary to practise. Even amongst trained non-medical acupuncturists there are splits at an individual and organizational level over such issues as the type of classical acupuncture favoured (Fulder 1988) and the terms on which incorporation into medical orthodoxy would be acceptable should attempts to gain state registration prove successful (Saks 1985). In addition, significant rifts exist between acupuncturists with and without orthodox medical qualifications in relation to questions like the appropriate length and content of acupuncture training programmes and the terms on which its practitioners should operate (see, for instance, Marcus 1992). Indeed, there are even divisions within the small band of acupuncturists in the medical profession – involving a majority group who wish to restrict acupuncture to a limited range of applications within orthodox neuro-physiological thinking and a minority who are more sympathetic to classical theories of acupuncture and wish to apply the technique to a broader span of maladies (Saks 1985).

It does seem possible, moreover, that splits of this kind could explain why the medical establishment has not taken a more positive view of acupuncture given the weakening effect which fragmentation has had on the acupuncture lobby in the politics of health care. That such divisions are worthy of serious consideration as an explanation of the fate of the method in modern Britain is accentuated by the fact that internal lines of cleavage in specific fields of alternative medicine in this country often seem to have been key factors in their continuing marginalization. As Fulder and Monro relate:

> The authorities, government and the professions are much more likely to give credence to a therapy if it is represented by a single well-organised body. Efforts to gain statutory recognition for therapies in the past have been hamstrung by divisions and infighting among several organisations in each therapeutic field. For example, when Joyce Butler M.P. put forward a motion in Parliament for the statutory recognition and registration of osteopaths, it was weakened by the failure of some osteopaths to support it. The same was true of the more recent action by the British Committee of Natural Therapeutics . . . when it helped to represent the rights of practitioners of natural therapies to give injections. The British Committee of Natural Therapeutics then fell apart itself as the organisations within it could not work together.
>
> (Fulder and Monro 1981: 25)

However, there are significant counter-arguments to this account of the medical response to acupuncture in contemporary Britain. In the first place, it underplays the cohesion which actually exists amongst acupuncturists, notwithstanding the dissonance in their ranks. Members of individual acupuncture organizations with predominantly lay recruits, for example, tend to be bound together not only by a common pattern of socialization and codes of practice, but also by such classic devices for maintaining group solidarity as fee-setting and prohibitions on advertising which diminish intra-group competition (Saks 1985). There are also strong and increasing ties between the non-medical acupuncture bodies, as highlighted in the 1980s when the four major associations in this field – the BAA, TAS, IROM and the RTCM – united under the umbrella of the CFA, which serves as a forum for discussion and cooperation on professional issues (Saks 1992b). The relationship between medical and non-medical acupuncturists has also been eased by the fact that the International Society of Acupuncture, which had previously restricted its membership to doctors, has opened its doors to anyone whose knowledge of acupuncture is up to acceptable standards (Saks 1985). This epitomizes the developing mutual respect that exists between different groups of acupuncturists internationally, even though powerful fragmenting influences remain as far as the medically and non-medically qualified in Britain are concerned.

There seems no compelling reason, though, why the impact of lingering rifts should have resulted in the persisting marginality of acupuncture in this country as they have not prevented both individuals and organizations making forceful pleas on behalf of the method in the modern period – at a time when the overall trend in the alternative therapies has also been towards greater, if not yet complete, institutional unity (Saks 1994). Comparative evidence on the response of medical orthodoxy to other forms of alternative medicine sheds additional doubt on claims about the destructive consequences of internal splits for acupuncture in the contemporary British context. Whilst rifts in osteopathy, for example, between medically qualified osteopaths, lay osteopaths with a more medical approach and lay osteopaths adopting a predominantly naturopathic orientation are often held to have retarded orthodox acceptance of the technique in Britain (Fulder 1988), similar divisions do not seem to have prevented osteopathy being incorporated into establishment medicine in the United States (Inglis 1964). This suggests that unity may not be a *sine qua non* for orthodox acceptance of unconventional therapies – a view which is supported by the failure of the long-established field of herbalism to gain a strong foothold in orthodox medicine in this country, despite being represented for over a hundred years by only one highly regarded association – the National Institute of Medical Herbalists (Fulder and Monro 1981). Indeed, if lack of unity is seen as the key to the largely unfavourable medical response to acupuncture, awkward questions arise as to why there has been a greater degree of professional interest in the method in recent times in countries like France and the United States where divisions within acupuncture have been no less substantial than in Britain (see Bouchayer 1991; Chow 1985).

But if divisions in the acupuncture movement cannot constitute an adequate explanation of the marginal position of the technique in twentieth century Britain, this is an even less satisfactory rationale for the climate of medical rejection in the nineteenth century in this country. Whilst contributors like Lavier (1966) have argued that differences of opinion about acupuncture played a major part in the decline of the method in a number of European countries by the end of the nineteenth century, the divisions which existed in this area in Britain at this time were much less marked than in the modern era; the growth of a plethora of acupuncture organizations taking different positions and the emergence of debates about the relative merits of Western as opposed to classical Oriental philosophies of medicine had not occurred at this stage. Although, as has been seen, there were disputes over the scope of application of acupuncture, these were not really thrown into relief until the emergence of Baunscheidtism following the establishment of the negative climate of medical reception of acupuncture (Saks 1985). Nor, indeed, does it seem that the disagreements which existed over the explanation of acupuncture at this time were fundamental given the stress placed on pragmatism in medicine, especially in the first half of the nineteenth century (Porter 1987). The only important split in the ranks of acupuncturists in this early period seems therefore to have been between those who held orthodox medical qualifications and those who did not (Haller 1973). But since this did not inhibit key proponents of acupuncture – such as Churchill and Elliotson – from putting a powerful case for the method in the nineteenth century in much the same way as their medical and non-medical counterparts in the latter half of the twentieth century, it is difficult to see why this division should have seriously restricted the growth of acupuncture.

It is hard to believe, therefore, that fragmentation within the acupuncture world has been the major factor in the marginalization of this technique in British medicine over the past two hundred years. It is ironic, though, that even if such splits were of greater significance, this would not necessarily be incompatible with the notion that the predominantly negative medical response to acupuncture is primarily a function of professional self-interests – for the divisions amongst acupuncturists could be seen as diluting their power against that of a self-interested medical orthodoxy. On this note, a further potential alternative explanation to that of professional self-interests will now be considered – namely, that of the power of the drug companies. This will enable the analysis to address Marxist concerns about the need to consider the wider influences of financial and industrial capital on health care in capitalist societies (see, for instance, McKinlay 1977; Navarro 1986).

CAPITALISM AND THE POWER OF THE DRUG COMPANIES

The power of the drug companies has frequently been invoked in the modern Anglo-American setting to explain the marginality of alternative medical therapies like chiropractic (Wardwell 1966) and herbalism (Inglis 1980). This explanation is also worth exploring in the sphere of acupuncture where Luh and Wilson (1978) argue that the method threatens drug company profits because it is a fairly cheap treatment which could dramatically reduce the amount of drugs prescribed.

In support of this explanation, drug companies have certainly shown little interest in promoting acupuncture at an overt level in recent years in Britain (Saks 1985). There are also no doubts about the enormous scale of the financial resources possessed by multinational drug companies over the past two or three decades (Bodenheimer 1985). These resources, moreover, have been used in ways which could have prejudiced the response of medical orthodoxy to acupuncture in this country. Around 15 per cent of the drug companies' turnover is spent on promoting their wares – including expenditure on sales representatives, advertising and free samples (Pietroni 1991). Whilst there is evidence of some cynicism amongst doctors about the gifts they are given by the industry, the overall impact of the promotional campaigns of the pharmaceutical companies may well induce a range of medical consciousness more compatible with the use of drugs than therapies such as acupuncture (Breckon 1972). Drug houses may also help to sustain this consciousness through the substantial funding they provide for medical conferences and research activities (Gould 1985), as well as the influence that they bring to bear on the editorial policy of the medical press given the dependence of the major medical journals on advertising revenue for their survival (Stacey 1988). Testimony to the power which the drug industry wields in practice, furthermore, appears to be provided by the large number of highly profitable drugs which have been introduced in Britain without entirely convincing evidence that they are more efficacious than their competitors or even that they lie within acceptable limits of safety – despite the existence of the Committee on Safety of Medicines which was set up to monitor the activities of the pharmaceutical companies (Collier 1989).

Nonetheless, although there are grounds for arguing that the drug companies have self-interestedly obstructed the development of acupuncture in this country in recent times, care needs to be taken in arriving at this conclusion. The power of the pharmaceutical companies in Britain can all too easily be inflated – as indicated by the ease with which competing treatments like electroconvulsive therapy have been incorporated into mainstream medicine in this country (see Mowbray 1959). There are also strong countervailing interest groups – even within capital itself – to rival the power of the drug companies in the health care arena. Of particular relevance in this respect are the manufacturers of medical equipment (Stacey 1988) who potentially have much to gain from the acceptance of acupuncture, not least because of the electronic equipment which, as has been seen, is increasingly associated with the technique. It is not surprising, therefore, that a growing number of companies are now involved in making acupuncture equipment and advertising their products in relevant professional journals (Saks 1985). This provides a useful check on glib statements about the omnipotent role that drug companies have played in shaping events in the health field in general and the medical response to acupuncture in particular – as, indeed, does Illich (1976: 82) who highlights the restrictions on their powers by noting that the global scale of use of medically prescribed drugs 'seems to have little to do with commercial promotion; it correlates mostly with the number of doctors, even in socialist countries where the education of physicians is not influenced by drug industry publicity and where corporate drug-pushing is limited'.

A further reason for casting doubt on the claim that the financial self-interests of the drug companies have blocked the development of acupuncture in modern Britain is that, even if they had the power to do so, it is not clear that acupuncture actually seriously threatens their economic interests. Central to this argument is the fact that major companies in this area have diversified their production policies to include other types of medical supplies and non-medical items like soft drinks and cosmetics, as well as drugs, thereby diminishing the threat of acupuncture to the industry's profits (Saks 1991a). As Stanway (1986) says, in face of the increasing popularity of such non-drug-orientated alternative therapies, these companies can soon find ways of replacing lost revenue from the marketplace. One of the ways in which they might achieve this end in the current climate is through the exploitation of acupuncture technology itself. But if this serves to minimize the financial challenge posed by acupuncture to the companies concerned, so too does the fact that alternative therapies like acupuncture are used most often as a supplement to orthodox medicine (Thomas *et al.* 1991). The threat presented by acupuncture, therefore, has not created an all-or-nothing situation for the drug companies. This point is accentuated by comparative evidence (see Saks 1985) which suggests that drug expenditure per capita is generally higher in Western countries where acupuncture has most strongly taken root – such as France and the United States – as compared to Britain where it continues to face an at best equivocal medical reception. From a comparative perspective, moreover, explanations of the largely negative contemporary medical response to acupuncture in this country based on the interests of the drug companies also founder because there is no clear association between the power of the pharmaceutical sector in specific societies as judged by drug pricing and the acceptance or rejection of acupuncture; thus drugs seem to be more expensive in nations like the United States and Japan where the method has attracted more favourable orthodox attention, than in Britain where prices are lower.

Claims about the role of the drug companies in explaining the medical reception of acupuncture in Britain in earlier times are also flawed by the fact that the rise of the highly organized multinational pharmaceutical industry did not begin until early in the twentieth century (Gould 1985) – well after the climate of rejection of acupuncture had been established by the medical profession. Admittedly, the roots of the patent medicine business stretch back to the early nineteenth century (Duin and Sutcliffe 1992). However, at this time the drug industry was not only operating on a much smaller scale, but was also far from being a power unto itself as the imposition of the Inland Revenue stamp duty on secret remedies amply demonstrates (Vaughan 1959). It is difficult too to believe that the producers of patent medicine would have been strongly opposed to acupuncture since they supplied the irritative oils which were applied to the skin after the administration of the Baunscheidt variant of the technique that grew in popularity from the 1840s onwards (Haller 1973). Nor is it likely that the pharmaceutical industry could have independently induced the medical profession to perpetuate the climate of rejection of acupuncture in the first half of the twentieth century as at this stage the medical profession seemed to be gaining the upper hand in the relationship – as indicated by the passing of the 1917 Venereal Diseases Act, the 1939 Cancer Act and the 1941 Pharmacy and Medicines Act, all of which restricted the kinds of illnesses which manufacturers of patent medicine could claim to treat (Vaughan 1959).

Yet even if one of the primary factors which Marxist writers see as shaping medical developments under capitalism – namely, the powerful multinational drug companies – can be ruled out as a major influence on the rejection of acupuncture in nineteenth- and twentieth-century Britain, this does not necessarily mean that the generally fairly icy medical reception of the method is unconnected with capitalism. It is also possible to argue that acupuncture has not been warmly received by the medical profession because it was incompatible with the newly dominant bourgeois individualistic ideology associated with the rise of capitalism, paralleling the explanation put forward by Wright (1979) for the rejection of astrology in the seventeenth century.

In his discussion of astrology, Wright notes that this bourgeois ideology stressed the need in medicine for, amongst other things, intervention to control nature, as opposed to acquiescence in nature and notions of universal harmony; individual consultations between doctor and patient for instrumental, curative, purposes; and an individualistic aetiology of disease, in contrast to one rooted in wider structures and forces. In these terms, the links of acupuncture in its traditional Oriental mould with theories of harmony and preventative medicine (Mole 1992) assuredly do not readily fit with capitalist ideological concerns. However, the contrasts with astrology are more instructive than the similarities – not least because, as has been seen, at the time of its rejection in the nineteenth century acupuncture was not practised in its classical form, but rather as a pragmatic device for dominating nature within the framework of a one-to-one relationship between practitioner and patient. And, even if it is accepted that Britain in the twentieth century can still be defined as a capitalist society, the ideological dissonance explanation of the more recent ambivalence of the medical establishment to acupuncture remains wanting. Although classical acupuncture – which has now become more widely known and practised in this country – has been the most strongly rejected element of the technique, this variant is still based primarily on an individualistic aetiology of disease and interpersonal consultation. It is also difficult within the ideological dissonance theory to understand why the more limited form of acupuncture couched in terms of Western medical science should also have been so tentatively received in modern British medical circles – not to mention why the medical profession in such an apparently archetypical capitalist society as the United States should have taken a more favourable stance on this subject than its counterpart in this country.

In sum, then, the notion that the predominantly negative response of the British medical profession to acupuncture in the nineteenth and twentieth centuries can be explained with reference to ideological currents bound up with the rise of capitalism seems even less viable than the view that it is related to the power of the drug companies. This leaves one final superficially plausible alternative explanation to that of professional self-interests to be considered – namely, the claim that acupuncture has been persistently shunned by the medical profession in Britain because of the influence of nationalism.

THE INFLUENCE OF NATIONALISM

Nationalism certainly seems as worthy of consideration as the previous factors examined since it has historically been an important factor in the development of this country (Greenfield 1992) and is often used to explain resistance to medical innovations. Youngson (1979), for example, found that national sentiment – embodied in English–Scottish rivalry – served to increase medical resistance to both Lister's concept of antiseptic surgery and Simpson's method of chloroform anaesthesia in nineteenth-century England. Nationalism, moreover, has occasionally been put forward as an explanation of the unfavourable climate of reception of acupuncture itself. Thus, Luh and Wilson (1978: 71) argue that the reasons for the early medical neglect of acupuncture in Britain and certain other Western societies 'lie in the cultural chauvinism of the Westerners who brought their own scientific methods to China in the last century'. The importance of analysing the influence of nationalism in this context is also underlined by the fact that acupuncture came under attack in both the Meiji era in Japan and the Kuomintang's period of dominance in China as part of the drive for modernization as waves of nationalistic fervour swept these countries in the nineteenth and twentieth centuries respectively (Powell and Anesaki 1990; Hillier and Jewell 1983).

However, nationalism *per se* ultimately falls down as an explanation of the response of the British medical profession to acupuncture. Few problems seem to have beset the introduction of other externally inspired innovations in medicine in the period under consideration – even when they derived from Britain's closest competitors, as in the case of aspirin which was developed at the tail end of the nineteenth century by the Bayer Company in Germany and speedily adopted in this country thereafter (Breckon 1972). And, at a more general level, there have also been many occasions in the past when scientific knowledge has spread from the Orient and achieved a ready acceptance in Britain. This is well exemplified by the early diffusion of information about gunpowder from China (Rogers 1962). But perhaps the most obvious reason for challenging the nationalism explanation in its own right is that it fails to account for the initial enthusiasm shown for acupuncture in some medical quarters in Britain early in the nineteenth century, as well as for the more recent resurgence of interest in the method amongst a small section of the British medical profession.

It could be argued, though, that a more sophisticated explanation is required – and, more specifically, that the climate of medical rejection of acupuncture was established in this country as a result of a combination of both nationalism and the perceived cultural inferiority of the Chinese. This is far more convincing in so far as it provides a rationale for the periods when the medical response to acupuncture was rather more favourable in Britain; these fall on either side of the humiliating experiences China underwent at the hands of the Western imperialist powers in the nineteenth and twentieth centuries, in which this country was eclipsed as a major power. As Haller says:

China's decline among the world powers in the nineteenth century and her subsequent partition into spheres of European influence . . . made her medicine appear quaint, if not anachronistic, compared with that of the more advanced nations of the world.

(Haller 1973: 1213)

Following the more general pattern of relationships between imperial powers and subject nations in the medical field (Doyal 1979), China was dealt with in one-sided fashion as a centre of archaic paganism whose medical system was inferior and in need of radical reform – until its fortunes revived after the mid-twentieth century (Huard and Wong 1968).

Nonetheless, for all its apparent plausibility, the addition of the concept of cultural inferiority to nationalism also fails to provide the explanation sought. In the first place, this rationale for the medical response to acupuncture in Britain does not square fully with the temporal sequence of events in the nineteenth century, as acupuncture in this country was strongly rejected before China's first symbolic defeat by the West in the 1840s – for it was only with the signing of the Nanking Treaty in 1842 following the first Opium War that the real decline and humiliation of China began (Vohra 1990). The claim that acupuncture was rejected on the grounds of the perceived cultural inferiority of China, moreover, is inconsistent with the vogue for 'chinoiserie' which swept many European societies, including Britain, in the later years of the nineteenth century (Davis 1975). And if nationalism coupled with China's diminishing credibility as a world power were important influences on the fate of acupuncture in British medicine up to the mid-twentieth century, it is hard to explain why the method continued to be used by doctors in the United States in this period and why there was a revival in acupuncture in French medical circles from the 1930s onwards – especially since the population of these countries could scarcely be claimed to be any less nationalistic or imperialistic than the British as far as China was concerned (Bowers 1974). It is puzzling too within this frame of reference why the British medical establishment should not have drawn on Japan's long tradition of acupuncture practice in the nineteenth and early twentieth centuries if the cultural inferiority of China was a stumbling block to the incorporation of the method into orthodox medicine for Japan was not only one of the Oriental societies from which acupuncture had originally spread to Europe, but also a country which had managed to modernize effectively without the stigma of direct imperialist intervention (Hane 1992).

This modified explanation is weakened further in the modern era in so far as acupuncture has largely remained an unorthodox therapy in this country – at a time when Britain has declined as a force in world politics, whilst China has emerged as a world power in international affairs (Mancall 1984). The contemporary credibility of this explanation has also been reduced by the fact that Britain has become culturally more cosmopolitan than ever before, both in general terms and in the medical arena in particular – as illustrated by the growth of the multinational trade in drugs and surgical supplies (Collier 1989). With an increasing number of viable sources of knowledge of acupuncture apart from China – including that of one of Britain's closest allies, the United States – even the more sophisticated nationalism explanation of the none too positive medical response to acupuncture collapses in the modern period, just as in earlier times. The influence of nationalism, therefore, must be discounted as a major factor influencing the medical reception of acupuncture in nineteenth- and twentieth-century Britain.

CONCLUSION

A wide range of plausible alternative explanations to that of professional self-interests for the predominant climate of medical rejection of acupuncture in Britain over the last two hundred years has now been appraised. As has been seen, none of these is at all convincing in itself and, for this reason, it also seems highly unlikely that even in combination the various factors assessed in this chapter could have played a major role in evoking the overridingly negative medical response to acupuncture. This strengthens the professional self-interests account, although the influence of such interests on the fate of the method in this country cannot, of course, be firmly established exclusively in this way. As yet, therefore, the notion that the vested interests of the medical profession, or at least powerful segments thereof, have been responsible for the generally unfavourable medical reaction to acupuncture is only based on evidence by default. An assessment is now needed as to whether there is any more positive support for the professional self-interest claim. This is the task of Chapter 6, which will illustrate further the application of the research framework outlined in Part I of the text for evaluating the altruism of professional groups.

6 Acupuncture and British medicine
The influence of professional power and interests

To move nearer to a convincing assessment of the extent to which the medical profession has acted altruistically in establishing a predominantly negative climate of reception of acupuncture from the early nineteenth century onwards in Britain, more direct evidence on the influence of professional self-interests is clearly needed in this field. As will be recalled from the theoretical and methodological framework set out earlier in this book, two further prerequisites need to be met before the central role of such interests in decision-making can be accepted. First, it must be established that the professional group under consideration had sufficient political resources to influence the direction of decision-making in its favour and that it deployed these resources accordingly. Second, the interests of the group must be shown to be compatible with the policy followed in the case being scrutinized. The extent to which these prerequisites have been met will now be examined to evaluate how far the vested interests of the British medical profession – or sub-sections thereof – can be seen to have played a major part in the medical response to acupuncture, starting with the question of whether key elements of the profession have both possessed the power to relegate the method to a tangential position in the health care system and employed such power to this end.

THE POWER OF THE BRITISH MEDICAL PROFESSION

The contents of Chapters 4 and 5 have already suggested that the power to impede the development of acupuncture in British society appears to have not only broadly lain in the hands of the medical profession since the beginning of the nineteenth century, but also been concretely used with this goal in mind. It is argued in this chapter that such a view is further reinforced when considered in greater depth and in a more focused way. Since the ability of the profession to limit the availability

of acupuncture has varied over time, this claim will be more systematically documented for each of the chronological stages delineated in
Chapter 4 for outlining the response of medical orthodoxy to acupuncture in this country. The analysis will centre on two levels of power
throughout – namely, that of the medical profession as a whole over
outsiders in general and lay practitioners of unorthodox medicine in
particular, and that of the elite of the profession over deviant insiders
with an interest in alternative medicine. These powers were quite weak
in the period between the sixteenth and eighteenth centuries for at this
time orthodox doctors formed a highly fragmented group with little
control over the practice of the large number of unregulated healers
(Saks 1992a) and the leaders of the prestigious RCP were barely able
to influence the work of those within their own ranks (Berlant 1975) –
still less that of other, lower-order, medical practitioners (Wright 1979).
However, the power of the medical profession, including its elite,
expanded after the turn of the nineteenth century over both internal and
external medical affairs – thereby strengthening the plausibility of
the professional self-interests explanation of the marginality of acupuncture in British medicine over the past two hundred years.

Early to mid-nineteenth century

As far as the period from the early to mid-nineteenth century in Britain
is concerned, though, the medical profession still did not possess
sufficient political resources to limit drastically the practice of acupuncture by outsiders. To be sure, its power over unregulated practitioners did increase as compared to earlier times as a result of the
growth of professional unity between the surgeons, apothecaries and
physicians who sought to present a united front in face of strong anti-
monopolistic feeling in the wider society (Berlant 1975), the cam-
paigning of the influential reform movement centred on the PMSA
which called for a single register of medical practitioners and sanctions
against unscrupulous quacks (Parssinen 1992), and the development of
medical journals which proved a valuable addition to the popular press
in the war of words against the fringe (Jewson 1974). But this power
was weakened by disputes between medical organizations over such
matters as appropriate standards of education and the supremacy of the
RCP (Stevens 1966) – not to mention the continuing difficulties which
the Royal Colleges and the Society of Apothecaries (SA) faced in
prosecuting unlicensed practitioners operating within their jurisdic-
tions, mainly because of the reluctance of juries to find for the plantiffs
in an era in which individual liberty was extolled (Parssinen 1992).

Nonetheless, although the medically qualified did not have enough political influence to prevent the unlicensed panacea usage of acupuncture from growing, they did have some power over lay therapists, largely through the medical press which was employed to the full against rival practitioners (Vaughan 1959). The exercise of this power, moreover, as was seen in Chapter 4, certainly seems to have restricted the growth of non-medical acupuncturists – if only by acting as a deterrent to both doctors and patients in cooperating with them.

The viability of the professional self-interests explanation of the limitations on the availability of acupuncture in the first half of the nineteenth century, however, is more strongly reinforced when the political resources possessed by the elite of the medical profession in Britain are considered; these resources were plainly sufficient to have brought about substantial restrictions on the use of acupuncture within the profession – including the sharp decline in the characteristically more limited application of the method by doctors after the end of the 1830s. The elite to which reference is made in this period consisted not only of the traditionally dominant leading members of the RCP, but also increasingly those of the fast-advancing RCS and, to a lesser degree, those of the SA and the PMSA (Saks 1985). Whilst the internal authority of this elite was adversely affected by its lack of cohesion – since each of the three main licensing organizations had its own separate corporate body controlling education and entry to the profession and the PMSA was in dispute with the Royal Colleges (Inkster 1977) – the position improved as the mid-nineteenth century approached with the emergence of the general practitioner and moves to establish a greater degree of homogeneity in the profession (Stacey 1988). These trends, together with the demise of the patronage system and the rise of hospital medicine, had the effect of paving the way for a more developed system of collegiate control in which senior members of the profession were increasingly able to impose a monolithic consensus in medicine (Jewson 1976).

The political resources available to this elite in the first half of the nineteenth century for generating such a consensus in the profession and suppressing deviant therapeutic beliefs centrally included control over entrants to medicine; although this social control mechanism was weakened by the plethora of licensing bodies in existence even as late as the 1840s, marginalized practitioners could be excluded from the most prestigious training posts in medical corporations like the RCP (Forsyth 1966). Further checks on the spread of marginal practices in the profession also became available as the well-worn system of informal social pressure exerted on deviant medical practitioners from above (Youngson 1979) was supplemented by increasing, albeit in-complete, elite regulation of the medical curriculum as the leaders of the profession gained progressive control over the content of medical education and training programmes were increasingly developed on a standardized basis (Holloway 1964). As the distribution of resources and rewards in the profession came to depend more on recognition by professional peers than the satisfaction of the patient, even greater opportunities arose for this elite to use its expanding control over careers in medicine to discourage those with interests in unorthodox therapies – as Elliotson found to his cost when, as has been seen, he was forced to resign his chair at University College in London because he refused to refrain from giving public demonstrations of mesmerism (Parssinen 1992). Finally, of course, the control by the medical elite of the major medical journals enabled it to impose a commitment to common theoretical assumptions and technical procedures in medicine, at a time when such journals were becoming ever more important to practitioners in building a career and as a source of medical knowledge (Jewson 1976). The power of this elite against unorthodox insiders, though, was far from total, even by the mid-nineteenth century. This is best illustrated by the case of research, over which those at the apex of the profession had relatively little direct control as it largely remained a non-specialized, spontaneous activity that had yet to be recognized as warranting substantial institutional and financial support (Thomson 1973). However, there is no doubt that the emerging medical elite had accumulated enough power by the late 1830s to limit much of the interest in acupuncture in the fast-developing profession – despite its weaknesses in combating the practice of the method by outsiders at this time.

This conclusion clearly supports the professional self-interests ex-planation of the growing climate of medical rejection of acupuncture which developed from the 1840s onwards. There is, of course, a distinction between having power and exercising it, but, as was seen in Chapter 4, there is ample evidence that the power of the elite was increasingly used against medically qualified acupuncturists as the first half of the nineteenth century wore on. At first, it will be recalled, the Royal Colleges appear simply to have sneered at or completely ignored deviant medical practitioners of the method. At a later stage, though, a range of social control mechanisms were brought to bear in this area; aside from the continuing exclusion of the method from the evolving orthodox medical curriculum, acupuncturists and other practitioners of unorthodox remedies in the profession were treated as moral outcasts by the leading medical journals, with all the deleterious implications that this carried for their future careers. Whilst a handful of acupuncturists within the profession still used the method despite these pressures, their experiences belie the claim in the *PMSJ* (1843) that it was much more difficult to deal with quackery practised by insiders than outsiders in medicine; in the first half of the nineteenth century professional power was even more successfully employed against the former than the latter, as far as acupuncture was concerned.

The central involvement of the elite in limiting the availability of acupuncture in the period before the mid-nineteenth century is reaffirmed by the finding in Chapter 5 that the medical response to the method at this stage was not heavily determined by either the drug companies or the dominant ideology associated with the rise of capitalism. As such, the independent influence of the medical profession as a whole and its leaders in particular seems to have been largely responsible in a causal sense for the fate of acupuncture up to the mid-nineteenth century – including, as was noted in Chapter 4, not only restrictions on the number of medical and non-medical acupuncture practitioners and the form in which the method was employed, but also by extension class and regional inequalities in access in an essentially private market structure.

Mid-nineteenth to mid-twentieth century

Much the same can also be said of the time span from the mid-nineteenth to mid-twentieth century in Britain, by the latter half of which acupuncture therapists had virtually become extinct. This was certainly true of non-medical acupuncturists, who fell into decline after a flurry of enthusiasm in the period leading up to the turn of the century. This decline came precisely at the time when the power of the medical profession over marginal practitioners as a whole was increasing. The pivotal event was the 1858 Medical Registration Act that firmly placed doctors in control of the medical arena through the establishment of the GMC which was heavily dominated by leading figures in the medical corporations and, at a later stage, also by representatives of the BMA (Forsyth 1966). The founding and development of the GMC had the effect of unifying the profession since it laid the basis for the compilation of a common register of all medically qualified practitioners and enabled the medical elite to increase further the cultural and educational homogeneity of registered practitioners around the principles of allopathic medicine (Inglis 1980). This served to strengthen the power of doctors as a collective group against outsiders – as did the terms of the 1858 Act, under which only those on the medical register could sue for fees or be employed by the state. At first, as Berlant says, licensing on such terms simply

> gave registered practitioners a psychological advantage over others by providing them with apparent state approval; that is, the prestige of the state was thrown behind members of the organized medical profession. The prospective patient might be more likely to select a state-approved practitioner than one with only a good community or professional reputation.
>
> (Berlant 1975: 156)

But with the passing of the 1911 National Health Insurance Act, which made health insurance for lower-paid workers compulsory, doctors gained a vital economic advantage over unlicensed alternative therapists because general practitioners were to be the exclusive suppliers of treatment under this scheme (Levitt and Wall 1992). The financial advantages of the monopoly which accrued were also paralleled in the first half of the twentieth century by the growth of professional unity based on the newly forged alliance between general practitioners and hospital specialists through the referral system (Stevens 1966) – as well as the relative freedom from public control that doctors were granted by the state (see, for instance, Klein 1973).

Yet if these changes strengthened the hand of the profession against alternative practitioners, so too – as previously documented – did the introduction by the GMC of a restrictive ethical code prohibiting cooperation between doctors fringe therapists; the continuing control of the leading medical journals by the medical profession which was used to step up attacks on alternative therapies from the mid-nineteenth century onwards; and legislation enacted in the first half of the twentieth century which limited the treatment of certain diseases to medical practitioners. To be sure, the power of the medical profession was still weakened by divisions within its own ranks – particularly between the Royal Colleges and the BMA over questions of style and influence (Berlant 1975) – and the continuing right of lay practitioners to practise under the common law. However, there is no doubt that the medical profession possessed greater political resources than had existed in earlier times to restrain non-medically qualified practitioners in general and unlicensed acupuncturists in particular. That doctors as a collectivity had the power to relegate the latter to a tangential position in the health care system is highlighted by the minimal challenge that alternative therapies presented to the profession from the 1920s to the mid-twentieth century (Inglis 1980) and the substantial level of control maintained by doctors over such specialized occupational areas as orthoptics and radiography which were admitted to the orthodox fold between the Wars (Larkin 1983).

There is, moreover, sufficient evidence to suggest that such power was employed to constrain the specific provision of acupuncture by outsiders and that the medical profession, in consequence, was mainly responsible for its almost total demise by the start of the twentieth century. As was noted in the previous chapter, trends in client demand cannot readily account for this demise as they are too closely associated with the expanding power of the profession itself in this period. It was also evident from Chapter 4 that the political resources which increasingly became available for use against marginal practitioners were employed against lay acupuncturists, especially in the crucial phase leading up to the turn of the century in Britain – as epitomized by the content, and pattern of appearance, of items on acupuncture in the leading medical journals which were scarcely designed to foster the broad-ranging applications of the technique favoured by non-medical acupuncturists (Saks 1991b). And although the medical response to lay acupuncture in the first half of the twentieth century is probably best described as one of 'implicit rejection' (Collins and Pinch 1979) in so far as the practice of the method by outsiders was rarely referred to in contemporary medical discourse, the professional silence about this technique in an era of growing medical dominance can be seen as being as indicative of the use of power against unregistered acupuncturists as the most forthright verbal critique of those operating in this field.

Additional support for the professional self-interests account is also provided when power relations within the profession are analysed in the period from the mid-nineteenth to the mid-twentieth century. Such an analysis shows that the elite of the profession had enough power to have ensured that there were very few medical practitioners of the method by the turn of the century in Britain. Crucially, the medical elite – comprised mainly of prominent representatives of the Royal Colleges and the BMA – was more cohesive than it had been in the first half of the nineteenth century because of the founding of the GMC and the growing emergence of laboratory medicine which formed the basis of the new orthodox medical consensus. Whilst the transition to laboratory medicine served to divide the elite into research workers and practitioners (Jewson 1976), it was sufficiently united to be able to impose its opinions on rank-and-file members – as in other developing scientific areas, in which Dolby (1979) argues that dominance by a small number of the most expert increasingly inhibited insiders from expressing contrary views.

The main channels through which the medical elite could control lower-order personnel in the period under consideration were extensions of the mechanisms available for this purpose in the first half of the nineteenth century. Control over entry to the profession, for instance, was increased by the growing centralization in elite hands of the previously fragmented licensing system, facilitated primarily by the 1858 Act. This Act also stiffened the effectiveness of medical education as a means of social control, as it prescribed that the elite-dominated GMC was henceforth to preside over standards of the undergraduate curriculum (Stacey 1992). In this way, the leaders of the profession were able to impose a degree of educational uniformity, mirroring that prevailing in many other evolving scientific fields (Mulkay 1972) – even if, as Stevens (1966) notes, there were still varying requirements for postgraduate medical training, as between the more traditional RCS and RCP and the relatively newly established Royal College of Obstetricians and Gynaecologists. Equally, social pressure linked to ostracism and patronization within the profession became a greater deterrent to the take-up of unorthodox practices by insiders, as colleagues rather than clients became the main reference group for doctors (Jewson 1976). Similar comment can be made about the growing elite control of the career structure – which seems to have restrained even Sir Thomas Horder from following up his recommendation that further research be conducted into radiesthesia in his controversial inquiry into this area in the 1920s (Inglis 1980). After the 1858 Act, though, such control in medicine took on formal as well as informal dimensions, as senior members of the profession could restrict deviance amongst insiders through disciplinary action. As Berlant observes,

> the state empowered the GMC to enforce legally the traditional internal controls of the medical profession. A registrant found guilty by the GMC of 'unprofessional conduct' or convicted of a crime could be stricken from the register. The purpose of the GMC, then, was to be a final authority on the conduct of practitioners.
>
> (Berlant 1975: 161)

That this power was real is illustrated by the case of Axham, who was struck off the medical register for acting as an anaesthetist to Barker, the famous bonesetter, in the early years of the twentieth century (Inglis 1980). The potential for elite control of deviant insiders was further augmented in the period from the mid-nineteenth to mid-twentieth century by the gatekeeping role of the editors and referees of the leading journals – whose part in socialization and career mobility was becoming more significant in science generally (Mulkay 1991). The increasing importance of elite domination of key research-funding organizations like the MRC as scientific inquiry was given greater weight in medicine

(Austoker and Bryder 1989) should finally be emphasized, because such bodies were generally reluctant to finance research into marginal therapeutics, even when conducted by qualified doctors (Saks 1985).

However, although the power of the elite over insiders was also enhanced by the growing legitimacy it was accorded as the complexity and content of knowledge expanded with the rise of laboratory medicine and other scientific developments (Mulkay 1979), its resources could still not ensure blanket conformity amongst rank-and-file members of the medical profession. This point is underlined by the way in which medical homoeopaths were able to block efforts by the medical elite to allow universities to refuse to award degrees to those intending to practise alternative methods on qualification (Nicholls 1988). Nonetheless, the power of the leadership of the British medical profession over fringe insiders undoubtedly escalated in the years spanning from the mid-nineteenth to the mid-twentieth century, to the point where it could not only stem the spread of acupuncture within the profession, but also more or less eliminate it from the orthodox medical repertoire. There is ample evidence, furthermore, that this power was employed against doctors drawn towards practising and/or researching acupuncture in the period under consideration. As will be recalled, the method found no sustained place in the medical curriculum, nor was there significant establishment funding of projects on acupuncture, even after the turn of the century when finance became more readily available for research within the profession. Elite control of the medical journals also entailed that very few items were published on the subject, particularly in the first half of the twentieth century, and those which did appear were none too positive about its medical applicability, especially as a panacea.

These points, documented more fully in Chapter 4, lead to the inexorable conclusion that the British medical profession in general, and its elite in particular, played a greater role in restricting the development of acupuncture – both in its wider and in its more limited forms and inside and outside the ranks of medicine – in the period from the mid-nineteenth to the mid-twentieth century as compared to the first half of the nineteenth century. This view is reinforced by the fact that such broader influences as the growth of the multinational pharmaceutical industry again do not seem to have fundamentally shaped the medical response to acupuncture in this time span. Accordingly, it would appear that the medical profession, or at least dominant segments thereof, must be seen as having primary responsibility for limiting the availability of acupuncture to such an extent that questions about class and regional inequalities of access to the technique paled into insignificance by the early twentieth century. But if this conclusion is clearly compatible with the professional self-interests explanation of the predominant climate of medical rejection of the method, this is also true of the contemporary era on which this book focuses – even if acupuncture has become more freely available and hard-line medical attitudes towards the technique have gradually begun to soften.

Mid-twentieth century to the present day

There is certainly little doubt that in the modern period the power of the medical profession against outsiders has grown still further in Britain as compared to earlier times. Although it is sometimes suggested that the establishment of the NHS in the late 1940s reduced professional control over medicine, the power and autonomy of the profession generally seem to have expanded in the British context – not least because such state involvement made the doctor–patient relationship more independent of the patient's ability to pay for medical treatment (Elston 1991). The power of doctors over medical affairs in Britain is also accentuated, for all the twists and turns in health policy since the War (Klein 1989), by the continuing pattern of professional dominance over state-funded research (Saks 1987) and the medical curriculum (Stacey 1992) – as well as the persisting professional control of the editorial policies of the leading medical journals and the fact that the authority of the medical profession over paramedical groups has been consolidated through legislative reform (Larkin 1983).

The medical profession has been remarkably successful, moreover, in resisting the growing pressure for a more democratically managed health system in Britain. From the outset of the NHS, doctors established a high level of representation on bodies like the Regional Hospital Boards and Hospital Management Committees and exercised considerable influence over wider-scale medical policies through traditional professional advisory channels (Klein 1989). And whilst there was a more formal attempt to introduce the notion of participatory democracy into the health sector through the creation of Community Health Councils, little attention appears to have been paid to their views (Harrison *et al.* 1990). The newly forged managerial tiers of the NHS following the 1974 and 1982 reorganizations, furthermore, remain strongly populated by representatives of the profession, leaving the structure of medical dominance at these levels more or less intact (Ham 1992). Of course, the government has introduced over the last decade a series of important measures seemingly aimed at reining in this power, including the concept of general managers and the internal market

(Baggott 1994). But there is as yet very little evidence that such changes have had a significant impact in this respect – indeed, they may have ironically increased the opportunity for key sections of the profession to participate in decisions about the use of resources (see Cox 1991; Elston 1991). All this, together with the fact that – notwithstanding *The Patient's Charter* (DoH 1991a) – the machinery for processing complaints against doctors has remained heavily peer-based and little more effective than in the first half of the twentieth century (Klein 1989), points to the continuing power of the medical profession as a collectivity in the contemporary era. The profession thus seems to have possessed sufficient political resources to exercise substantial levels of control over acupuncturists operating outside its boundaries since the mid-twentieth century in Britain.

This is confirmed when the availability of such resources and the way in which they have been employed against non-medically qualified alternative practitioners are considered in the period under discussion. Fringe therapists were clearly placed at an even greater competitive disadvantage when the NHS was established since it allowed doctors – and allied professional groups – to extend their monopoly over a greater range of practice. This brought direct financial benefits to the medical profession, as well as the perpetuation of the exclusive right to sue for fees and to claim to treat a wide spectrum of illness (Huggon and Trench 1992). In this context, the power of the profession is highlighted by its central role in the rejection of applications from lay osteopaths and chiropractors to become professions supplementary to medicine (Fulder and Monro 1981). The continuing ability and propensity of the profession to exclude alternative practices from the orthodox medical curriculum and to denigrate them in the mainstream medical journals should also not be underrated, given the potential restrictive impact on referrals to outsiders (Saks 1985). Nor should the significant control by the medical profession over research funding be neglected as a resource for stifling fringe practice in view of the acute shortage of financial support in this area (Fulder 1988). The power of the medical establishment to limit the growth of alternative practitioners, moreover, has been sharpened by the splits which, as was seen in Chapter 5, have divided marginal medicine in general and lay acupuncture in particular over the past few decades.

The power of the medical profession in relation to non-medically qualified alternative therapists, though, should not be exaggerated in the contemporary period any more than in earlier years. The government certainly has not always toed the line formally adopted by the medical profession in relation to fringe practitioners. This is illustrated by the decision of the Minister of Health to overrule the objections of the BMA to spiritual healers having access to NHS hospitals in the 1950s and 1960s (Inglis 1980) and, more recently, by the designation of junior ministers with specific responsibilities for alternative medicine, including the practice of those outside the orthodox health care professions (Saks 1991a). Such examples – coupled with the continuing right of non-medically qualified therapists to operate under the common law – underline that doctors still do not possess monolithic power over outsiders. There are also occasions in which the power of the profession may not have been used to the full against the non-medically qualified – as arguably witnessed by the decision of the GMC in the mid-1970s to relax its prohibitive ethical code on medical cooperation with fringe practitioners (Fulder and Monro 1981). Having said this, though, the medical profession in contemporary Britain still seems to have had the political resources at its disposal to contain substantially the growth of fringe practice and to have generally used these resources to this end. Indeed, the fact that consultations with orthodox doctors still far outnumber those with lay therapists despite the popularity of alternative medicine (Sharma 1992a) testifies to its current influence.

As has been seen in Chapter 4, moreover, there is much evidence that such resources have been applied to non-medical acupuncturists with real effect from the mid-twentieth century onwards – notwithstanding the rapid expansion in numbers of lay practitioners of the technique over the last two decades. It is clear from this evidence that non-medically qualified acupuncturists have been detrimentally affected by, amongst other things, the exclusion of the method from the standard medical curriculum at undergraduate and postgraduate levels; the hostility of the mainstream medical journals; the lack of availability of orthodox funding for research activities; and the generally negative stance of the medical profession on cooperation with lay practitioners. In addition, the profession must, as part of its social gatekeeping function, bear some responsibility for the continuing exclusion of lay practitioners of acupuncture – and other alternative therapists – from a secure role within the NHS, which has adversely affected the provision of the method in this country (Saks 1985).

This is not, of course, to absolve non-medically qualified acupuncturists themselves from responsibility for retarding their own position. They certainly could have moved faster to satisfy public demand for acupuncture, as suggested by the length of waiting lists in this area, and they have also yet to apply formally to join the professions supplementary to medicine (Fulder and Monro 1981). Neither of these instances, though, can be fully separated from the negative response of the medical profession to fringe acupuncturists; this response has not encouraged the non-medical practice of the method and has led to a sense of fatalism over the outcome of any application to become part of medical orthodoxy (Saks 1985). The profession therefore must assume the major share of responsibility for restricting the availability of the typically wider-ranging practice of lay acupuncture in modern Britain both inside and outside the NHS, together with its associated implications for class and geographical inequalities of access. This conclusion is reinforced by the fact that its power seems to have been exercised relatively autonomously; as will be recalled from Chapter 5, neither the drug companies nor capitalism at a broader ideological level seem to have greatly influenced the medical response to acupuncture in contemporary British society.

But if the medical profession as a whole can be treated as a quasi-independent group in this case, so too can the elite of the profession in its handling of acupuncturists within its own ranks. This elite is even more clearly definable than in the period prior to the mid-twentieth century, again consisting primarily of the leading members of the expanding number of Royal Colleges and the BMA who are strongly represented on bodies like the GMC which play a major part in medical policy-making (Stacey 1992). Its influence, moreover, is magnified by the increasing cohesion which has developed in medical leadership circles in the modern era (Saks 1987). That this now mature scientific elite has had the power to exercise control over insiders is suggested by the relatively small proportion of the medically qualified who have become members of the Medical Practitioners Union and other ginger groups in the profession (Watkins 1987). This potential for control seems to have extended to acupuncture where the professional elite has had the capacity to restrict considerably the involvement of medical insiders with alternative therapies in recent times, in face of growing popular demand.

The potential for such control within the profession from the mid-twentieth century onwards is highlighted by the continuing ability of the medical elite to regulate entry to the profession by excluding 'undesirable' applicants – including likely sympathizers with unortho-dox views – from professional programmes of study (Widgery 1988). Equally, the power of the elite to determine the content of the medical curriculum at undergraduate and postgraduate level has remained an important method of social control over medical insiders (Moran and Wood 1993). Its significance is brought home by the predominantly allopathic basis of conventional medical training (Inglis 1980) and the difficulties that doctors can experience in obtaining orthodox financial support for courses in alternative medicine after qualification (Saks 1985). These elite controls have been supplemented, as in earlier times, by informal social pressure on deviant practitioners – which perhaps explains the reluctance of the doctors who joined the SMN in the 1970s to allow their names to be publicly released (Eagle 1978). Elite control of the career structure in medicine has also helped to ensure that doctors remain within the orthodox fold, especially in the hospital sector where there is growing competition for top specialist posts and distinction awards (Levitt and Wall 1992). The potential for control over insiders has been reinforced by the retention by the GMC of the power to take formal disciplinary action against doctors cooperating with lay therapists on illegitimate terms – even though its ethical guidelines in this area have now been diluted (Stacey 1992). The elite also still influences the publication policies of the mainstream medical journals, which appear to be as biased against the medically qualified as the unqualified in relation to alternative therapies (Inglis 1980). Meanwhile, persisting elite control over research funding in the public and much of the private sector has accentuated its potential leverage over doctors taking up alternative medicine – in an area in which even the orthodox profession has been poorly funded over the period under consideration (West 1992). This elite power, moreover, has been reflected at a local as well as a national level, where research proposals from doctors for clinical trials of such practices as traditional flower remedies and radionics have been turned down by medical committees (Eagle 1978).

It is therefore clear that the leaders of the British medical profession have, if anything, increased their power to restrain the development of alternative methods within their own ranks from the mid-twentieth century onwards. Admittedly, this power is again still far from total, a point highlighted by the growth in the number of doctors interested in alternative medicine in recent years and the fact that successive governments have continued to resist pressure to exclude what little medical provision there is of therapies like homoeopathy from the NHS (Nicholls 1988). Nonetheless, internal controls have given the medical elite sufficient power to have largely held in check the pressure which has been building up to incorporate fringe methods more fully into the orthodox repertoire as a result of rising public demand (Saks 1991a). Just as in the case of the power of the profession as a whole over lay acupuncturists, moreover, the political resources of the leaders of the profession, as was seen in Chapter 4, seem to have been actively used against medically qualified acupuncturists, despite the moderation of the hard-line stance taken by this elite since the beginning of the 1970s. As will be recalled, the medical establishment has yet to include acupuncture as an integral subject in its basic medical curriculum and official postgraduate training programmes. Macdonald (1982) believes that this omission has played a crucial part in fostering sceptical attitudes about acupuncture in general and traditional acupuncture in particular – a point which is accentuated by the difficulties of obtaining orthodox funding for attending courses on acupuncture outside the conventional system of medical education. And whilst the stigma associated with acupuncture inside the profession has been declining in recent times, it still seems likely that the career prospects of at least some doctors have been jeopardized by their involvement with this technique. As was seen earlier too, elite control of the mainstream medical journals has not been used to promote the method in a wholehearted way – even though acupuncture was treated more positively after the 1950s and 1960s, albeit in its non-classical form. Equally, elite-dominated research-funding bodies like the MRC have greatly restricted expenditure on acupuncture, with the result that its medical exponents have been placed in a similarly disadvantaged position to that of other medical practitioners of alternative therapies in research terms.

This should not be taken to suggest that the elite of the profession must shoulder complete responsibility for the marginal position of acupuncture within the ranks of orthodox medicine in the period following the mid-twentieth century in Britain. The relative infrequency with which items on acupuncture appear in the mainstream medical journals and the comparative rarity of research awards in this area, for example, may be linked to the low number and standard of submissions (Saks 1985). However, care is needed here as it is no less difficult to disentangle the behaviour of medical acupuncturists from the response of the leaders of the profession to the method than in the case of the alleged self-inflicted marginality of lay acupuncturists. Thus, explanations of marginality based on the pattern of submissions to medical journals and research bodies must be weighed against the possibility of commissioning specific articles and pieces of research. Similarly, any reluctance of doctors to apply for grants to study acupuncture should in part be related to a lack of confidence in outcomes, given the at best ambiguous attitude of the medical establishment to this subject in the period under scrutiny. The medical elite in Britain must still therefore be considered to have played a central role in restricting the spread of acupuncture inside the profession following the mid-twentieth century – and hence also to have diminished the general availability of medical acupuncture to the public, with all the concomitant class and geographical inequalities in access to this form of provision.

This conclusion, coupled with that concerning the power which the profession as a whole has possessed over, and used against, the broader-ranging practice of acupuncture by outsiders, is plainly consistent with the professional self-interests explanation of the marginality of this technique in modern Britain. As such, it has now been established that the medical profession in general and its elite in particular possessed the political resources to have severely restricted the development of acupuncture in this country over the past two centuries and that such power has been exercised, for the most part, to this end. But before moving on to consider more specific evidence on the self-interest hypothesis, it is worth noting that comparative analysis further supports the claim that prime causal responsibility for the marginal position of acupuncture in the nineteenth and twentieth centuries in Britain has lain in the hands of the medical profession.

PROFESSIONAL POWER AND THE FATE OF ACUPUNCTURE: A COMPARATIVE PERSPECTIVE

More precisely, this claim is reinforced by comparative data which suggest that acupuncture has tended to be more strongly incorporated into orthodox medicine in societies outside the Oriental culture area where the power of the profession and its elite has been substantially weaker than that of Britain in determining the extent to which acupuncture is included in its work. This is particularly evident in the two European countries where acupuncture has come closest to becoming part of conventional medicine – namely, Russia and France. As was seen in Chapter 4, in both of these societies in recent years the number of medical personnel involved in practice and research in this field indicate that acupuncture is on the verge of gaining full orthodox acceptance. At the same time, Russian and French doctors have had only partial control over the therapeutic content of their work, albeit for differing reasons. In the former case, the professional power and autonomy of doctors was significantly abrogated under state socialist policies in the Soviet Union following the Bolshevik takeover in 1917 (Davis 1989). The relative weakness of doctors as a group in relation to acupuncture in this context is highlighted by the way in which medical interest in the method mirrored the party line on Sino-Soviet relations in the period before the demise of the Soviet political system. More specifically, acupuncture first emerged from obscurity in the 1950s with the development of political links between China and the Soviet Union, then disappeared from the limelight as ideological divisions widened in the 1960s and was finally resurrected in the 1970s as an 'Eastern', rather than 'Chinese', form of medicine, to avoid sacrificing ideological purity in a climate of continuing Sino-Soviet antagonism (Kao 1973). In the very different political milieu of France, on the other hand, where acupuncture has been even more favourably received by medical orthodoxy, doctors have had to be open to the method because the health care system has for many years been extensively based on private health insurance and fee-for-service arrangements which have encouraged doctors to cater for patient demand (Rodwin 1989) – not least in relation to alternative medicine in general and acupuncture in particular (Bouchayer 1991).

The relative weakness of the power of doctors in countries outside of the Orient where acupuncture has come closest to becoming part of medical orthodoxy is well illustrated too by the case of the United States – the main source of comparative example in this book. The persistence of medical interest in acupuncture in the crucial years following the mid-nineteenth century in America seems to have been strongly related to the climate of anti-elitism dominated by the frontier spirit (Stevens 1971) – in which the predominantly fee-for-service system coupled with a high degree of public acceptance of a range of alternative practices considerably limited the power of doctors to exclude such methods from their repertoire (Wallis and Morley 1976). Similar comments apply to the upsurge in the number of doctors practising and researching acupuncture after the 'ping-pong' diplomacy in the early 1970s (Duke 1972), although this resurgence of medical interest must also be seen in the context of the financial support provided by the federal authorities in this area as a consequence of the policy of detente with China (Davis 1975) – funding which has recently been paralleled with the establishment of the National Institutes of Health Office for the Study of Unconventional Medical Practice in the United States (Eisenberg *et al.* 1993).

It would seem, then, that in the three non-Oriental societies in which acupuncture has gained the greatest degree of orthodox acceptance – whilst still remaining an alternative therapy – doctors have been far from omnipotent in determining the nature of their therapeutic role. This contrasts with the position of the British medical profession which has been far less vulnerable to the pressures of consumer demand than its counterparts in France and the United States, given the distinctive pattern of state intervention in health care. Such state involvement in Britain has in turn been much less erosive of professional power than in the Soviet model (Freidson 1970). This broad brush comparative picture further sustains the notion that the British medical profession has been centrally responsible for the marginal position of acupuncture in this country over the last two hundred years.

The control that doctors possess over the content of their professional work is not, of course, the only factor which has influenced the fate of acupuncture in countries outside the Orient. This is accentuated by the variation in the reception currently given to acupuncture by the medical profession in Western European countries with insurance-based fee-for-service medical systems – ranging, as has been seen, from the more positive response of doctors in Finland, Austria and West Germany to the icier reception in Italy and Sweden – when a universally less hostile line on acupuncture might have been anticipated in view of the relatively high recent levels of public demand for alternative medicine within the market arrangements for health care in such societies (Sharma 1992a). This discrepancy raises important questions about the conditions under which acupuncture has come to be more or less strongly rejected by the medical profession internationally. Comparative analysis suggests that the nature of the professional response to acupuncture is also strongly related to the extent to which countries have enforceable laws restricting the use of the method to the medically qualified. As Stanway (1986) observes at a broader level, when doctors in Western societies have effective legal restrictions which exclude the lay practice of alternative medicine, they are more likely to respond favourably to public demand for such therapies – and this, of course, will be particularly apparent when professional control over the therapeutic content of medical practice is relatively weak.

In countries where doctors have taken a more favourable stance on acupuncture, therefore, restrictive legislation tends not only to exist, but also to be stringently enforced against unorthodox practitioners in general and lay acupuncturists in particular. As Fulder (1988: 91) notes, in France 'the law has deterred laymen from careers in complementary medicine, thus leaving it open for French doctors to add a good deal of complementary medicine to their exclusive domain'. Much the same can be said of the legislative position in Finland and Austria where medical acupuncture has also been expanding of late (Stanway 1986). And whilst West Germany superficially differs from the general pattern because acupuncture has been favourably received by medical orthodoxy despite the fact that both doctors and non-doctors are formally allowed to practise the method, the picture changes when it is appreciated that lay practitioners of acupuncture can only operate under very strict statutory control (Macdonald 1982). The United States fits into this template too, in so far as the contemporary growth of medical interest in acupuncture has been accompanied by legislation in the majority of states placing this technique under the exclusive control of licensed physicians and doctors of osteopathic medicine (Chow 1985). On the other hand, societies where the medical profession has taken a fairly hostile stand on acupuncture tend to either lack restrictive legislation or fail to police it effectively as far as non-medically qualified practitioners are concerned. Thus, in Sweden, where there is little medical involvement with acupuncture, lay acupuncturists can practise without infringing the law (Fulder 1988). This parallels the case of Britain where there has been an at best equivocal and at worst antagonistic medical response to acupuncture in a situation in which, as has been seen, anyone may practise acupuncture and other forms of alternative therapy under the common law.

Leaving aside the issue of how far the development or otherwise of legislation creating professional monopolies over alternative medicine in general and acupuncture in particular reveals a further dimension of the power of the medical profession, the foregoing analysis clearly raises the question as to why there should be a link between legislation effectively restricting acupuncture practice to doctors and the degree of incorporation of the technique into medical orthodoxy in countries outside the Oriental context. One possible explanation of this relationship is that the strategy employed by doctors is based on the self-interests of the profession in obstructing the take-up of acupuncture in its own ranks where there are no legal restrictions on the activities of outsiders because of the dangers of further popularizing the method and legitimating the practice of fringe acupuncturists in a manner likely to threaten the established medical reward structure. This hypothesis cannot be examined fully here in an international context, but it does lead the inquirer smoothly into the next phase of the chapter, in which more direct evidence is considered on the influence of professional self-interests on the medical reception of acupuncture in nineteenth- and twentieth-century Britain.

THE ROLE OF PROFESSIONAL SELF-INTERESTS IN THE RECEPTION OF ACUPUNCTURE IN BRITAIN

As will be recalled, if the self-interests of the medical profession – or leading segments thereof – are to be seen as centrally accounting for the marginal position that acupuncture has occupied over the last two hundred years in Britain, it is not enough simply to show that this group has both possessed the requisite power and used it to this end. It is also necessary to establish that the policies adopted by the profession on acupuncture since the early nineteenth century have broadly been consistent with professional self-interests. In assessing how far this has been the case, the compatibility of such interests with, first, the policies of the medical profession in general towards the lay practice of acupuncture and, second, those of the narrower professional elite towards medical insiders involved with the technique will be analysed in chronological stages, beginning with the period from the early to the mid-nineteenth century. As noted in Chapter 3, interests will be regarded as being advanced only in situations in which the balance of gains accruing to an individual or group exceeds losses in relation to specific policies, with primary reference to power, prestige and wealth. In framing the analysis, it should also be stressed that, in Chapter 5, the seemingly most plausible alternative explanations to professional self-interests have already been considered and found unconvincing.

Early to mid-nineteenth century

Clearly, in assessing professional self-interests as a possible explanatory factor in the marginalization of acupuncture in the first fifty years of the nineteenth century, two events are critical – the attack which the medical profession launched on lay practitioners of acupuncture and other fringe therapists, particularly during the 1840s, and the growing hostility of the developing medical elite towards insiders engaged in marginal practices such as acupuncture at the tail end of this period. But before their compatibility with professional self-interests is directly examined, the reasons why the method began to be more widely used in the early nineteenth century – especially by the small group of doctors who employed acupuncture on an occasional basis in the years up to the 1830s – should first be explored.

The appeal of acupuncture to some medical practitioners at least in this period is easy to understand given, as has been seen, the apparent simplicity of the technique, its seeming capacity to produce immediate results in a narrow range of conditions and the fact that there was a sporadic market for this and other forms of marginal medicine in the private sector – not least amongst the middle and upper classes (see Belcombe 1852; Parssinen 1992). The existence of such a market would have been particularly financially attractive to the expanding band of general practitioners at this time who often earned only very modest incomes, as well as to physicians and surgeons with positions at hospitals and medical schools, the greater part of whose income still came from private practice, in a highly competitive situation (see Waddington 1984; Porter 1989). That several of the medical pioneers of acupuncture in this country, including Elliotson and Churchill, were relatively young when they began to use the method (Saks 1985) also testifies to the interest which lower-ranking doctors had in risking such involvement to gain the rewards of wealth, status and power that often accrue to successful innovators (Rogers 1962). It is not surprising, therefore, that some qualified medical practitioners joined the limited number of lay exponents of the technique – for whom the method would also have had a strong financial appeal, especially given their usage of it as a panacea – in employing acupuncture in the early decades of the nineteenth century in Britain.

However, as has been seen, although both of these groups came under increasing attack from the medical establishment from the late 1830s onwards, this was most accentuated in relation to unqualified outsiders. The attack by the profession here seems to be explicable in terms of a similar pattern of market-based interests to those that initially may have led unlicensed therapists to adopt such methods. More specifically, the congruence between the interests of the profession as a collectivity and the policy it pursued towards lay acupuncturists and other non-medically qualified practitioners appears to reflect the long history of competition for patients that existed between such groups and the difficulties facing the medical profession in enforcing restrictive legislation against the far greater numbers of unlicensed practitioners (Waddington 1984). In this light, the attempt to limit the practice of fringe therapists by, *inter alia*, waging campaigns against them in the popular press and medical journals, could only have advanced the general interests of the profession – even if, as will be recalled, the results of this activity did not reap dramatic rewards immediately in fields such as acupuncture, due to the relative lack of power of the medical profession in the first half of the nineteenth century.

This conclusion is reinforced when the nature of the challenge that unlicensed outsiders presented to the interests of the medically qualified in Britain is analysed in more detail. As Nicholls (1988) suggests, the threat posed by unqualified practitioners in the early part of the nineteenth century was amplified when they employed therapeutic methods – like acupuncture – that were safer than the heroic therapies which doctors normally used to treat illness at this time. But if this sharpened the challenge that lay acupuncturists, amongst others, presented to the wealth, status and power of doctors by throwing into question the exclusivity of their knowledge base, so too did the conflict between contemporary medical theories and the theoretical underpinnings of fringe acupuncture in the period under consideration. This is because the mainly holistic *modus operandi* on which lay acupuncture was predicated significantly departed from more orthodox medical thinking about the causes of health and illness – and in particular from the localized pathology model which was in the process of supplanting traditional systems theories of disease by the mid-nineteenth century (Parssinen 1992). As a result, the lay practice of acupuncture further endangered professional authority over the production and transmission of medical knowledge.

The biggest threat to the interests of qualified doctors as a whole in the first few decades of the nineteenth century, though, was probably posed by the numerous unqualified 'empirics' who denied the need to understand why remedies worked before employing them (Vaughan 1959). The main reason why these elements of the fringe, who were also prevalent amongst lay acupuncturists (Haller 1973), offered such a powerful challenge to orthodox doctors was because they questioned not just the content of medical education, but also whether any systematic training was necessary for practice – at a time when medical orthodoxy was stressing the need for a greater degree of scientific understanding in medicine (Saks 1991b). Since the successful pursuit of this latter strategy helped to bring about an increase in the power and status of doctors, by reducing the ability of the public to evaluate their performance and by raising the standing of the growing numbers of general practitioners whose skills were still linked with the lower-level crafts and trade, it is not surprising that so much attention was devoted to the denunciation of 'empirics' by the leaders of the medical profession at this time (Parssinen 1992) – including in the field of acupuncture where, as has been seen, there was considerable debate about its underpinning rationale, even in the ranks of orthodox medicine.

The view that professional self-interests were compatible with the increasingly negative stance of the medical profession towards the fringe in general and lay acupuncturists in particular in the period leading up to the mid-nineteenth century appears even more plausible in light of the common application of marginal therapies like acupuncture as cures for all ills by unlicensed practitioners (Camp 1973). This form of practice, by broadening the threat to the power and status of doctors, may help to explain why Renton (1830: 101) wrote that, in the medical community, the utility of acupuncture was 'very readily suspected, when its infallibility is given out for the removal of too many diseases'. The antipathy of the medical establishment towards such claims by fringe practitioners, however, is also consistent with the economic interests of the profession, in so far as the non-medical employment of such techniques as acupuncture on a panacea basis directly challenged the financial security of doctors in an era when the demand for fringe therapies was sufficiently strong to attract substantial numbers of patients away from more orthodox medical provision (Parssinen 1992). The scale of this challenge at all levels of the medical hierarchy should not be underestimated because of both the relative impoverishment of many doctors and the wealth of some of the fee-paying clientele siphoned off by lay practitioners of acupuncture and other medical heresies in the first half of the nineteenth century (Waddington 1984).

But if the medical profession as a collectivity at this stage had a strong interest in publicly condemning practitioners of marginal thera-pies – and especially the panacea practice of the 'empirics' – it is also important to note that the profession was not an undifferentiated entity, and that the relative balance of gains and losses associated with this policy varied between groups within the medical fold. This is well illustrated by the small minority of medical practitioners of acupuncture at this time; those who distanced themselves from the fringe by applying the technique to a limited range of conditions and by relating their practice to mainstream medical theories could only have benefited from the campaign against unlicensed practitioners since this restricted external competition, whilst the few medical acupuncturists who en-gaged in 'empiricism' and used the method as a panacea could scarcely avoid their association with outsiders offsetting any competitive market advantage gained (Saks 1985). Medical acupuncturists, of course, came under increasing fire after the late 1830s from the developing elite of the medical profession which used its growing power to undermine the interest-based incentives of doctors to take up acupuncture. The main issue here, though, does not so much concern the effects of the actions of the professional elite as the extent to which its policy of reducing the involvement of insiders with acupuncture and other marginal therapies, through its control over such spheres as the medical journals and the medical curriculum, advanced the interests of doctors in general and the leadership of the medical profession in particular.

In this respect, there is little doubt that the more successful policy of the medical elite of restraining the activities of deviant insiders was highly consistent with professional interests in the period leading up to the mid-nineteenth century in Britain. To have overlooked the medical practice of fringe therapies like acupuncture – particularly in the case of colleagues whose involvement with marginal medicine came closest to mirroring that of the non-medically qualified – risked legitimating the work of lay therapists which, as has been seen, the profession had a strong stake in suppressing. In addition, the hostility of many orthodox doctors towards medical practitioners of alternative medicine is readily explicable in terms of the growing competitive threat that such deviant practitioners posed to their livelihood in an era when there was still much popular demand for fringe therapies (Parssinen 1992).

The link between professional interests and medical efforts to control doctors engaging in unconventional practices like acupuncture, however, is most apparent in the critical period from the late 1830s onwards, when licensed practitioners were striving to reform the medical profession. Too close an alignment with marginal practices at this time could have jeopardized the drive for increasing professionalization and thus have thwarted attempts to consolidate and extend the power, prestige and financial rewards associated with orthodox medicine (Parry and Parry 1976). The reasons for this are twofold. First, the continuing proliferation of medical practitioners of the unorthodox perpetuated pre-existing divisions amongst the medically qualified at a stage when internal unity was a key political resource in the struggle to achieve fully-fledged professional standing (Saks 1985). Second, the existing relationship between medical orthodoxy and the fringe weakened the case for professional monopoly rights based on exclusionary closure in a situation in which medical practitioners needed to develop a distinct identity and a spotless reputation (Inkster 1977). These arguments are accentuated by the fact that a unified and self-governing medical profession was ultimately only established in 1858 after 17 medical bills were introduced in Parliament over a twenty-year period – in large part because doctors were not held in very high public regard at this time and the opponents to reform 'continued to insist on the right of every Englishman to select his own brand of medical treatment, without the interference of laws and licensing bodies' (Parssinen 1992: 111–12). Against this background, it is easy to see why leading reformers sought to purge acupuncturists and other unorthodox practitioners from the profession in the first half of the nineteenth century, as this was the strategy most compatible with the long-term self-interests of both the medical elite and doctors as a collectivity in the British context.

In this sense, the policy of marginalizing acupuncture practitioners, both inside and outside the medical profession, was certainly more attractive than the wholesale medical incorporation of the method, given the potential benefits associated with the successful reform of the profession and the limits on public demand for medical acupuncture as doctors progressively gained more control over the content of their work. This argument is reinforced by the fact that the method came closer to being incorporated into orthodox medicine in the United States than in Britain after a similar initial period of medical interest in the early nineteenth century. This can be explained in terms of self-interests by the greater incentives for physicians in the former society to respond to client demand in view of the stronger emphasis placed on *laissez-faire* and anti-elitist principles in the 1840s and 1850s which inhibited the establishment of professional monopoly rights in American medicine (Rosenberg 1977). In these circumstances, the strategy most consistent with medical interests in the United States was not to reject the method as in Britain, but to continue with the restricted medical application of the method whilst condemning at every opportunity the practice of this and other marginal therapies by lay practitioners.

Having said this, the vested interests hypothesis as applied to Britain in the first half of the nineteenth century has been disputed. Quen (1975b: 153) has attacked the claim that the medical rejection of acupuncture in this period can be explained with reference to simple selfish economics because, although the reaction of some practising physicians may have been influenced by the threat that acupuncture posed to their livelihood, the concept of self-interests 'was not mentioned in contemporary correspondence, and it could not have been a significant factor for the nonphysician scientists'. Such objections, however, do not stand up. Taking first the claim about 'nonphysician scientists', this group was not of great importance in this period, which pre-dates the rise of laboratory medicine where the research worker became more central (Jewson 1976). And since medical research was typically undertaken in the free time of practising doctors in the early years of the nineteenth century (Holloway 1964), such scientific investigators as there were generally shared common interests with medical practitioners as regards acupuncture – and not just in relation to narrow economic definitions of interests, but also those based on status and power. Furthermore, to argue that the absence of references to interests in the contemporary medical literature on acupuncture indicates that they carry little explanatory weight is to ignore that 'it may be the operation of such interests which has been responsible for their very invisibility' (Shapin 1979: 140); it would be surprising indeed if references to the self-interests of doctors appeared in orthodox medical publications of the day on the rejection of acupuncture for their exposure could have tarnished the public image of the profession at a critical stage in its development. Questions can also be raised about how far the mention of subjectively identified interests in the literature in any case forms a viable basis for interpreting the direction of the self-interests of doctors – especially in light of the argument pursued in Chapter 3 about the pitfalls of conceptualizing this notion in terms of overtly expressed wants and the advantages of more objective means of assessment.

The adoption and implementation of a more objective approach to the consideration of interests therefore casts great doubt on Quen's reservations about the influence of professional self-interests on the medical reception of acupuncture in the first half of the nineteenth century in Britain. At the same time, it also avoids the self-fulfilling assumption that all decisions can ultimately be traced back to interests, whether or not these are referenced in the contemporary literature (Webster 1991). But whilst medical self-interests, at a variety of levels, seem to have been highly congruent with the increasing orthodox rejection of acupuncture as the mid-nineteenth century approached, what of the period leading up to the mid-twentieth century?

Mid-nineteenth to mid-twentieth century

If the influence of professional self-interests on the medical response to acupuncture after the mid-nineteenth century in Britain is to be demonstrated, it will need to be shown that such interests were consistent with the medical policies that substantially contributed to the almost total demise of the lay practice of acupuncture and the virtual elimination of interest in this method within orthodox medicine by the first half of the twentieth century. As regards the non-medical practice of acupuncture in Britain, incentives for outsiders to treat patients using the method initially remained up until the turn of the century. As will be recalled, lay practitioners of acupuncture and other marginal therapies retained their right to operate under the common law and this, together with the persisting demand for unorthodox remedies in the latter half of the nineteenth century, gave a relatively straight-forward and seemingly efficacious technique like acupuncture continuing appeal to the medically unqualified – albeit on a lesser scale than more traditional methods like hydropathy and herbalism (Inglis 1980). The picture, however, changed progressively thereafter in the wake of the intensified medical campaign against fringe practitioners, following the success of the medical reform movement. A key question here is whether this campaign was fully compatible with professional self-interests.

In this respect, it is difficult to argue anything but an affirmative case. Whilst the profession managed to consolidate and extend its mono-polistic position by the mid-nineteenth century through the 1858 Medical Registration Act, there was a danger that the privileges so gained could have been rescinded in face of 'the levelling forces of liberalism and egalitarianism' which continued to prevail in British society (Berlant 1975: 167). For this reason alone, lay practitioners of alternative therapies like acupuncture still posed a real threat to the medical profession in the second part of the nineteenth century – despite their falling numbers as the end of the century approached – because of the challenge they presented to its exclusive knowledge-claims on which the wealth, status and power of the profession had by now come even more strongly to rest. As in the early nineteenth century, this challenge took two main forms. In the first place, professional privileges were threatened by unorthodox practitioners who subscribed to thera-peutic explanations radically conflicting with those underpinning con-ventional medicine, which was increasingly rooted in the allopathic principles associated with the rise of first hospital and then laboratory medicine (Jewson 1976). In the case of lay acupuncture in the second half of the nineteenth century this threat was based on the newly conceived Baunscheidt device, the use of which – like many marginal methods of the day – was centred on the previously dominant, and competing, systems approach to disease (Haller 1973). The interests of the medically qualified as a whole were also again challenged through the widespread existence of 'empirics' on the fringe (Vaughan 1959), not least in the field of acupuncture (Haller 1973). Such practitioners continued to place the exclusive knowledge claims of the profession in jeopardy because of the questions their pragmatism raised about the need for the lengthy periods of training on which orthodox medicine was by then firmly founded (Stacey 1988).

It is easy to understand from the standpoint of medical self-interests, therefore, why the profession 'did not approve of the lenient treatment of quacks' (Jones 1981: 20) and strengthened its attack on lay practi-tioners in the latter part of the nineteenth century. The link between medical interests and policy in this period becomes even clearer, however, in view of the opportunity that the profession possessed at this time to align itself more fully with the prestigious mantle of science; whilst doctors were assisted in this quest by the decline of the patronage system in which the wishes of patients had constrained them 'to cure disease, and do naught else' (Jewson 1974: 381), the activities of outsiders cast the scientific credentials of the profession into doubt. Such lay practitioners challenged not only the existing medical reward structure, but also that of the future – for the adoption of a scientific ideology extolling the impartial search for truth subsequently enabled a number of professional groups significantly to advance their position in the Anglo-American context (Mulkay 1991). This interpretation of the direction of the interests of both medical practitioners and the gradually expanding numbers of medical researchers with regard to lay practice is underlined by the widely held view at this time that progress in medical science was slipping behind that of the other physical sciences (MacLaren 1976). In consequence, there were parallels in the second half of the nineteenth century in Britain between the condemnation by university scientists of amateurs involved in practices like spiritualism and that by the medical profession of lay practitioners of acupuncture and other marginal therapies; both served to diffuse the threat which outsiders posed to scientific credibility (Palfreman 1979).

The interest of the medical profession in suppressing fringe medicine in general and fringe acupuncture in particular in the period up to the late nineteenth century is reinforced by the continuing panacea application of such techniques by their unlicensed practitioners (Lu Gwei-Djen and Needham 1980), which heightened the challenge to the knowledge-claims of medical orthodoxy. This style of lay practice also broadened the direct threat to the livelihood of doctors, despite the professional market advantages gained through the 1858 Medical Registration Act. This is illustrated by the fact that, whilst this legislation meant the Poor Law Commissioners were able to insist that candidates for appointments must be qualified doctors, some commercial bodies offering medical services in return for regular payment still employed unlicensed practitioners (Jones 1981). Direct competition between doctors and lay practitioners of alternative medicine, though, was probably greatest in the fee-for-service sector where the patients of the non-medically qualified continued to be drawn from the richer as well as the poorer sections of society, at a time when the incomes of many members of the profession remained relatively low (Porter 1987).

By the beginning of the twentieth century in Britain, however, the interests of the non-medically qualified in practising alternative therapies were much diminished as public demand for unorthodox treatment sharply decreased largely, as has been seen, because of the growing power of the medical profession – most strongly epitomized by the 1911 National Insurance Act, which substantially improved the market position of doctors as against fringe practitioners. These trends in demand, it will be recalled, were especially marked in the case of acupuncture where the consequent fall in numbers of lay practitioners effectively eliminated any threat posed to the profession. The almost complete demise of non-medical acupuncture practice highlights the depressed condition of the fringe as a whole at this time; Inglis (1980: 70) claims that Barker, the bonesetter, was the only unlicensed practitioner 'who disturbed the peace of mind of the medical profession in Britain in the years before the outbreak of the First World War' and that medical orthodoxy subsequently had no serious rivals before the revival of public enthusiasm for alternative therapies in the 1950s and 1960s. In these circumstances, the move towards a lower-key medical response to lay acupuncturists in the first half of the twentieth century seems perfectly explicable in terms of professional self-interests; as both medical researchers and practitioners began to reap the rewards of the successful defence of scientism and professionalism, there was little to be gained by tilting at windmills as far as their interests were concerned. This is not, of course, to suggest that the medical profession was averse to acting when its interests were directly threatened – as it did, for instance, in blocking the attempt by lay osteopaths to obtain registration as an autonomous health profession in the 1930s which challenged the controlling position of doctors in the health care division of labour (Larkin 1992). But such interest-linked action appears to have been more defensively than offensively oriented than was the case in the second half of the nineteenth century, as marginal medicine declined as a force in Britain.

It is important to remember, though, that some doctors also occasionally used acupuncture as well as lay practitioners in the years stretching from the mid-nineteenth to the mid-twentieth century – at least in the early phases of this period. Such doctors still had incentives to employ the method at this time – just like many other exponents of marginal therapies – because of the continuing public demand for this technique in a competitive marketplace. However, its medical appeal was tarnished by the even more negative stance of the professional elite towards insiders involved with acupuncture following the success of the medical reform movement. This perhaps explains why the few doctors who took up the method seemed less likely to be drawn from younger practitioners as compared to the period before the mid-nineteenth century, as opportunities to build a professional reputation from an association with acupuncture diminished. Those entering this field in fact appear to have belonged mainly to the two groups in the medical profession who had least to lose from a career viewpoint – namely, higher-order hospital doctors using acupuncture on an experimental basis and established general practitioners with extra income to gain from employing the method (Saks 1985). It is understandable in terms of interests, moreover, why such medical acupuncturists, as has been seen, usually practised the more limited form of the method and sought out acceptable theories of its *modus operandi* in an age in which empirically-based panaceas were held in increasing disregard by the medical elite.

This professional elite, however, was successful in virtually eliminating orthodox involvement with marginal medicine in general and acupuncture in particular by the beginning of the twentieth century. In this respect, its restrictive policies – which shaped the pattern of the medical take-up of acupuncture and undermined the demand-led incentives for doctors to use the method – also seem to accord with professional self-interests. Clearly, medical practitioners of acupuncture could not be seen as a substantial threat to the livelihood of more orthodox doctors before the turn of the century, in view of their generally limited use of the technique and their relatively small and diminishing numbers, paralleling those of other medical practitioners of marginal methods (Inglis 1980). But they still threatened to legitimate the position of rival lay practitioners and challenged professional unity, a key political resource in the process of professionalization. This helps to explain why it was in the self-interest of the leaders of the profession to continue to suppress deviant insiders following the 1858 Act. Indeed, the hard-won privileges of the profession might well have been put under further pressure had not doctors maintained their distance from fringe therapies, a point that was not lost on the medical elite which was already becoming 'explicitly engaged in a programme of recruitment from exclusive high-status social backgrounds' to improve the public image of orthodox medicine (Parry and Parry 1977: 121).

Whilst this also accounts for the particular hostility the elite displayed towards doctors applying acupuncture in the broad-ranging manner of the non-medically qualified, the challenge to the wealth, status and power of the medical establishment by deviant insiders as a whole faded considerably after the turn of the century – just as for the wider profession in relation to fringe outsiders – as marginal medicine fell into decline. In this context, it is easy to understand in terms of interests why the leaders of the medical profession should have held back from overtly attacking medical practitioners and researchers of acupuncture in the first half of the twentieth century; as previously noted, the medical employment of the technique had virtually died out by this time and the elite was in a powerful position to control future developments, should the situation in this or other fields of medical unorthodoxy slip out of hand. In this vein, it is not surprising that the appointment of a medical homoeopath as royal physician in the 1920s 'caused wry amusement, rather than wrath, in the medical profession' (Inglis 1980: 93).

But if the link between medical policy on acupuncture and professional self-interests was as close from the mid-nineteenth to the mid-twentieth century in Britain as in the first half of the nineteenth century, this conclusion is underlined by the comparison with the United States, which highlights that the exclusion of acupuncture, rather than its incorporation into the orthodox repertoire, remained the most viable option in Britain over this time period from the viewpoint of professional self-interests. This may seem an anomalous claim, given that acupuncture continued to be employed by American physicians in the years between 1850 and 1950, despite the fact that the method was still practised by outsiders in the early twentieth century (Rosenberg 1977) and the medical profession had by then 'succeeded in having state licensing boards, dominated . . . by representatives of the state medical societies, established in every state' (Berlant 1975: 234). However, it will be recalled that the American medical profession did not gain exclusive rights over the practice of acupuncture until after the mid-twentieth century and that doctors in the United States had a stronger interest in being responsive to consumer demand for acupuncture and other alternative therapies in a predominantly fee-for-service system than in the evolving state-based system in Britain in which the profession exercised greater control over such demand. There was therefore less incentive for the medical profession in Britain to incorporate acupuncture in face of competition from lay practitioners of the technique than in America where it remained in the interests of some physicians to practise acupuncture whilst the profession as a whole strove to distance itself from lay competitors (Burrow 1963).

Since Quen's reservations about the lack of explicit reference to professional interests in relation to acupuncture are no more applicable to this period than earlier times and it is still difficult to separate the interests of the increasing numbers of 'nonphysician scientists' from those of medical practitioners on this issue, the compatibility of professional interests and the medical reception of acupuncture seems clear up to the mid-twentieth century in Britain. Lest this be seen as an overly cynical interpretation of the medical response to acupuncture, it should be stressed that vested interests have been widely implicated by sociologists in the historical response by scientists to innovation (Webster 1991). This is exemplified in relation to medicine by Youngson who highlights the role of professional interests in generating medical resistance to Lister's system of antiseptic surgery in the latter half of the nineteenth century because this concept

> brought with it the likelihood . . . of extensive and in part unforeseeable changes in the practice of surgery, and could thus be viewed as a fundamental threat to the qualifications, attainments, earning capacity and social position of all who were expert in the 'old' surgery.
>
> (Youngson 1979: 217)

After analysing a number of developments in medicine ranging from Jenner's principle of vaccination to Semmelweiss's theory of contagion,

Stern (1927) went so far as to argue that the innovations which are the most threatening to the professional self-interests of doctors are the least likely to be accepted. This theory certainly fits the historical past of acupuncture, but how far are such interests commensurate with the modern medical response to acupuncture in Britain, on which the case study is primarily centred?

Mid-twentieth century to the present day

It is argued here that such professional self-interests were still compatible with the predominantly negative stance which doctors in general and the medical elite in particular continued to take towards acupuncture at least up until the mid-1970s in Britain. This claim is also not far removed from the spirit of recent social scientific work on the contemporary medical response to innovations where professional self-interest has frequently been seen as having a significant influence on events – not least in the reception given to alternative medicine (see, for instance, Fairfoot 1987). The specific case for a linkage between medical interests and the continuing rejection of acupuncture after the mid-twentieth century, however, cannot be assumed, but requires careful examination.

Turning first to consider the hostile medical response to lay acupuncture in the period under scrutiny, the analysis should again begin by accentuating the reasons for the appeal of acupuncture to the outsiders who increasingly took up the method from the 1950s onwards. Despite the escalation of the medical attack on fringe acupuncturists and other such practitioners of alternative therapies, as well as the growing appreciation of the complexity of the theories underpinning traditional acupuncture at this time, lay therapists had a stronger interest in taking up the method than they had done in the preceding half century; expanding knowledge about the breadth of its application and rising demand for such treatment together combined to extend opportunities to establish successful private practices in this field (Saks 1985). Although this led, as has been seen, to a gradual acceleration in the numbers of non-medical acupuncturists – outstripping in scale those prevalent in the nineteenth-century heyday of the technique – this growth was not consistent with the interests of the profession as a whole. That this was so, and that the policy of the medical profession of continuing to deploy its resources more overtly against fringe therapists in general and lay acupuncturists in particular in the period from the mid-twentieth century to the early 1970s was compatible with such interests, is thrown into focus by the classic framework outlined by Wardwell for assessing the threat posed by marginal practitioners to members of the orthodox profession in modern industrial societies.

Wardwell (1976: 63) argues that the most serious threat to the privileged position of the contemporary medical profession is presented by outsiders who 'challenge some of the basic assumptions of orthodox medicine and attract patients with a wide variety of conditions'. Non-medical acupuncturists in the period up to the mid-1970s in modern Britain assuredly fell into the former category, for the philosophical basis of mainstream medicine was challenged by the competing classical Oriental theories on which much of the lay practice of acupuncture became focused. Whilst this threat to medical orthodoxy – which has parallels in other areas of alternative medicine – was accentuated by the small, but diminishing, group of untrained 'empirics' who also practised acupuncture (Saks 1985), it is particularly highlighted by the challenge that fringe acupuncturists presented to orthodox knowledge-claims by applying the method to a wide range of conditions at a time when the effectiveness of conventional medicine was being radically questioned on a number of fronts. Aside from further endangering professional claims to possess an extensive body of esoteric knowledge, the broad-ranging approach of most fringe acupuncturists and other unorthodox therapists was beginning by the early 1970s to challenge the incomes of doctors in private practice (Saks 1992b). The force of the threat posed is brought out by contrasting the extent to which professional interests were jeopardized in this period by lay acupuncturists as compared to members of the professions supplementary to medicine and limited practitioners like opticians and dentists who did not typically adhere to conflicting theories of medicine, subscribe to pragmatic views of healing, apply their techniques in blanket fashion to disparate conditions or formally compete with medical practitioners for patients (Martin 1969).

Nonetheless, lay practitioners of acupuncture did not challenge the basic income and security of the majority of doctors, who were working in the NHS and less extensively engaged in private practice than in earlier times (Allsop 1984). The threat that non-medical acupuncturists posed to the profession, however, was far from minimal. Wardwell argues that the degree to which any particular irregular group threatens medical orthodoxy in the modern context varies according to

such . . . conditions as: (a) the number of marginal healing groups in existence at a given time; (b) the relative size, popular support, and political influence of each; (c) the degree of solidarity or fragmentation within the unorthodox practitioner group; (d) the effectiveness of the group's leadership; and (e) whether the unorthodox group is seeking to maintain independence and distance from orthodox medicine or striving for some kind of acceptance, toleration or even incorporation within medicine.

(Wardwell 1976: 64)

On these criteria, lay acupuncturists represented an important and expanding challenge to the interests of the profession by the mid-1970s in Britain, despite the by now considerable medical power base. This is evident from the number of non-medical acupuncture groups in existence by this time – ranging from the BAA to the IROM – and the mushrooming growth of alternative therapies more generally (Inglis 1980). The threat of lay acupuncturists to the medical profession was further enhanced, moreover, by the developing links between such practitioners and other fringe therapists (Webster 1979) and their rising numbers, public support and political impact – as illustrated in the first half of the 1970s by the existence of over one hundred practising members of the BAA alone and the increasing frequency with which questions were asked in Parliament about the availability of the method (Saks 1985). Whilst, as noted in Chapter 5, lay acupuncturists and other fringe therapists were split by internal divisions in this period, their organizations had sufficiently strong internal cohesion and leadership to mount effective lobbies (Fulder and Monro 1981). The most significant danger posed by lay acupuncturists to the medical profession on Wardwell's criteria, however, was that most of these practitioners showed little desire to be incorporated into orthodoxy on subordinate terms. As such, they formed a greater challenge to orthodoxy than groups like radiographers and physiotherapists who had exchanged subordination for official recognition in the health care division of labour (Larkin 1983). Indeed, by the early 1970s medically unqualified acupuncturists were more threatening to the profession than many of their unorthodox counterparts – as, for example, Christian Scientists whose religiously centred practice limited the competition with orthodox medicine in an increasingly secular society (Nudelman 1976) and osteopaths who were progressively moving away from using their technique as a distinct system of medicine (Eagle 1978).

In sum, then, lay acupuncturists constituted a growing threat to the interests of the British medical profession from the mid-twentieth century to the mid-1970s, in so far as they challenged its hard-won status, power and wealth. The challenge to the status and power of the profession in general and its elite in particular is epitomized, as was seen earlier, by the increasing number of consultations with non-medical acupuncturists in this period. Admittedly, some of these were last-resort cases, many of which were drawn from low-prestige areas of medicine like geriatrics – attracted by the promise of acupuncture in chronic and degenerative disorders (Inglis 1980). Yet this should not mask the threat to the economic interests of the profession of the claim by lay acupuncturists to succeed where orthodox medicine had failed, including in the more prestigious specialisms of medicine like cardiology and neurology characterized by higher than average levels of private practice (see De Santis 1980; Klein 1975). The economic challenge to general practitioners was less significant, given their more restricted involvement with private medicine and the monopoly on state employment afforded by the existence of the NHS – which in fact provided an incentive to off-load troublesome patients to acupuncturists and other marginal practitioners (Strong 1979). When judged overall, though, the economic threat of lay acupuncturists to the medically qualified by the mid-1970s was substantial enough, especially in view of the middle- and upper-class origins of a significant part of their clientele in a competitive medical market (Saks 1985). Nor should it be forgotten that in the modern era such alternative practitioners have challenged the position of orthodox medical researchers as well as medical practitioners. The threat from lay acupuncturists in this sense is encapsulated in a reply by a leading non-medical acupuncturist to a critical article on acupuncture by Professor Wall, the head of the cerebral functions unit at University College in London, who expressed 'sympathy for Professor Wall, having spent a lifetime researching into physiology, to now find that so much of his work needs to be rethought, restudied and substantially amended' (Rose-Neil 1972: 309).

While the action taken by the British medical profession to restrict the growth of lay acupuncture in the years leading to the mid-1970s was therefore generally compatible with its own self-interests, the attack on non-medical acupuncturists in this period was even more consistent with the interests of the small, but growing, number of doctors who took up acupuncture after the Second World War. Such non-medical practitioners challenged their status and power even more than orthodox doctors as they often had a lengthier training in, and a deeper classical knowledge of, acupuncture (Saks 1992b). They also more directly threatened the earning capacity of doctors in this field who, as has been seen, were primarily concentrated in the private sector. But if these factors – together with a desire to win respectability within the profession – help to explain why the few medical exponents of acupuncture at this time should have so willingly joined in the attack on the fringe, they do not account for their decision to employ such a marginal form of therapy in the first place. This too seems amenable to an interest-based explanation, given both the financial benefits to medical acupuncturists in a lucrative area with a fast-expanding public demand and the opportunity that acupuncture presented for successful practice with a relatively short period of training (Saks 1985).

The appeal of acupuncture to insiders, though, was limited in the period up to the early 1970s by the strong professional obstacles set up by the medical elite to those engaging in acupuncture research and practice. These ensured that, in terms of interests, acupuncture was primarily attractive to general practitioners with no real stake in the career hierarchy and an expanded world of private practice to gain in an otherwise fairly barren segment of the market (Saks 1992b). But even here the balance of advantage was tenuous, given the stigma associated with the technique. It is therefore not surprising that few doctors should have employed acupuncture at this time and that those that did were primarily generalists – paralleling the latter half of the nineteenth century, with the caveat that they were more likely to be drawn from lower-order medical strata and less reticent about employing acupuncture as a broad-ranging therapy than their predecessors a century earlier (Saks 1985). However, as will be recalled, the scope of application of medical acupuncture was progressively narrowed down by the beginning of the 1970s, by which time medical exponents of the method more commonly subscribed to orthodox neurophysiological accounts of acupuncture than traditional explanations of its *modus operandi*. This trend is readily explicable in terms of the self-interests of medical acupuncturists in remaining within the outlying boundaries of the profession at a time when fringe competitors were beginning to mount a greater challenge to their security. But this still leaves open the critical question of to what extent the interests of the leaders of the profession were compatible with their policy of stifling the growth of medical acupuncture in the two and a half decades following the mid-twentieth century in Britain.

In this respect, the continuity between medical interests and action is also evident. Doctors practising acupuncture and other marginal therapies increased the economic competition in private practice for the profession in a similar, if scaled down, manner to that of the fast-expanding fringe. In addition, deviant insiders challenged the status and power of the medical establishment by claiming to possess superior knowledge in selected areas of research and practice – a challenge highlighted by the unwillingness of consultants to refer even last-resort patients to general practitioners using alternative therapies such as acupuncture in the period under discussion (Saks 1992b). And whilst professional solidarity was hardly the vital political resource for the profession that it had been during the previous century, the formation of groups like the MAS and, at a broader level, the SMN in the 1960s and early 1970s could only have diminished its collective power. The main challenge to the profession and its leadership from such deviant insiders, though, was that medical involvement in this field, while still limited, could legitimate the growing lay practice of alternative therapies. This helps to explain why the leaders of the profession were most concerned about doctors using marginal methods like acupuncture as broad-ranging remedies underpinned by unorthodox theories which offered encouragement to fringe outsiders (Saks 1985). The potential benefits to the profession and its elite of restricting the medical employment of acupuncture and other alternative methods therefore were not only substantial, but also far outweighed the costs in the years leading up to the mid-1970s in Britain – particularly since, in the acupuncture field, lay practitioners had not yet achieved enough support for an American-style model of professional incorporation to be contemplated in terms of medical self-interests at this stage (Rosenberg 1977).

Nonetheless, whilst the attempt of the British medical establishment to constrain the development of acupuncture within its own ranks was as consistent with professional interests as the attack which it launched against lay acupuncturists from the mid-twentieth century to the beginning of the 1970s, it will be recalled from Chapter 4 that thereafter the medical profession began to move in an incorporationist direction; although acupuncture retained its standing as an alternative medicine, the numbers of doctors involved in this field rose steadily at the same time as the medical elite softened its hard line on the method. Larkin has observed that:

> Strategically the medical profession may be said to seek dominance amongst health occupations, but tactically it varies its approach according to (a) changing perceptions of its own role, and (b) the degree and character of the perceived threat from without.
>
> (Larkin 1978: 845)

How far, though, does the recent shift in medical strategy continue to mesh with professional self-interests in British society?

Before considering the rationale for this apparent shift towards a more incorporationist policy, it should be remembered that the medical profession broadly maintained its attack on lay acupuncturists and other fringe practititoners from the mid-1970s onwards through the medical journals and other channels. This hostility towards non-medically qualified acupuncturists, who had every incentive to continue to take up the method in a situation in which public demand for the therapy was still expanding, was even more consistent than in earlier years with the interests of the profession because of the increasingly powerful challenge that they presented to its security from the latter half of the 1970s to the early 1990s, given the wider development of alternative medicine in Britain. This is clear if the basic template established by Wardwell (1976) for assessing the threat posed by marginal practitioners to the medical profession is applied to this time span. In this regard, as has been seen, non-medical acupuncturists maintained their challenge to the philosophical basis of contemporary biomedicine and continued to treat a broad range of conditions, in line with their general commitment to classical theories of acupuncture. The growing scale of the threat posed by such practitioners, however, is best gauged by examining their position against the more detailed list of criteria that Wardwell lays down to evaluate the degree to which particular types of irregular therapists endanger medical orthodoxy.

In this sense, the number of lay acupuncture groups has continued to expand, along with those representing other fringe practices – to such an extent that even by the early 1980s there were estimated to be some 54 associations and 44 training establishments for alternative medicine in Britain (Fulder and Monro 1981). The threat of lay acupuncturists to the medical profession, moreover, has been increased by the consolidation of linkages between these practitioners and other fringe therapists – not least through the ICM, the CCAM and most recently the British Complementary Medical Association (Langford 1992). This raises the spectre that the floodgates may open if non-medically qualified exponents of acupuncture gain comparable state recognition as a profession. This spectre looms large, given the spiralling client demand for such practitioners which is now met by a growing number of lay acupuncturists surpassing that for most other specific alternative therapies and comprising part of a total of tens of thousands of alternative practitioners across the country (Fulder 1988). The challenge to medical orthodoxy has been further underlined by the expanding political influence of non-medical acupuncturists and other unorthodox therapists from the mid-1970s onwards, supported by individual patrons and generally favourable media coverage as well as the recently established all-party Parliamentary Group for Alternative and Complementary Medicine (Sharma 1992a). It has also been amplified by the increasing internal cohesion amongst many groups of fringe therapists including lay acupuncturists, as epitomized by the formation of the CFA in 1980; although disputes do still occur, unity rather than discord is progressively becoming the keynote at a time when effective leadership is not lacking (Saks 1992b). The medical profession, moreover, cannot be reassured by the fact that lay acupuncturists, like many other fringe therapists, have been seeking independent state registration – as signposted by the passage of the Osteopaths Act which grants osteopaths effective closure of title and lays down the basis for self-regulation (Standen 1993) – in a field in which new ministerial responsibilities have been created and government officials have shown themselves not always to be slavish adherents of orthodox medical opinion (Saks 1991a).

In this light, non-medically qualified acupuncturists have come to represent a fundamental threat to the status and power of the medical profession over the last two decades in Britain, as more and more patients seek treatment from unorthodox practitioners of this and other alternative therapies. Admittedly the majority of these consultations are currently used as a supplement to orthodox medical treatment or for a narrowly circumscribed range of conditions (Thomas *et al.* 1991). However, this should not diminish the significance of the economic threat that broad-ranging lay practitioners of acupuncture present to doctors in private practice, particularly since alternative medicine still seems to be disproportionately used by the more affluent sections of society (Sharma 1992a). The economic challenge to the profession by lay therapists, though, has not just been restricted to private practice, but has now spread to encompass medical practitioners and researchers in the state sector. This is mainly because of the threat of systematic encroachment by outsiders like lay acupuncturists on the sacred territory of the profession in the NHS – a threat accentuated by a 1989 MORI poll which showed that some three-quarters of the population wanted acupuncture and longer-established forms of alternative medi cine more widely available in the state health system (Saks 1991b). Accordingly, the mainly negative stance of the medical profession towards fringe therapies in general and lay acupuncture in particular since the mid-1970s has been highly compatible with professional self-interests, as it has struggled to contain the rising tide of fringe practitioners. This conclusion is especially pertinent as regards medical acupuncturists who have continued to have an additional stake in suppressing the rivals who most directly endanger their interests in a common area of practice – both financially in the fast-expanding market in alternative medicine and in terms of status and power, given the typically shorter training received by medical acupuncturists as distinct from their lay competitors (Saks 1991a).

But if the adoption of such a negative stance by medical acu-puncturists towards lay outsiders is now even more consistent with their interests, the reasons for the enhanced appeal of acupuncture to the rapidly growing band of doctors who have entered this field since the mid-1970s clearly requires explanation – given the persisting position of acupuncture as an alternative therapy, with the limitations that this has imposed on the prospects of its medical exponents building a successful orthodox career. Plainly, medical interest in acupuncture has continued to be fostered by such factors as spiralling client demand and the increasing crisis of confidence in allopathic medicine. These have enhanced the opportunities for private practice at a time when the range of short training courses for the medically qualified in the technique has expanded (Saks 1985). Acupuncture has also become more appealing to medical researchers with the recently identified connection between the effects produced using this method and endorphins and other neuroactive substances which figure in orthodox medical theories. This has facilitated the search for interesting and rewarding problems by scientists engaging in a process of 'intellectual migration followed by the modified application of existing techniques and theories within a different area' (Mulkay 1972: 34).

Acupuncture in Britain, though, has not proved uniformly attractive to all groups within the medical profession since the mid-1970s, any more than in earlier periods. Like certain other contemporary areas of alternative medicine (Eagle 1978), the method seems to have been most frequently adopted by general practitioners and a small, but steadily expanding, higher-order group of more senior hospital specialists (Camp 1986). This pattern differs a little from the years immediately following the mid-twentieth century when generalists almost exclusively dominated the ranks of medical acupuncturists, but again seems closely linked to the respective interests of the parties involved – as discussed in more detail by Saks (1985). In terms of the balance of costs and benefits, it is easy to see why more senior members of the medical profession have entered the acupuncture field; the gains from simply conforming are limited and any risks are minimized by their position in the professional pecking order, particularly since the most characteristic recent form of involvement with acupuncture at consultant-level has been part-time, within the parameters of conventional neurophysiology. That general practitioners should have continued to practise the method most substantially in recent times is also not surprising since, just as in the immediate postwar period, acupuncture has provided increasing opportunities to build a reputation and to engage in private medicine, in a field where career prospects have hitherto been distinctly limited. This contrasts with the position of middle-ranking medical specialists who have had the greatest incentive to shun techniques like acupuncture because of the threat which non-conformity poses to their more extensive promotion chances and the value of their existing skills based on a lengthy period of training and experience (see, for example, Stephens 1983).

Perhaps the key factor, though, which has led more doctors from a wider range of backgrounds into the acupuncture fold is that the stance of the leaders of the profession has become decidedly less hostile towards medical acupuncture – as witnessed, for instance, by the decreasing stigma associated with the technique and the improved chances of obtaining small amounts of official funding for training and research in this field, recounted in Chapter 4. This shift in stance cannot be separated from the pressures that led to the intensification of the attack on lay acupuncturists and other non-medically qualified practitioners after the mid-1970s. More specifically, there is still a strong case for arguing that the gradual incorporation of the method into the orthodox medical repertoire over the past two decades in Britain has served the interests of both the profession as a collectivity and its elite by countering the growing threat of non-medical outsiders to the profession (Saks 1992b). Nonetheless, this case is not completely clear-cut in so far as the expanding number of acupuncturists within the profession, as in the period prior to the mid-1970s, has increased the competition for orthodox doctors in private practice; challenged the status and power of those subscribing to more conventional medical theories and techniques; acted as a fragmenting influence on the profession; and, most important of all, raised the prospect of damaging the interests of the profession by further legitimating the work of fringe competitors.

These costs, however, have been more than offset by the terms on which the medical profession has so far incorporated the method. As seen earlier, the power of the medical elite has been used to deter doctors involved in the field from employing acupuncture in its classical form and to encourage them to apply it mainly to pain-related conditions, supported by orthodox neurophysiological explanations of its *modus operandi*. This has much reduced the extent of the competitive threat to more conventional practitioners and researchers from insiders using acupuncture, especially given the limitations of the challenge in its two primary areas of application. In relation to anaesthesia, the threat has been defused because the practical anaesthetic capabilities of acupuncture 'are considered so inferior to conventional anaesthesia that there is little possibility of its being used extensively for surgery in . . . Britain' (Webster 1979: 134). In the more promising case of pain itself, moreover, medical acupuncturists have not strongly challenged the rest of the profession, given the large size of the potential client group and the relative lack of prestige associated with this area (Saks 1985) – not to mention the fact that their contribution has helped to restore the tarnished credibility of the profession in this field (Taylor 1985). The threat posed by such acupuncturists specifically to the medical elite has also been attenuated by the gradually increasing involvement of higher-order specialists with the technique, which has mainly been employed on the basis of theoretical knowledge drawn from mainstream medicine to which the leaders of the profession have the most convincing claim to expertise. This suggests too that the divisive effects of the increasing adoption of acupuncture within the profession can be overstated (Saks 1985).

The dangers presented by fringe practitioners to doctors as a collectivity as a result of the gradual trend towards incorporation in this country over the past two decades have also been greatly diminished by the restricted way in which acupuncture has been adopted by the medical profession, with its delimited areas of application linked to orthodox theorizing reducing the degree to which lay acupuncture therapy is legitimated. As Webster notes,

> the gradual definition of acupuncture as a limited analgesic and therapeutic technique represents the process of reducing the cost of entry into the area for allopathic groups, where 'cost' is measured in terms of the scientific capital required for entry.
>
> (Webster 1979: 130)

The practice of giving minimum encouragement to non-medical acupuncture whilst incorporating the method into the profession has also been supported by the continuing exclusion of the method from mainstream medical education and research programmes and the provision of post-registration short courses in acupuncture solely for doctors (Saks 1992b). The distancing of non-medically qualified acupuncturists involved here has been further underwritten by the persisting emphasis of the profession on the hazards of independent lay acupuncture practice and the merits of confining the use of the technique to doctors or subordinated groups such as nurses and physiotherapists within the health care division of labour (Marcus 1992) – following the classical professional strategy of absorbing threatening techniques through a process of delegation to maintain orthodox hegemony (Strong 1979). This strategy has become especially important in terms of professional self-interests following the recent confirmation by the government that lay therapists can now be subcontracted into the new market-oriented NHS (DoH 1991b).

Given that the risks to the profession associated with the incorporation of acupuncture from both insiders and outsiders have been significantly reduced by the terms on which the British medical profession has adopted the method since the mid-1970s, the balance of costs and benefits has clearly favoured an incorporationist strategy from the standpoint of medical interests – particularly since this has enabled the profession to turn challenge into opportunity by creating more fertile conditions for the medical colonization of acupuncture, in face of growing public demand (Saks 1992b). The greater degree of control that the medical profession in Britain continues to possess over the content of its work and the less stringent legal restrictions that exist on the practice of acupuncture as compared to the United States also help to explain in terms of interests why incorporationist tendencies in this country have not gone as far as in America (Saks 1985). It has nonetheless been in the interests of doctors in both countries in recent times to endeavour to limit the use of the method to insiders – in much the same way as in relation to homoeopathy in the contemporary Anglo-American context (Nicholls 1988; Coulter 1985). From the viewpoint of medical interests, this has been preferable to the absorption of outsiders into mainstream medicine because of the increasing scale of the challenge that lay acupuncturists and other alternative therapists have posed to the wealth, status and power of the medical profession on both sides of the Atlantic (Saks 1991a; Eisenberg *et al.* 1993).

But if the specific pattern of incorporation of acupuncture that has begun to emerge in Britain since the mid-1970s is compatible with medical self-interests, this should not be taken to imply that lay acupuncturists have simply been the persecuted victims of the ego-centric policies of the medical establishment, either contemporaneously or historically. Vested interests also seem to have been a strong influence on the operation of non-medically qualified acupuncturists themselves since the early nineteenth century – and not just in terms of the incentives possessed by such practitioners to take up the method at various points over the past two centuries. This is well exemplified by the explicit attempt of the BAA in the 1970s to set up an official register for all qualified acupuncturists and to purge 'charlatans and imitators' in acupuncture, a stance which not only echoed the nineteenth-century monopolistic strategy of the medical profession itself, but also promised to advance the interests of non-medical acupuncturists, had parallel state support been forthcoming (Saks 1985). It should be stressed, however, that the main focus here has been on the interests of the medical profession and its relevant constituent sub-groups, rather than those of outsiders. As has now been seen, such interests have been broadly consistent with medical policy on acupuncture over the past two centuries in Britain.

CONCLUSION

This chapter has shown both that sufficient power has existed in the hands of the British medical profession in general and its elite in particular to influence the direction of decision-making about acupuncture since the early nineteenth century and that this power has been deployed in a manner compatible with the medical interests concerned over this period. Taken in conjunction with the unconvincing nature of alternative explanations of the predominant climate of medical rejection of acupuncture explored in Chapter 5, it must therefore be concluded that professional self-interests seem to have been primarily responsible for medical policy in this area in nineteenth- and twentieth-century Britain – including the recent tentative steps towards incorporation. The time has now come to examine in more detail the extent to which such interests have been consistent with the public interest in the medical response to acupuncture in order to complete the illustration of the theoretical and methodological framework for assessing the altruism claims of the professions outlined in Part I of this book. This task will be undertaken in Chapter 7, following an exploration of the ideologies surrounding the medical reception of acupuncture which form a further intriguing aspect of the interplay between professional interests and the public interest in this field.

7 The medical reception of acupuncture in Britain

Professional ideologies and the public interest

Whilst the medical response to acupuncture as a form of alternative medicine in nineteenth- and twentieth-century Britain has now been argued to be largely based on professional self-interests, the negative implications of the predominant policy of rejection for the availability of this procedure to the public as a whole and to specific social class and regional-based groups in particular should not be forgotten. Such problems of access pinpointed in Chapter 4 raise the question of whether the response of the medical profession to acupuncture has matched its own public interest ideology. Before turning to analyse this crucial issue in the case study, though, it is worth noting that the claims so far sustained about the role of professional self-interests in the medical reception of acupuncture are reinforced by the ideological stance taken by medical orthodoxy over this procedure.

PROFESSIONAL IDEOLOGIES, INTERESTS AND ACUPUNCTURE

In making this judgement, it should be recognized that there is little agreement about the definition of the contentious concept of 'ideology' in the social sciences (Heywood 1992). However, the controversies can be readily circumvented by noting the rationale for employing the concept in this context – namely, to consider the consistency of the ideological positions adopted by the medical profession, or segments thereof, with professional self-interests in the reception of acupuncture. Definitions of 'ideology' which posit an invariable relationship between ideology and interests must therefore be ruled out, to avoid self-fulfilling conclusions. This being the case, the notion of 'ideology' is viewed in a minimalist sense as 'a set of closely related beliefs or ideas, or even attitudes, characteristic of a group or community' (Plamenatz 1971: 15). This usage also side-steps the common association of ideology with distortion and falsity (Heywood 1992); as Ryan (1970: 221) says, 'talk of ideology is . . . talk about those ideas which are selected and held for their effects on the converted, not for their truth'. Whilst this remark should doubtless encompass the effects of ideas on the non-converted too, the concept of 'ideology' delineated here clearly allows the link between professional ideologies and interests to be explored without unnecessary definitional presumption in studying the relationship between medical orthodoxy and acupuncture. This task will now be undertaken, starting with a consideration of the first half of the nineteenth century and concluding with a particular focus on the contemporary era in Britain.

Early to mid-nineteenth century

There is little doubt that there was a high degree of congruence between medical interests and professional ideologies in the period leading up to the mid-nineteenth century in Britain. As will be recalled, the interests of the medically qualified at this time lay in minimizing the extent of the practice of outsiders, including lay acupuncturists. It is not surprising, therefore, that medical publications of the day frequently referred to fringe practitioners of acupuncture and other unorthodox therapies as frauds and linked their work to that of the discredited mountebanks of the seventeenth and eighteenth centuries who hawked their wares at fairs and carnivals (Parssinen 1992). Nor is it difficult to understand why doctors should have publicly given such strong emphasis to the financial self-interests of outsiders by referring to them as mere 'money-grubs' (*Lancet* 1845) and drawing attention to 'the enormous income and bloated wealth of many of them' (Flood 1845b: 203). This coupled with the stress in medical journals and pamphlets on the gullibility of clients of such practitioners – in a situation in which public ignorance and the profusion of quackery were claimed to be intimately allied (*PMSJ* 1843) – served as a potential deterrent to self-respecting patients who might otherwise have forgone the ministrations of orthodox doctors and sought treatment from their fringe competitors. The direction of medical interests in this situation also helps to explain why doctors propagated the belief that lay acupuncture was largely based on magic and superstition (Rosenberg 1977) – in much the same way as, for example, the unorthodox practice of mesmerism (Parssinen 1992) – with all the retrogressive associations which this conjured up with traditional systems of healing in Tudor and Stuart times (Larner 1992).

Paradoxically, such attacks on the fringe also enabled medical practitioners to accentuate their own virtues as against outsiders – a point illustrated by the great emphasis placed by doctors on their high 'scientific repute' (*London Medical Gazette* 1844) and their concern not with superstition, but with 'the deep truths of science' (Flood 1845a). This contrast, which was particularly congruent with medical interests as doctors began to organize systematically from the 1830s onwards to enhance their collective standing through the reform of the profession, also achieved indirect expression in the pronouncements on the relative safety of patients in the hands of the medically qualified as compared to those of lay practitioners. Although this was not a central part of the profession's stance on acupuncture, one contributor to this theme observed that the work of lay therapists as a whole represented 'a fearful and yet legalized carnage . . . rivalling the ravages of war' (Flood 1845b: 203) – against which medical practitioners were able to use their position to advance their own claim to a more extensive professional monopoly by arguing that, if the public was to be protected, no one should be able 'to undertake the management of disease whose competence to do so had not been duly tested and legally certified' (*PMSJ* 1843: 491).

Nor should one overlook the negative statements about the medical practice of acupuncture that emanated from within the profession in the years immediately preceding the mid-nineteenth century – especially in relation to doctors whose use of the method most closely mirrored that of lay acupuncturists. Whilst such practitioners were not usually taken to task for the risks that they presented to their patients, any success they achieved in applying the technique to a broad range of conditions was typically ascribed to chance, even by other medical acupuncturists who employed the method in a more limited manner (Elliotson 1850). Medical practitioners of unorthodox therapies, just like their counterparts on the fringe, were frequently attacked too for being mercenary and dishonourable and for preying on the ignorance of the public (Parssinen 1992). Indeed, the leaders of the profession also accused unorthodox medical practitioners of fraudulence – a classic case being that of Professor John Elliotson, the acupuncture pioneer, whose experiments with mesmerism were denounced as trickery in the 1830s by the editor of the *Lancet*, Thomas Wakley (Bartrip 1990). Since, as was seen in Chapter 6, it was in the interests of the medical establishment to put its own house in order as well as to restrict the practice of outsiders at this sensitive stage of professional development, these ideological components of the medical reponse to acupuncture were also highly compatible with professional self-interests.

Mid-nineteenth to mid-twentieth century

Much the same appears to have been true of the period between the mid-nineteenth and mid-twentieth century in Britain – when prevailing medical ideologies about exponents of marginal methods both inside and outside the ranks of the medically qualified were also consistent with professional group interests. In relation to the medical interests and ideologies surrounding the lay practice of acupuncture and other alternative therapies in the years leading up to the turn of the century, it will be recalled that it was to the advantage of doctors as a collectivity to sustain their attack on the non-medically qualified, because of the threat the latter posed to the growing power and privileges of the profession. It was therefore clearly again compatible with the interests of the medical profession for it to condemn such practitioners at the ideological level by, for instance, commenting on the 'crass stupidity of persons who, when anything is the matter with them, place themselves in the hands of men who rob their victims of both money and life' (*Lancet* 1871: 598). As such, doctors continued to reaffirm their own credentials as representatives of a profession safeguarding the health of the public by focusing on the dangers of quackery, not least in relation to lay acupuncture (Dudgeon 1872). The ideology of scientism was also regularly employed to distinguish the rationality of the medically qualified from fringe practitioners who were at best disparagingly referred to as being engaged in the 'so-called science of healing' (*Lancet* 1889).

The consistency between these ideological currents and medical self-interests persisted well into the first half of the twentieth century as far as fringe therapists were concerned. Although the threat of practitioners such as lay acupuncturists receded markedly in this period, it was still not in the interests of the profession, as has been seen, to encourage their development. This was reflected in the fact that the dominant professional ideology remained antagonistic to the medically unqualified, even though it was less frequently overtly expressed at this time. When this ideology did emerge in debate, however, its staple elements were all too familiar – including, amongst other things, equating lay practitioners with irrational superstition (*Lancet* 1934); highlighting the risks associated with the practice of the medically unqualified (*Lancet* 1938); and drawing attention to the frauds perpetrated by outsiders, whose excessive fees were also condemned (Vaughan 1959).

Comparable links between ideology and interests in orthodox medicine are evident too when the stance of the medical establishment towards doctors employing alternative therapies is scrutinized in the latter half of the nineteenth and first part of the twentieth century in this country. In the former period, as will be recalled, the profession in general and its elite in particular had a strong interest in suppressing such activities – especially where conflicting theories and wide-ranging applications of the methods concerned were involved, largely because of the legitimacy that this might bestow on their lay competitors. It is not surprising, then, that the importance of eliminating the use of alternative therapies such as acupuncture within the profession was emphasized in medical publications (*Lancet* 1864) and accompanied by continuing claims about the ignorance and non-scientific orientation of unorthodox insiders (*BMJ* 1863; Donkin 1880). Related comments in the leading medical journals, moreover, about the discrediting influence of alternative practice within the profession – as exemplified by the observation in the *Lancet* (1880: 889) that fellows and licentiates of the RCS consulting with the fringe should 'think more of the dignity of the College they are connected with' – are equally compatible with an interest-based account of the response of the medical profession to acupuncture and other marginal therapies. However, as the threat of doctors employing alternative medicine declined following the turn of the century, references to their compromised position in the profession became less common. But when such medical practitioners were discussed in orthodox circles, they were usually again dealt with in terms of the negative rhetoric of fraudulence and humbug and seen as remaining in practice only because of the credulity of the public (Parker 1921; *BMJ* 1945), thus reaffirming the connection between professional ideologies and interests in the years leading up to the mid-twentieth century in Britain.

Mid-twentieth century to the present day

There seems no reason to suppose that doctors in more recent times have been any less prone than other scientists to 'select descriptions and justifications from the available vocabulary in accordance with their interests' (Mulkay 1979: 113). Despite claims that such ideo-logical linkages are now rarely forged because scientific orthodoxy is based on the pursuit of objective truth, many social scientists believe that ideology and interest remain closely connected in contemporary science (Webster 1991). In this respect, Collins and Pinch (1979) provide a general framework for categorizing the ideological strategies adopted by scientific orthodoxy in rejecting deviant knowledge-claims in the modern era. These include a blank refusal to believe; the skilful use of semi-philosophical rhetoric; associating unorthodox methods with unscientific beliefs; accusations of triviality; attacks on the methodological precepts underpinning competing sets of ideas; making unfavourable comparisons with canonical versions of the scientific method; levelling accusations of fraud against unorthodox practitioners; *ad hominem* arguments; and the magnification of anecdotal evidence.

The use of some of these devices to advance medical self-interests in relation to alternative medicine in general and acupuncture in particular in the hundred and fifty years preceding the mid-twentieth century has, of course, already been illustrated. The focus in the case study, however, is more on the present than the past and in this sense such ideological components not only have been in evidence in the reaction of the medical profession to alternative therapies as a whole, but also seem to have been deployed in a manner closely corresponding to professional self-interests. This is very apparent in the medical response to the challenge from lay practitioners in this country up to the mid-1970s. At this time, the scientific credentials of fringe practitioners of spiritual healing, for instance, were cast into doubt by claims in mainstream medical publications that they were engaged in 'hocus pocus' and that any apparent success could be ascribed to spontaneous remission and suggestion – paralleling accusations of fraud made in the mainstream medical literature about lay exponents of techniques like radiesthesia (Inglis 1980). The small number of doctors who took up alternative therapies, moreover, were also open to such charges in this period, as Eagle (1978: 67) notes with reference to orthodox attacks on medical homoeopathy on the grounds that 'it is unscientific, that the evidence for its efficacy is anecdotal and that it has not been subjected to the rigours of contemporary scientific evaluation'. Interestingly too, although orthodox ideological assaults on alternative medicine in all its forms continued after the mid-1970s – drawing on the familiar imagery of 'irrationality', 'charlatanism' and 'quackery' (*BMJ* 1985; Skrabanek 1986) – these have generally been moderated in more recent times as far as doctors are concerned, as the gradual incorporation of such therapies into medical orthodoxy has become more compatible with professional self-interests. Nowhere is this better highlighted than in the apparent shift of position between the two latest BMA reports on alternative medicine, in which the outright condemnation of alternative therapies linked with 'superstition, magic and the supernatural' (BMA 1986) has been transformed into a concern with the most appropriate means of regulating these therapies from the viewpoint of the profession (BMA 1993).

Such associations between professional ideologies and interests in the medical response to alternative medicine in modern Britain have been strongly reflected in the case of acupuncture, just as in earlier times. This is certainly true in the period up to the early 1970s when, as has been seen, it was in the interests of the profession as a whole to ensure that both the lay and medical employment of acupuncture was restricted. Whilst the degree to which acupuncturists challenged ortho-dox practitioners and researchers at this stage should not be overstated, the interests of the latter groups were undoubtedly compatible with the dominant medical ideology set out in the few items that were published on acupuncture in the 1950s and 1960s. This ideology included the recurring theme that classical acupuncture had no objective basis and was connected with witchcraft – indeed, in the *BMJ* (1968) the method was equated with snakes' blood and crocodiles' teeth as a remedy for illness. This emphasis on the unscientific nature of acupuncture – especially in its traditional form – was complemented, moreover, by both medical criticisms of the methodology employed in acupuncture research which threw into question the favourable results achieved in this field and a refusal to accept that genuine acupuncture points existed which provided a convenient rationalization for the medical estab-lishment to refrain from subjecting the method to the research tech-niques that it so extolled (Ewart 1972).

The links between medical interests and ideology became even closer, however, as the popularity of acupuncture grew in the years from 1970 to 1975. Given the enhanced professional interests in restraining acupuncture that this entailed, it is understandable that the mainstream medical journals in the early 1970s stressed the lack of safety of the method, particularly in unqualified hands – mainly as a result of the risks of the transmission of disease through insufficiently sterilized needles and needle insertions damaging vital internal organs (Webster 1979). Medical interests at this stage were also consistent with the complaints of orthodox specialists in leading medical publications that 'traditional acupuncturists did not abide by the norms of openness and impartiality, relying instead on popularisation and sensationalism to attract support for their technique' (Webster 1979: 133) – claims about the unscientific nature of lay acupuncture which were epitomized by the reference of the *BMJ* (1973a) to their classical practice as 'intuitive nonsense'. The nature of the contribution made to the ideological war against lay exponents of the method by medical acupuncturists, whose position was most strongly challenged by fringe developments, can be understood in terms of interests too. This helps to explain why medical pioneers of acupuncture like Moss were able to suggest that lay practitioners of this technique 'could do a lot of harm . . . [and] would be taking money under false pretences from sick and unhappy people' (Ewart 1972: 115).

The compatibility of professional ideology and interests is also evident in the British medical response to insiders employing acupuncture in the first half of the 1970s. In this respect, the prevailing medical ideology in general and that of the medical elite in particular was again adverse. Whilst relatively little attention was given to the dangers of the medical application of the method, medical acupuncturists in the early 1970s, like their non-medical counterparts, were often faced with a stubborn refusal to believe that the technique could work, even in its more limited form as an analgesic. Thus orthodox doctors were reluctant to accept that lung reflation could occur without assisted ventilation in operations in which the chest wall was opened under 'acupuncture anaesthesia' (Karols 1972), despite clear evidence to the contrary (see, *inter alia*, Hamilton 1972; Gustafsson 1973). Occasionally too such reticence was expressed rhetorically, as when one medical contributor responded to Chinese reports that the number of needles used in surgical analgesia was progressively being reduced by asking 'whether this technique would still be successful if the final reduction were made and no needles inserted' (Ramsay 1972: 233). Such trivialization of acupuncture was echoed by MacIntosh (1973: 455) from the Nuffield Department of Anaesthetics who wrote that 'acupuncture needles bear a similar relationship to ether as does a bottle of coloured medicine to penicillin in the treatment of septicaemia'. This aspect of medical ideology was also intertwined with destructive methodological attacks on pain studies by medical acupuncturists which were predicated on the assumption that, if acupuncture was found to work, there must be a flaw in the research procedure (Mumford and Bowsher 1973). In addition, the employment of acupuncture in surgery was frequently associated with chicanery by medical orthodoxy (*Lancet* 1972) – not least because its apparent analgesic effects were viewed as largely being due to the prior administration of sedatives and local anaesthetics (Saltoun 1973). Members of the orthodox profession also often dismissed the analgesic application of the method by ascribing its influence to such mechanisms as hypnotism, the placebo effect and cultural stoicism (Wall 1972, 1974) thereby linking even medical acupuncture to 'pre-scientific' health care practices (Porter 1987).

In the early 1970s, therefore, an inextricable connection between orthodox medical ideology and professional self-interests continued to exist which was to the advantage of most elements of the profession, as it restricted the competitive threat from both insiders and outsiders in this field. However, whereas the ideological stance of the medical establishment on lay acupuncturists was consistently antagonistic in the period from 1970 to 1975, the position was less clear as regards medical acupuncturists, particularly since a small, but increasing, number of mainstream journal items began to appear defending the employment of the technique by doctors – not least by rebutting the charge that 'acupuncture anaesthesia' was a hoax based on political indoctrination (Brown 1972), and presenting positive evidence for the application of acupuncture for pain (Andersson *et al.* 1973). This signalled the beginning of the gradual shift of medical interests towards the incorporation of acupuncture in Britain. As such, there were strong parallels with the United States at this time, where ideological claims denying the importance of acupuncture and connecting its practice with brainwashing and deception coexisted with sympathetic support for its limited use as an analgesic within the ranks of orthodox medicine (Duke 1972). Whilst there were distinctions between Britain and the United States in terms of the medical ideologies espoused – the most obvious being that the American profession initially took a more favourable position on the employment of acupuncture by insiders in view of its differing balance of interests (Rosenberg 1977) – they have since come further together as the interests of the British medical profession have swung in the direction of incorporation.

But if the interests of the British medical profession in general and its elite in particular have lain in incorporating acupuncture since the mid-1970s, these interests have been reflected in the less hostile ideological stance taken towards medical acupuncturists who pose the least threat to the wider profession – namely, those who practise the technique in restricted form and subscribe to more orthodox explanations of its *modus operandi*. As will be recalled, the mainstream medical journals have generally subscribed to a more positive view of the analgesic application of acupuncture by doctors – especially when legitimated by orthodox neurophysiological theorizing – even though the more challenging employment of traditional acupuncture has largely been seen as lacking both rationale and utility. Although acupuncture has received rather more acceptance in its limited form than certain other alternative therapies, the ideology underpinning this acceptance has restricted its medical impact, even in what is regarded as its most productive area of application in orthodox terms. This is highlighted by a recent Working Party of the RCS (1990: 23) which, whilst acknowledging its increasing use in the treatment of pain, concluded that acupuncture 'may have a role as an adjunct to conventional treatment but it is not likely to be useful as the sole technique for the treatment of moderate to severe pain after surgery'. Medical acupuncture has also continued over the past two decades to have ideological opponents in the medical journals who have variously regarded the method as a political myth (*Lancet* 1981), criticized acupuncturists for their 'select-ive inattention' to studies showing the technique to have no scientific validity (Skrabanek 1984) and attacked the methodological precepts of research supporting its use (*Lancet* 1990).

In line with the changing interests of the medical profession, however, such ideological assaults on acupuncture have mainly been reserved for lay acupuncturists and the classical variant of the technique with which they are so strongly associated – as witnessed, for instance, by the previously documented emphasis in recent orthodox medical publications on the dangers posed by lay acupuncturists and the absence of a scientific basis for their practice. This ideological stance has broadly meshed with professional interests in keeping unorthodox practitioners in check in a situation in which the lay challenge to allopathic medicine has been mounting. Predictably enough – given the special stake which medical acupuncturists have in restricting competition from outsiders – doctors practising the method have again been the most vociferous in the ideological condemnation of fringe acupuncturists. In this sense, medically qualified acupuncturists have not only equated traditional acupuncture treatment by the medically unqualified with 'ancient fairy tales' (Roberts 1981), but also warned against consultations with such therapists without prior medical referral because of their lack of clinical expertise (Marcus 1992). Professional self-interests too seem to account for the fact that medical acu-puncturists have sought both to distance themselves from the 'mumbo jumbo' underpinning the traditional yin-yang theories of acupuncture linked with practitioners outside their ranks (Stephens 1983) and to cultivate a scientific ideology to differentiate and legitimate their own involvement with the technique – the main components of which include a commitment to orthodox methodologies for investigating acupuncture (Cahn *et al.* 1978) and more conventional accounts of its operation, such as those involving endorphins (Campbell 1987).

Yet if medical interests and ideologies have been broadly compatible, even in the recent drift towards the medical incorporation of acu-puncture in Britain, such self-sustaining ideologies are not the exclusive property of the medically qualified. Similar degrees of congruence between interests and ideologies are also found amongst fringe practi-tioners in general and lay acupuncturists in particular. This is well illustrated historically by the way in which Christian Scientists gained credibility in the nineteenth century by drawing on the prestigious mantle of 'science' (Lee 1976), paralleling the manner in which some non-medically qualified acupuncturists employed the self-styled title of 'professor' to expand their clientele earlier in that century (Churchill 1822). In the modern era groups like scientologists and chiropractors have similarly increased their legitimacy in Britain by drawing on the symbols and technical hardware of orthodox medical science, whilst osteopaths have sought to turn the tables on doctors by accusing them of acting against the interests of patients with musculo-skeletal problems by treating symptoms rather than causes (Saks 1985) – a similar charge to which they themselves have been subjected by the medical profession (Larkin 1992). Scientism has also been a key element of the ideology advanced in defence of the interests of lay acupuncture – including the stress placed by the BAA (1982) on the claims that the meridians of acupuncture contain DNA and that Qi, the life force, can be conceptualized in terms of electro-magnetic energy. Paradoxically, however, the scientific impartiality of the medical opponents of traditional acupuncture has also been questioned in a manner furthering the interests of the BAA, as highlighted by the following reply by its then Chairperson to a medical attack on acupuncture in the early 1970s: 'Professor Wall "guesses" that acupuncture does not have the pain inhibiting effect claimed. The Chinese have successfully concluded about 800,000 operations and Professor Wall takes a "guess". How scientific are we?' (Rose-Neil 1972: 309).

The scope of the ideology of lay acupuncturists today, of course, extends far beyond a preoccupation with scientific symbolism and encompasses, amongst other things, a positive stress on the distinctively holistic aspects of traditional acupuncture as compared with orthodox biomedicine and an attack on medical acupuncturists who have only taken short courses in the subject for having insufficient knowledge to practise (Mole 1992). This can be seen as part of the professionalizing strategy of non-medically qualified acupuncturists. As Webster (1979: 132) says, 'both allopathic and marginal groups deploy a variety of normative principles that champion . . . universalism, impartiality, and disinterestedness . . . [which] can be seen to be primarily associated with specialist and professionalist interests'. The main focus here, though, has been on the interests and ideologies of doctors and in this respect the high degree of consistency between the two reinforces the argument that the medical response to acupuncture in nineteenth- and twentieth-century Britain – and, in particular, the predominant climate of medical rejection of acupuncture which has developed over this period – has been largely inspired by professional self-interests. But if the primary determinant of the fate of acupuncture in this country does indeed seem to have been, in the words of Webster

(1979: 134), 'the specialist and professional strategies deployed by the dominant allopathic groups, both internally among their number, and externally, against the marginal traditional acupuncturists', have such self-interested strategies, which have undoubtedly limited the availability of the method, served the public interest?

THE MEDICAL PROFESSION, ACUPUNCTURE AND THE PUBLIC INTEREST

In considering this question in depth to round off the case study – and conclude the demonstration of the empirical applicability of the research framework outlined in Part II of this book for evaluating the extent to which altruism prevails in the professions – it should be stressed that showing that a professional group has acted in a self-interested manner over a specific issue does not necessarily imply that the interests of the public have been undermined; as will be recalled from Chapter 3, a number of permutations exist, including the possibility that the pursuit of self-interests has retarded or advanced the common good. As such, no assumptions can be made about the compatibility or otherwise of orthodox medical policy on acupuncture with the public interest over the past two centuries on the basis of the arguments so far put forward about the role of professional interests in the reception of acupuncture in this country.

Having said this, the ideology of the British medical profession from the early nineteenth century onwards has explicitly emphasized that its largely negative response to both acupuncture in particular and alternative medicine in general – especially in the hands of the medically unqualified – has been in the public interest. Certainly, the campaigns launched against quackery in the 1830s and 1840s by the *Lancet* and the *PMSJ* were held to be inspired by the desire 'to protect the public' (Parssinen 1992; Bartrip 1990), whilst later in the century 'the interests of the general public' and 'the people's welfare' were also frequently invoked in the medical press in the attack on fringe therapists such as acupuncturists (see, *inter alia*, O'Sullivan 1875 and *Lancet* 1889). In more recent years, medical acupuncturists themselves have been the most outspoken element of the profession in this respect, as illustrated by Roberts (1981) who contrasts traditional acupuncturists with 'meaningless qualifications' with medically qualified practitioners operating in the 'public interest' and Marcus (1992) who believes that allowing lay acupuncturists to advertise runs contrary to 'the best interests of patients'. This trend is paralleled in the United States where the medical profession responded to the new wave of consumer interest in the method from the early 1970s by claiming that 'for the safety of the community acupuncture should be taken over by the medical profession' (Inglis 1980: 131). Such ideological emphasis in the Anglo-American context is not too surprising given that, as was highlighted in the Introduction, claims to serve the public interest have been commonly expressed by doctors on both sides of the Atlantic over the last two hundred years, representing a long-standing and increasingly central part of their professional codes.

The public interest aspect of the altruistic ideology of the medical profession in Britain, however, cannot simply be taken on trust. As will be recalled from Chapter 1, there is much debate between sociologists of the professions over the extent to which the self-proclaimed col-lectivity orientation of such occupational groups can be seen as a guide to practice. This debate has been reflected in the acupuncture arena, where medical claims to be protecting the common good in establishing a predominant climate of professional rejection of the method have been opposed by acupuncturists. Thus, Rice (1972: 262), for example, has protested that attacks by the medical establishment on the technique 'can only do great harm . . . to the majority of people in our country'. Such counter-claims underline the key point in this book that, if the degree to which professional groups have acted altruistically in specific policy areas is to be investigated adequately, assertion must be replaced by empirically-based argument within a carefully delineated theoretical and methodological research framework. This applies no less to the question of the direction of the public interest in relation to acu-puncture, which will now be examined from this vantage point.

It is first necessary to recall the definition of the public interest developed in Chapter 2 as part of the framework for assessing the altruistic orientation of the professions. A case was then made for conceptualizing this notion relativistically in terms of the basic values of the community under consideration – which in the British setting would be the social principles of the liberal-democratic state. These principles are essentially those of promoting the overall welfare, seeking justice and ensuring an appropriate level of liberty for all citizens. Policies compatible with the public interest in relation to acupuncture in Britain, therefore, are those which advance or at least do not conflict with these principles. It is important to remember, though, that the notion of the public interest as here defined only takes on full meaning when considered in a particular time and place – for it is only in such a clearly specified setting that the substantive content of the various social principles and the balance that is struck between them can be discerned. This being said, the extent to which the policy of the

British medical profession on acupuncture was compatible with the public interest in the first half of the nineteenth century can now be assessed.

Early to mid-nineteenth century

At this time the framework of values on which the public interest can be taken to rest in Britain was more firmly rooted in the libertarian, as opposed to egalitarian, mould on the range of values that Donabedian (1973) outlines as prevailing in differing species of liberal-democracy – in so far as the right to individual freedom was given greater emphasis than social justice and the collective welfare in a situation in which the philosophy of minimizing state interference with the market principle was politically favoured (De Swaan 1990). Whilst a completely *laissez-faire* system did not exist in the period from the early to the mid-nineteenth century in British society, it was widely felt that the pursuit of unfettered individual self-interest would produce efficient outcomes which would ensure progress and advance the public interest and that 'the unseen hand of the market' should be given primacy over the extension of state provision to meet basic needs and guarantee any more than formal equality before the law (Heywood 1992). These dominant values, moreover, found strong expression in the health arena in the early Victorian era where the idea of public responsibility for health was very limited and individuals were largely left to their own devices to obtain health care on a fee-for-service basis (Levitt and Wall 1992). It should also be stressed that, as noted in Chapter 2, there are strong parallels between this period in Britain and the United States in the twentieth century in relation to the individualistic, anti-collectivist values prevailing at the broadest political level and the manner in which these were applied – especially in the preservation of the client's right to decide how to spend his or her money on health care and the restriction of government intervention in this sphere.

This explication of the public interest is vital for interpreting the extent to which the medical reception of acupuncture in Britain in the early decades of the nineteenth century was in the common good. On this interpretation, the initial occasional and limited use of acupuncture by doctors can be seen to have served the public interest because, even though this practice did not receive the wholehearted support of the emerging profession, its medical exponents were positively responding to the sporadic consumer demand in the marketplace for a method which appeared to be relatively effective and safe for a restricted range of conditions, as compared to other more traditional remedies of the day. As such, the medical response to acupuncture in Britain up to this point could be viewed as upholding individual freedom of choice in health care and furthering the overall welfare of the population. This also may be seen to apply to the response of doctors to lay acupuncturists up to the 1830s, which was not as adverse as it was later to become, at a time when there were very real limitations on the resources available to members of the developing profession to control outsiders.

However, all this was to change in the period from the late 1830s onwards when a strong climate of rejection of acupuncture developed as doctors sought to achieve a more extensive, legally underwitten position of professional closure. That this militated against the public interest is indicated – as was seen in Chapter 5 – by the apparent therapeutic advantages of this technique, even in its rudimentary form, over the procedures which made up the emerging new medical orthodoxy in at least some areas of practice. Such a view is reinforced by the fact that factors like the absence of a satisfactory explanation of the *modus operandi* of acupuncture and nationalism also do not seem to have been genuine obstacles to the medical acceptance of the method at this stage. It is further accentuated by the previously documented widening of social class and geographical inequalities of access to acupuncture that occurred as a result of the changing stance taken towards the technique by the medical profession in general and its elite in particular. These growing inequalities in the availability of the medical variant of the method should not be given excessive prominence in the assessment of the direction of the public interest in early Victorian Britain because the reduction of inequality was not yet a major item on the political agenda – as underlined by the wide social divisions more broadly prevalent in health care in this period (Stacey 1988). Nonetheless, it is still clear that doctors in Britain increasingly acted against the public interest in relation to acupuncture as the mid-nineteenth century approached, for the medical rejection of this method not only infringed the principle of individual liberty which was such an important part of the philosophy of the liberal-democratic state, but also adversely affected the welfare of many sections of society.

These comments about the implications of the negative response of the medical profession to acupuncture in the period immediately before the mid-nineteenth century in Britain – which contrasted with the more positive reaction to the technique by doctors in the United States at this time in face of consumer demand for what appeared to be a useful therapeutic procedure – apply not only to the extremely limited adoption of acupuncture by insiders from the late 1830s onwards, but also to the intensified attack that the medical establishment launched against fringe practitioners of this and other methods. The action increasingly taken by the medical profession against fringe acupuncturists ran counter to the public interest because it restricted the use of the procedure by outsiders, in a situation in which, as will be recalled, claims about the relative dangers of quackery associated with acupuncture carried scant credibility and lay acupuncturists were virtually the only source from which its broad-ranging form was available – in spite of expanding public demand following the advent of Baunscheidtism.

It might, of course, be argued that the medical attack on lay practitioners of acupuncture at this time, if not merited in its own right, was justified by virtue of the broader struggle of the profession with the fringe as a whole – given the overtly expressed concern of doctors to protect the public interest by suppressing the wider abuses associated with quackery. This was certainly how the leaders of the profession defended the case for an extension of their monopolistic privileges. As the *Lancet* noted,

> every man has an abstract right to practise any wholesome art he pleases; but no man has a right to deceive, injure, poison, or mutilate the people; and, as medical skill cannot be always judged by the event of individual cases, nor always be distinguished from impudent, wicked pretensions, by the public, it is admitted by all writers on law and politics, that it is the duty of Government to see that every medical man into whose hands the life of any member of the community is committed, at any one time or other, possesses a competent degree of professional capacity and acquirement.
>
> (1840: 538–9)

Despite the subsequent state legitimation of the medical crusade against the fringe, though, it is still not clear that medical antipathy towards lay acupuncturists in Britain up to the mid-nineteenth century was compatible with the public interest. As was stressed in Chapter 2, the public interest as here defined is not necessarily synonymous with the wisdom of state officials for governments can make decisions which militate against the common good. The argument is also further diminished by the fact that, as previously discussed, it was very difficult to distinguish orthodox and non-orthodox practitioners in terms of the nature of their training and practice in this period.

Mid-nineteenth to the mid-twentieth century

Yet whilst the credentials of the British medical profession in serving the public interest can increasingly be challenged in relation to acupuncture before the mid-nineteenth century, much the same can be said thereafter. It should first be noted, though, that in the period up to the beginning of the twentieth century at least, the value structure of liberal-democracy against which the public interest is to be judged remained fundamentally libertarian (Donabedian 1973). To be sure, changes were gradually occurring: social justice and the collective welfare in particular were of increasing political moment, as reflected in the slowly growing body of legislation in the health arena involving the state meeting its public responsibilities (Ham 1992). Nevertheless, the emphasis on individual freedom remained paramount in a health system that was still primarily based on fee-for-service transactions, despite the rise of friendly societies centred on the concept of mutual self-support (De Swaan 1990).

Within this framework, the persisting climate of medical rejection of acupuncture, which was consolidated as the profession gained a position of closure through the 1858 Medical Registration Act, could be seen to have militated against the public interest up to the turn of the century. It was certainly difficult to justify the highly limited availability of acupuncture from the medically qualified in terms of the common good, given its apparent continuing practical advantages in fields such as pain control, even when compared to the new procedures associated with the rise of biomedical orthodoxy. Nor, as was noted earlier, could the negative medical response to acupuncture at this time be reasonably explained by factors like its lack of an adequate underpinning rationale or indeed the absence of market demand which persisted well into the latter half of the nineteenth century. The elite of the profession in limiting the practice of acupuncture by insiders in fact exacerbated social class and geographical inequalities of access to this technique, in an age in which social inequalities in health were beginning to become more politically sensitive (Stacey 1988).

But if this also seems to undermine the justification for the attempts by the medical profession to eliminate the popular lay practice of acupuncture in the name of the public interest before the end of the nineteenth century, the passing of the 1858 Act does not necessarily restore professional integrity on this score. Whilst any reforms extending the scope of state intervention in the Victorian era would have needed to be supported by very persuasive arguments to be consistent with the public good in what was still a predominantly market-based society, there do not seem to have been such grounds for the 1858 legislation – a point borne out by the protracted debates that surrounded its passage through a Parliament steeped in a *laissez-faire* philosophy (Jones 1981). Increased state intervention in the health arena was not, of course, precluded within the prevailing framework of political values, as illustrated by the various sanitary and housing reforms of the 1860s and 1870s which could be justified in terms of the overall welfare (Duin and Sutcliffe 1992). However, the actions of the state in extending the monopoly rights of doctors at this time were difficult to defend because, although some fringe practices may have been potentially harmful, as Freidson (1970: 51) observes, 'it was doubtful that the actual knowledge and skill of the university-trained practitioner in those days equipped him to practice any more effectively than his self-taught or apprenticed competitor'.

It might be argued, though, that parallel systems of occupational licensure – including medical licensure – widely exist today in the United States, a country which even in modern times shares a similar configuration of political values to those prevalent in the latter half of the nineteenth century in Britain. Yet, although such licensure has also been supported in America by medical arguments about protecting the public against the dangers of incompetent practice, its value has been challenged by authors such as Friedman (1962), who, as will be recalled from Chapter 1, believes that professional monopolies in medicine and other spheres have negative repercussions for the wider public. But perhaps the greatest difficulty of using the current situation in the United States as evidence that the suppression of lay acupuncturists and other fringe therapists in late nineteenth-century Britain was compatible with the public interest lies in the fact that at a comparable stage in American history, legislation like the 1858 Act was not seen as appropriate, as it would have impeded individual freedom at a time when the distinctive competence of doctors could not justify this. As Freidson (1970: 21) again says, it was only in the twentieth century in the United States that licensing in medicine was firmly established and this only when, with 'a sound technical basis to his training, the physician could win confidence and establish the justice of his claim of privilege'.

There seems little doubt, therefore, that the public interest was not well served by the legally reinforced climate of medical rejection of acupuncture established both inside and outside the profession from the mid-nineteenth century to the start of the twentieth century in Britain. Questions can also be asked about the public interest orientation of the British medical profession in the first half of the twentieth century when acupuncture was virtually unavailable in any form, mainly because of the negative attitude of the medical establishment as it became more unified and its power grew in the wake of further key legislative reforms in the health arena.

In Britain at this time the general framework of values underpinning the public interest in liberal-democratic societies was now beginning to move markedly towards the egalitarian end of the spectrum set out by Donabedian (1973) – in which greater weight was given to increasing social equality and the general welfare through collective action and correspondingly less stress was placed on ensuring the freedom of the individual to do as he or she pleased. These changes have been chronicled sociologically by Marshall (1963a) who describes how the civil and political rights established in the nineteenth century – which provided for individual freedom, equality before the law and more extensive public participation in the political process – were increasingly augmented by social rights in the twentieth century and the full realization of the conditions of citizenship. This theme is also taken up by Dahrendorf (1959) who notes that the growing establishment of universal suffrage in societies like Britain was progressively matched by a strong ideological commitment to expanding welfare intervention and diminishing the extremes of economic and political inequality found in nineteenth-century capitalism – developments seen more recently by De Swaan (1990) as part of a civilizing process designed to remedy the external effects of adversity and deficiency. Whilst such accounts are linked to contentious theories about the reasons for these changes and their effects on the nature of society, they usefully highlight the shift in the balance struck between the principles of the liberal-democratic state in this country in the first half of the twentieth century (Giddens 1981). The new emphasis given to these varying principles is reflected in the fact that by the end of this period, Bottomore was able to relate that:

> Laissez-faire capitalism . . . has more or less vanished; . . . there is some degree of central economic planning, some attempt to regulate the distribution of wealth and income, and a more or less elaborate public provision of a wide range of social services.
>
> (Bottomore 1965: 12)

In health care specifically this emerging ethos was centrally represented by the passing of the 1911 National Health Insurance Act and the 1946 NHS Act which promoted the values of equality and welfare at the heart of the notion of citizenship by restricting, to some extent at least, the principle of individual freedom and choice (Levitt and Wall 1992). But whilst these reforms are broadly in step with the changing conception of the common good in the years leading up to the mid-twentieth century in Britain, what of the medical response to acupuncture at this time?

It is again difficult to avoid the conclusion that the medical profession in general and its elite in particular contravened the public interest, given their part in almost completely eliminating the employment of acupuncture by both insiders and outsiders in this period. The major reason for this, though, was not the failure of the profession to let the market take its head through the demand mechanism in order to preserve individual liberty, as in nineteenth-century Britain – for the demand for acupuncture was virtually non-existent in the decades immediately following the turn of the century, not least because of the earlier negative response of the profession towards it. Rather, the public interest was jeopardized because the shifting balance of values in this period meant that the welfare principle positively enjoined the profession to encourage the expansion of acupuncture practice and research because, just as in the nineteenth century, the method appeared to continue to offer some benefit in terms of safety and efficacy as compared to contemporary biomedical procedures. Since these benefits were partially linked to the perceived success of acupuncture in treating the pain-related degenerative disorders of the growing proportion of elderly people in the population (Victor 1991), the case for increasing its availability in Britain was strengthened – especially because, as was seen in Chapter 5, arguments about the dangers of quackery and the difficulties of learning to administer the technique were not convincing. In assessing the direction of the common good in this context, it should finally be observed that considerations of social justice are of less significance here because, as was previously noted, the almost total lack of provision of acupuncture from doctors and non-doctors alike made class and regional inequalities of access peripheral, notwithstanding the growing centrality of egalitarianism in the complex of values for framing judgements about the public interest in the first half of the twentieth century.

The primary reason why the stance of the medical profession on acupuncture flew in the face of the public interest as the mid-twentieth century approached, therefore, lies in the apparently adverse implications for the general welfare of the persisting – albeit rarely overtly expressed – negative response of the medical establishment to this procedure. Despite the changing socio-political context, moreover, the response of the profession to acupuncture can be little more positively interpreted in the period from the mid-twentieth century onwards, even though its position has now started to shift from outright rejection to limited incorporation.

Mid-twentieth century to the present day

In order to locate the relationship between medical policy on acupuncture and the public interest in its appropriate frame of reference from the 1950s onwards, it needs to be emphasized that egalitarian, rather than libertarian, values continue to be given greater weight in modern Britain as compared to earlier times, alongside considerations of the general welfare. This is epitomized by the further development of the NHS – not only in the immediate postwar period, but also in more recent years (Levitt and Wall 1992). In this context, the failure of the British medical reception of acupuncture significantly to advance the public good can be highlighted through Cochrane's classic schema for assessing the outcomes of expenditure in the health sector. Cochrane (1972) argues that health spending in the modern era should be directed towards ensuring the maximum degree of effectiveness, equality and efficiency. Whilst he obscures the values on which these three yardsticks and the balance between them are centred by passing them off as neutral indicators of optimality, such criteria – situated in their relevant socio-political framework – form a useful basis for examining the public interest orientation of the medical profession towards acupuncture following the mid-twentieth century. Each of the criteria will now be considered in turn in relation to both the period of general medical rejection of acupuncture up to the early 1970s and the new phase of limited incorporation of the procedure thereafter.

In terms of effectiveness, acupuncture certainly seems to have remained a worthwhile method of treatment after the mid-twentieth century in Britain, as regards not only pain, but also a broader range of maladies. This point is accentuated, as will be recalled, by growing evidence on its safety and efficacy relative to orthodox medicine in a number of conditions – including chronic degenerative disorders and strokes which have been given high priority in such government publications as the pivotal *Report* of the Royal Commission on the NHS (1979) and *The Health of the Nation* (DoH 1992) during this time span. Acupuncture seems to be relevant too to the care of people who are disabled or terminally ill which has become a significant political priority. This is highlighted by the documented success of acupuncture in providing symptomatic relief where conventional therapies have failed, most notably when employed as an analgesic (Lewith 1982). Claims about the effectiveness of acupuncture in prevention (see, for example, Mann 1973; Mole 1992) also underline its potential importance in terms of the contemporary political agenda as illustrated by, *inter alia*, the government White Paper on *Prevention and Health*

(DHSS 1977) and the recent well-publicized campaigns of the Health Education Authority (Ham 1992).

In these circumstances, the negative response of the British medical establishment to acupuncture in the period up to the mid-1970s should be viewed as increasingly running counter to the public interest given the restrictions that this imposed on the availability of acupuncture in all its forms; the impact of rejecting such an apparently effective technique in an era in which knowledge of the method was expanding seems retrogressive in light of the mounting political stress placed on the general welfare and the less heavy emphasis given to the principle of preserving individual liberty at this time. A similar picture emerges in the period from the mid-1970s to the present day in Britain where, as has been seen, despite the slowly developing medical incorporation of the method, acupuncture has still to transcend its position as a marginal therapy – particularly as far as the broader practice of lay practitioners is concerned. As such, it is difficult for key medical institutions like the GMC and the MRC to claim to be operating in the public interest in the acupuncture arena, especially at a time when consumer demand for the method is rising and the freedom of the individual has re-emerged as a more prominent political issue (King 1987).

This interpretation of the direction of the public interest in the medical reception of acupuncture since the mid-twentieth century in Britain is reinforced when the second aspect of the framework employed by Cochrane (1972) for assessing the British health system is considered – namely, that of equality. In this respect, Cochrane argues that the health service in this country should be aiming, amongst other things, to diminish existing class and geographical inequalities, so that treatments of proven effectiveness are available to all who need them. This reflects the postwar emphasis on the value of social justice, which found powerful expression in the basic objectives of the NHS following the 1946 Act (Levitt and Wall 1992) and still carries significant weight today, notwithstanding the more divisive Conservative policies of the 1980s and early 1990s in the health arena (Ham 1992). Against this background, the largely unfavourable response of the medical establishment to acupuncture, which has now begun to shade into an incorporationist position, also seems to have undermined the public good. As has been seen, this stance ensured that from the 1950s onwards most acupuncturists – and particularly its classical lay exponents – were exclusively engaged in private practice, with all the associated consequences for class and regional inequalities of access to the technique. Although acupuncture is gradually becoming more available from orthodox practitioners in its restricted form in pockets of the public sector, contemporary British medical policy on this procedure appears to have done relatively little to enhance the disadvantaged position in health care of both the lower classes and those living in unfavoured geographical localities (Widgery 1988). Whilst such inequalities may have been more politically acceptable in the *laissez-faire* environment of much of the nineteenth century, they do not fully accord with the public interest in the latter half of the twentieth century; the central philosophy of the health service that access to the best health facilities available should depend primarily on 'real need' (Royal Commission on the NHS 1979) remains, despite the shifting climate of political values underpinning current government thinking in health and other fields (Riddell 1991).

The third criterion that Cochrane (1972) employs to evaluate the contemporary health service is that of efficiency based on the search for maximum effectiveness at minimum cost. Although widely used in the assessment of the NHS since its inception – as the early Committee of Enquiry into the Cost of the NHS (1956) highlights – this criterion has become even more pertinent in the new market-oriented structure (Ham 1990). Its application to acupuncture in Britain since the mid-twentieth century strengthens the view that the medical response to this method has run counter to the public interest in both its rejecting and its more recent incorporationist modes. Reference has already been made in this chapter to the apparent advantages of acupuncture over orthodox medicine in terms of its utility and safety in social priority areas. To these need to be added the relatively low costs of the method; as noted in Chapter 5, practitioners can be trained in its rudimentary form in a short time and the equipment required is relatively cheap when set against current spending on drugs and high technology in the NHS. In this light, the phased introduction of acupuncture into the public sector on a greater scale than hitherto in selected areas of application has for some time appeared more efficient – despite being fairly labour intensive – especially if undertaken at the expense of the orthodox therapies which are most vulnerable to challenge. Whilst not diminishing the need for more research into acupuncture, this point is sharpened by the fact that, as previously noted, the majority of the public currently believe that acupuncture and other more established alternative therapies should be more fully incorporated into the NHS. In the age of *The Patient's Charter* (DoH 1991a), which marks the resurgence of individual liberty as a key political parameter by elevating the importance of the consumer in health care, the predominant pattern of the medical reception of acupuncture again seems to have militated against the common good by unduly restricting its availability within the state sector.

This is not, of course, to say that acupuncture should be confined to the NHS; as was seen in Chapter 2, the existence of a limited private medical sector is important in liberal-democratic societies because it helps to maintain individual freedom. Nor is it suggested that the inclusion of this method in the NHS is the only way of advancing the public interest in this area. As the foregoing discussion indicates, the common good would also have been served in modern Britain by more rapidly transforming acupuncture into a staple part of mainstream medicine by, for example, increasing orthodox funding of acupuncture research, introducing the method more widely into the medical curriculum and giving it more extensive coverage in the mainstream medical journals. All this highlights the negative influence that key elements of the medical profession seem to have had on acupuncture in this country in terms of the public interest since the mid-twentieth century. This is very clear in the period of predominant medical rejection of the technique up to the mid-1970s. But it is no less so in the incorporationist phase thereafter because, whilst the medical profession has taken some positive strides in this area – for example, by enhancing the availability of acupuncture in medical practice – the forward movement involved has by no means kept pace with the imperatives suggested by, *inter alia*, the increasing depth of knowledge of, and demand for, this technique in all its guises within prevailing political parameters in the modern era.

This still leaves several specific issues unresolved as far as the nature of the current public interest is concerned – such as how much time should be devoted to acupuncture in the basic medical curriculum and what proportion of orthodox research funding should be spent on the evaluation of the technique. Such issues – whilst interesting – do not require detailed exploration here. One question, however, which is particularly significant from the viewpoint of the relationship between acupuncture and the public interest is that of which groups should be the standard-bearers for acupuncture in this country today – doctors, lay exponents of the method or a combination of the two? This question is thrown into relief by Dolby (1979) who notes three main ways by which a deviant science can come to be respected: for the ideas to be developed independently by orthodox scientists; for scientific orthodoxy to incorporate a deviant science on its own terms; or for deviant practitioners themselves to become part of orthodoxy.

In the case of acupuncture, it would clearly be in the public interest for doctors and other orthodox health personnel to be more substantially involved with the method in future, particularly given the foothold which it has now begun to establish within medical orthodoxy. As has been seen, this would at least allow acupuncture to be more extensively deployed by orthodox health practitioners at a basic level after a brief training. Greater existing medical involvement with acupuncture, moreover, would not only add legitimacy to the method and increase its availability inside and outside the NHS, but also help to ensure its safe practice from the standpoint of Western anatomy and physiology. This accentuates the gulf between the public interest and the contemporary policy of the medical establishment on acupuncture in Britain, which has not gone far enough in encouraging medical interest in the technique by, for instance, creating specific teaching posts in medical schools and investing in research in this field. What, though, is the most appropriate role for lay acupuncturists in the future in this country?

In this respect, the current right of lay acupuncturists to engage in private practice certainly seems compatible with the public interest; to deviate from this policy would not only deprive consumers in Britain of the main source of the broader-ranging traditional form of acupuncture, but also infringe individual freedom of choice which has for long been enshrined in health care in this country under the common law. Admittedly, clients may be put at risk by the seemingly very small, and decreasing, numbers of lay acupuncturists who operate without acceptable minimum levels of formal training. Yet even this risk, as will be recalled from Chapter 5, is offset by legal and other safeguards that exist against malpractice. Indeed, there is a powerful case for encouraging practitioners with appropriate education and experience from the major non-medical acupuncture organizations to become part of mainstream medicine – as both NHS practitioners and researchers – in view of the shortage of doctors with a wide knowledge of acupuncture and an ability to apply the method in both its narrow and its broader classical moulds. Their entry into the NHS would be likely to increase the overall welfare and advance the cause of social justice in a manner consistent with the public interest in modern Britain, with the costs offset as necessary by reducing state expenditure on orthodox procedures with less effective outcomes.

This raises the question, though, of how might such qualified lay acupuncturists be most usefully integrated into the health service in this country. As was seen in the last chapter, lay acupuncturists can now be contracted into the NHS by fund-holding general practitioners and other key players within the market-led state health sector. There is evidence that this is already starting to happen (Vickers 1994). However, whilst potentially helpful in the short-run, this mechanism is liable to leave such therapists in a situation in which they are operating under the authority of doctors. Although the referral principle can provide protection for consumers against the lack of clinical knowledge of lay practitioners (Eagle 1978), it may also work to their disadvantage because doctors may not always have the necessary understanding of alternative therapies to make appropriate referrals – as presently seems to happen in the parallel case of the professions supplementary to medicine (Larkin 1983). Placing such therapists in the position of limited practitioners like opticians may not resolve the situation in view of the wider applications of acupuncture and the characteristically tightly defined span of tasks associated with this category of health personnel (Turner 1987). Given too the professional interests involved, there is an argument in terms of the public interest for allowing lay acupuncturists to operate more independently in the sector – especially since, as was noted earlier, non-medical practitioners trained by the leading acupuncture organizations now generally possess a basic understanding of anatomy and physiology. The time may not yet quite be ripe for introducing such a scenario in light of current debates over the accreditation of lay acupuncturists and other alternative therapists. However, from the standpoint of the public interest, it may well represent a desirable future in the wake of the 1993 Osteopaths Act which provides for the statutory registration and self-regulation of British osteopaths, and which promises to serve as a model for the advancement of a number of the alternative therapies over the next decade (Standen 1993).

Having sketched out the nature of the public interest in relation to acupuncture in Britain in modern times, it should be added that claims about the contemporary value of a more pluralistic health system are also supported by wider international trends. A government commission in New Zealand recently decided, for instance, that chiropractors 'should, in the public interest, be accepted as partners in the . . . health care system' (Fraser 1981: 73), whilst the government in the Netherlands has begun actively to encourage a more fully integrated system of orthodox and marginal medicine (Visser 1991). These examples of pluralistic approaches to health care follow in the footsteps of Chinese health policy in which traditional practitioners, in the words of Lu Gwei-Djen and Needham,

> are working side by side with modern Western-trained physicians in full cooperation. . . . The two types of physicians have joint consultations and joint clinical examinations, and there is the possibility for patients to choose whether they will have their treatment in the traditional way, including acupuncture, or the modern way.
>
> (Gwei-Djen and Needham 1980: 3)

There are, of course, dangers in abstracting the discussion of the public interest in Britain from its socio-political moorings in view of the relativism of the concept of the common good employed here. These pitfalls, however, are countered by the fact that the trend towards pluralistic health care systems reflects the commitment of the WHO 'to promote the integration of proven valuable knowledge and skills in traditional and Western medicine' (Stanway 1986: 42). But if this supports the interpretation of the public interest in the specific case of acupuncture in modern Britain, so too does the absence of a convincing reason why the differing philosophical underpinnings of classical acupuncture and allopathic medicine should prevent the integration of this method into mainstream medicine, as discussed in Chapter 5.

Although individual medical practitioners have shown varying levels of receptivity to acupuncture in modern times, therefore, it would seem that the response of the British profession as a whole and that of the medical establishment in particular to this procedure from the mid-twentieth century onwards – despite recent shifts of position – has largely been incompatible with the public interest. To conclude this section, though, it is worth emphasizing that the definition of the common interest employed here, whilst defensible, is not universally agreed; contributors like Illich and Navarro, operating with different theoretical premises, would almost certainly dispute this account of the contemporary situation. Their divergent work will now be briefly examined in this context to highlight the essence of the central concept of the public interest applied in this case study and the rationale for employing it.

Illich (1975; 1976) holds that the medical crisis afflicting societies like Britain is due to the increasingly counterproductive clinical effects of the modern health care apparatus and the addictive dependency that it fosters, which is linked to the general problem of the overproduction of goods and services in the industrial world. Accordingly, for Illich, any attempt to expand the scope and equalize the availability of institutional medicine – in acupuncture and other fields – can only be health-denying. As Illich says of efforts to further the cause of alternative medicine as a whole in this way:

> The net effect of this kind of therapeutic pluralism might easily be more corporate medicine. Acupuncturists, Ayurveds, homeopaths, and witches can be assigned departments in a world-wide hospital for life-long patients. In a therapy-oriented society, all kinds of Aesculapians can share in the monopoly of assigning the sick role, but the more different professional cliques can exempt the sick from their normal obligations, the less people on their own define how they wish to be known and treated. Unless the disestablishment of the medical

corps leads to more access by the citizen to self-cure, it will reinforce rather than reduce sickening medicalization.

(Illich 1975: 79–80)

The public interest on this interpretation, therefore, lies in setting legally defined limits to growth in medicine and other areas of life and restoring individual autonomy and self-control – not in assimilating acupuncture, on whatever terms, into mainstream medicine.

Marxist authors like Navarro (1976; 1986) would also be sceptical about such an integrationist stance for advancing the common good as far as acupuncture in modern Britain is concerned, albeit for different reasons to Illich – who is criticized for failing to appreciate the full significance of capitalist social relations in his analysis of the contemporary health crisis (Richman 1987). The damage held to have been caused by these social relations leads such writers to suggest that health reforms based on a bourgeois individualist philosophy – as exemplified by the proposals for acupuncture advanced here which are predicated on an individualistic aetiology of disease and one-to-one consultations between client and practitioner – represent little more than ineffectual tinkering with an oppressive system. As Navarro observes,

> contrary to what Illich and others postulate, . . . the greatest potential for improving the health of our citizens is not primarily through changes in the behaviour of individuals, but primarily through changes in the patterns of control, structures, and behaviour of our economic and political system.

(Navarro 1976: 128)

Doyal (1979) concurs, using evidence on the ill-health created in capitalist societies through the physical processes of commodity production, the effects of commodity production and the nature of the commodities themselves to fuel her argument that the public interest lies in going beyond the demand for more state-organized medicine within capitalism and establishing a socialist health service within a radically different socio-economic system.

Such implied criticism of claims about the nature of the public interest sustained here, however, misses the mark primarily because it involves interpreting the common good in a manner far removed from current liberal-democratic structures and principles. Illich engages in a backward-looking association of the public interest with a return to what Horrobin (1978: 1) has described as 'some ill-defined past Utopia when things were different and better' based on a social order akin to a scaled-down and humanized version of capitalism. The Marxist interpretation of this concept, on the other hand, looks forward to a society in which capitalist social relations have been superseded by those of socialism. In both instances questions can be raised about the merits of conceiving the public interest in such a sweeping, non-incremental manner – not to mention whether the totalistic changes suggested would have the positive effects envisaged on health care (Hart 1985). But the main reason why these challenges are limited is because the visions of the common good on which they rest go beyond the purpose of the enterprise in this case study – namely, that of applying a notion of the public interest to the response of doctors to acupuncture in Britain against which their behaviour can be reasonably and usefully judged in its appropriate socio-political setting.

Whilst the analytically most productive conceptualization of the public interest for studying the medical response to acupuncture in this country in the modern era is therefore held to be focused on the complex of values underpinning the present British liberal-democratic state, it is worth stressing that the direction of the public interest in this sense varies between societies. In the United States, for instance, less emphasis would be placed on the desirability of state intervention to increase the availability of, and equality of access to, acupuncture than in Britain, given the long-standing political centrality of individualistic values in America noted earlier. In socialist countries like China and the previously constituted Soviet Union, on the other hand, as can be surmised from Chapter 2, collective action of this kind would be more strongly favoured. It should be emphasized, though, that the stance taken within socialist societies – just as in liberal democracies – can differ; lay acupuncturists with a lower degree of training, for example, would have been more likely to be employed within the state in the name of the public interest under Maoist policies in the 1960s Chinese Cultural Revolution than under Marxist-Leninist principles in the Soviet Union at this time where the perpetuation of hierarchical divisions between experts and the masses was favoured. The focus on international variations in the public interest, however, should not obscure the fact that British medical policy on acupuncture since the mid-twentieth century – just as in the previous one and a half centuries – has generally been inconsistent with the common good on the definition adopted here.

CONCLUSION

Whether the recent moves by the medical profession in this country to incorporate acupuncture are extended in a manner more consistent with the public interest in future will depend not only on the stance of the medical establishment towards acupuncturists operating within its own ranks, but also, as Inglis (1980: 199) says, 'on the willingness of the medical profession to forget its former passion for exclusivity, and to recognise the advantages of accepting the practitioners of traditional medicine as potential allies, rather than as rivals'. Despite the changing medical response to alternative medicine in recent years, it is not easy to be optimistic about this prospect – particularly as far as the higher echelons of the profession are concerned (Saks 1994). This view is reinforced by the acupuncture case study in which professional self-interests seem to have been the greatest impediment to the development of this procedure in postwar Britain.

This case study of acupuncture has not, of course, just dealt with the period from the mid-twentieth century onwards in this country, but also the years stretching back to the early nineteenth century. As such, the tension between professional interests and the common good has been shown to have been an enduring feature of the historical, as well as the contemporary, context in Britain. In this respect, the arguments presented in Part II of the book regarding the extent to which the medical profession has acted altruistically in establishing and perpetuating one of the more negative international climates of reception of acupuncture over the past two hundred years have indicated that professional self-interests have not generally been subordinated to the public interest. As was shown in Chapter 5, none of the more superficially plausible alternative explanations to that of professional self-interests appear to account for the largely unfavourable medical response to acupuncture in nineteenth- and twentieth-century Britain. But if this suggests that the vested interests of the medical profession, or at least dominant segments thereof, have had a decisive influence on events, this view was supported in Chapter 6 by evidence showing that the profession itself must assume primary responsibility for the fate of acupuncture throughout the period under consideration and that medical policies on the method have been compatible with professional self-interests. Since the medical response to acupuncture can now be seen not only to be ideologically consistent with this interpretation, but also to have contravened the public interest over the last two centuries in this country, it must be concluded that the altruistic claims of the British medical profession have not been translated into practice to any substantial degree in this sphere.

This is a significant finding in itself. But it is important not to lose sight of the central reason for engaging in this case study – namely, to illustrate the way in which the theoretical and methodological framework developed in Part I of the book for evaluating the altruism of professional groups can be empirically applied, all of a piece, to a specific issue area. This task has now been successfully accomplished in relation to acupuncture, a form of alternative medicine which has hitherto been little researched by sociologists in Britain.

Conclusion

The case study of acupuncture therefore highlights the lines along which a more rigorous examination of the degree to which professional groups pursue strategies serving their own interests at the expense of the public interest might proceed – and thus indicates how the deficiencies of existing work in the sociology of professions in Britain and the United States can be overcome in this area. Before considering the implications of the framework developed here for future research into the professions in the Anglo-American context, though, the specific relevance of this case study of alternative medicine for health policy in Britain will be briefly considered. In this respect, the most striking feature of the analysis of the medical reception of acupuncture in this country over the past two centuries is the doubt shed on the extent to which the response of the medical profession in general and its elite in particular has been characterized by altruism. This raises questions about the wisdom of leaving crucial decisions about health care in Britain under professional control. By extension, the value of professional self-regulation and monopoly in medicine in this country must also be queried, especially since the broader altruism claim has become one of the most central bases on which doctors and other professional groups justify their privileged location in the occupational structure (Dunleavy and O'Leary 1987).

Social scientists to date have taken a range of positions on this issue. One view is that the autonomy of the medical profession should be retained, but restricted to the more esoteric aspects of its work – with professional control only over scientific and/or theoretical matters in which doctors possess a special expertise. Thus Freidson (1970), for instance, believes that the public should play a greater role in devising health policy and determining the social and economic parameters of the medical task, but that the power of the medical profession should be retained in areas directly involving knowledge about the causes of illness and the procedures likely to cure, or alleviate the effects of, ill-health. This position is favoured by Freidson (1970: 371) in part because 'the profession's autonomy seems to have facilitated the improvement of scientific knowledge about disease and its treatment'. However, such improvements are by no means guaranteed, as the acupuncture case study demonstrates. Klein (1989) also notes that whilst the medical profession in Britain, as in the United States, has increasingly accepted peer group review as a means of evaluating performance in clinical areas, there are shortcomings – including the difficulties of ensuring that this becomes anything more than a voluntary educational mechanism within the profession and differentiating technical from social, economic and moral judgements.

It is not surprising, therefore, that some critics have taken a more radical posture on the question of professional autonomy in medicine, suggesting that the power of professions in such fields should be abolished. Friedman (1962), as has been seen, contends that consumer sovereignty and the market should reign supreme in health care and other fields to enable customers, not producers, to decide what will serve them best. Illich (1973: 34) has also called for the elimination of professional monopolies as part of the solution to the crisis of counterproductive growth in industrial societies – not least in medicine, where he claims that the time has arrived 'to take the syringe out of the hand of the doctor, as the pen was taken out of the hand of the scribe during the Reformation in Europe'. From such roots have come the increasingly influential contemporary advocates of consumer power who wish to curtail the restrictive practices of the professions in the market (Elston 1991). Support for the deprofessionalization of medicine has, of course, historically derived not only from the political right, but also from the political left (Parkin 1979); this is underlined by the previously documented attacks that socialist governments have made on the privileged position of professional groups like doctors – as epitomized by the progressive dissolution of independent centres of medical influence in the period up to the early 1920s in the former Soviet Union and the attempt to reduce medical mystification by encouraging mass participation in the construction and implementation of health policies in the wave of Maoist revolutionary fervour in China after the mid-1960s.

To some extent, however, the radicals have been overtaken by events given current claims – noted in the Introduction – that the deprofessionalization and proletarianization of medicine is already in process in the Anglo-American context. But such topical debates should not unduly divert the inquirer here for, as Larkin (1988) has cogently argued, whilst there may or may not have been a decline in medical dominance in the United States, Britain should be treated as a separate case, in part because of the stronger facilitative role that the state has played historically in expanding medical power in this country. Having said this, the more negative stance taken by the government in Britain on the professions over the past decade (Burrage 1992) indicates that the direction of state policy on the medical profession is not immutably set for the future. Some contributors in fact believe that the ideal course lies somewhere between that steered by the reformers' respect for professional expertise and the radicals' equally powerful irreverence for the professions. Thus Wilding claims that in medicine and other social welfare fields in Britain:

> No one would wish to see the professions totally subservient to the will and whims of the state. Equally, the autonomy to which the professions lay claim fits ill with a democratically agreed range of publicly provided and publicly financed social policies. There has to be an accommodation between the professions and the state, preserving the professions as independent critics of public policies while at the same time securing their subordination to agreed public policies and purposes.
>
> (Wilding 1982: 130–1)

This position is supported by Stacey (1992) who notes that, although there are arguments for dismantling the medical profession, the prospect of losing such a strong and independent body capable of defending the public against threats as diverse as salmonella and nuclear waste is undesirable.

The stance taken on the most appropriate means of regulating doctors in Britain will, of course, depend in some measure on the theoretical perspective of the inquirer. But, although the initial presuppositions of functionalists, neo-Weberians, Marxists and others will inevitably influence their conclusions (Saks 1985), this should not diminish the significance of empirical research in shaping policy outcomes in this field. Careful consideration is particularly needed of such issues as the circumstances under which the medical monopoly in this country has been both established and maintained, the extent to which the more esoteric, technical aspects of health care can be fruitfully debated by the public and the comparative success of differing methods of controlling doctors as a collectivity (see, for instance, Waddington 1984; Hoffman 1989; Freddi and Björkman 1989) – as well as the degree to which the British medical profession has operated altruistically in practice. This latter point brings the discussion full circle, serving as a reminder that, whilst it is important to be aware of the potential policy implications of the case study, it is premature to make firm recommendations about the future; aside from other consider-ations, the altruism of the medical profession in Britain has only been cast into doubt in one area in this book – in which the results may be atypical. Since, as indicated in Chapter 1, work on this topic by sociologists to date has largely proved inadequate, further analysis of a wider span of health issues within the theoretical and methodological framework set out in Part I of this volume should be conducted before definitive conclusions are reached about moderating the power of the medical profession in this country.

This is not to suggest that the case study of the medical reception of acupuncture in Britain is in any way peripheral for it has importantly shown that the research framework for investigating the existence of altruism in the professions can readily be operationalized. In this sense, the study has illuminated one way at least in which the self-validating positions of many of the more blinkered contributors to the sociology of professions in Britain and the United States can be transcended – by exposing claim and counterclaim in the altruism debate to systematic empirical scrutiny. Given that the theoretical and methodological tools outlined here provide a basis for filling a major lacuna in the field, it is hoped that they will be applied to a much wider terrain than that of medicine in Britain. As was seen in Chapter 3, doctors are not the only occupational group in this country to have achieved a position of exclusionary closure – so too have solicitors and barristers through their monopolies over the provision of legal services. In addition, there are a number of occupations in Britain like nursing and pharmacy which have not managed to accomplish full social closure, but which warrant research along the lines indicated because they possess some of the trappings of the classic professions (Turner 1987). Nor should the professions of medicine and law and the many other vocational groups – from accountants to architects – that have obtained occupational licensure through state legislation in the United States (Freidson 1986) be forgotten in view of the Anglo-American focus of this book. The investigation of the extent to which these groups subordinate their interests to the public interest is no less vital since, as noted earlier, the altruism claim is strongly emphasized by established and aspiring professions on both sides of the Atlantic and sociological research into this issue in the United States has been no more satisfactory than that undertaken in Britain.

The implementation of a more extensive research programme to examine the altruistic orientation of professional occupations is especi-ally important because of its broader policy relevance, given the previously discussed significance of the professional complex in the Western world in general and the Anglo-American context in particular. Such a research programme may provide crucial insights for policy makers in deciding how best to regulate professional groups as a whole. The importance of the altruism debate for public policy on the professions is underlined by the contemporary role of the state in creating and sustaining the privileged position of professions through the legislative process in Western Europe and the United States (Moran and Wood 1993), at a time when greater thought needs to be given to the most appropriate relationship between professions and society (Wilding 1982). This debate also has implications for countries outside the Western world – such as reformed Eastern bloc socialist states which now see independent professions as the key to their future (Field 1992; Heitlinger 1992).

But if the broad question of whether professional groups place greater stress on self-interests than the public interest has obvious practical as well as academic relevance, it is essential that more refined work is conducted into this area in future to inform the debate. The following questions, amongst others, could helpfully be addressed. How far are there variations in the extent to which professions engage in altruistic behaviour? Is there a significant difference between the degree to which professional and non-professional groups act altruistically? What is the relationship, if any, between the strength of the altruism claim in particular professions and professional practice? And is there a link between the emphasis placed on altruistic service by professions and the shifting socio-political milieu in which they find themselves or, indeed, their changing aspirations as professional groups? The latter question is especially compelling in light of recent sociological interest in the role of professional ethics – which are increasingly viewed not just as operational codes *per se*, but as a socially variable resource deployed in the politics of professionalization (Abbott 1983).

Whilst the consideration of such questions goes beyond the scope of this book, this should not inhibit discussion about an even more fundamental issue – namely, that of why there have been so many weaknesses to date in the Anglo-American literature on the altruism of professional groups across the range of perspectives in the sociology of professions. Drawing primarily on medical examples, Strong (1979) suggests that the main reason for misleading and distorted sociological accounts of the function and behaviour of professional occupations – including the extent to which such groups subordinate their own interests to the public interest – lies in the self-interested professional ambitions of sociologists themselves in Britain and the United States. The ensuing paradox, in which the professional self-interests of sociologists are claimed to have influenced the very subject they would study, is seen to account for the ascendance of both the 'conservative' taxonomic perspective and 'radical' neo-Weberian and Marxist approaches to the professions at differing points in time. Although Strong's assumption that sociology is a profession can be debated (Saks 1985), his intriguing argument about the self-interested double game played by sociologists in relation to the altruism debate has a significance which is worth exploring further. This exploration must, of course, begin with a more detailed elucidation of his position.

In this respect, Strong believes that the prevalence of the benevolent assumptions of taxonomic writers on the altruism of professional groups up to the 1960s – in which professional ideologies were generally taken on trust – is connected to the stake sociologists of the professions had in aligning themselves with dominant groups in Britain and the United States at this time. Although the degree to which sociology was subordinated to dominant interests is probably overstated, this interpretation follows Gouldner (1971) in seeing the compromised world views pervading sociology in this period as tied to the vested interests of sociologists in, *inter alia*, attracting research funds from more affluent sections of society and enhancing their power and prestige through professionalization. In his interest-based explanation of the recent shift of the sociology of professions in a more challenging direction through the development of neo-Weberian and Marxist perspectives on professional altruism, Strong notes that whilst sociologists in the immediate postwar era may have secured their position by allying with the powerful, they were only rewarded with a small 'piece of the action' which worked to the advantage of their professional rivals. Given that sociology had established itself academically on both sides of the Atlantic by the 1960s, he contends that the potentially greater benefits of a more critical sociological approach to the professions transformed this into the new orthodoxy. As Strong says,

> it is precisely because most forms of radical sociology have a greater imperial potential than any other type of theory that they have such great professional charm. By emphasising the social and thus political nature of those vast areas of life that are normally reified, they break down the conventional barriers which serve to exclude the professional sociologist and so make the whole of human existence our preserve.
>
> (Strong 1979: 202)

Yet although this argument helps to explain the radicalization of sociological opinion on the altruism claims of professions – and much of the blinkered thinking with which this is associated – Strong's analysis is also sufficiently sophisticated to explain the limited survival of the no less self-fulfilling taxonomic approach to the sociology of professions. In this respect, he argues that the minority appeal of the taxonomic perspective continued because of the advantages from the viewpoint of professional self-interests of a dual strategy involving alliances with both the powerful and the powerless, in which the stance of sociologists on particular professions varies according to such factors as the degree to which they have successfully penetrated the professional field in question, the extent to which this field is in crisis and the availability of a relevant body of theory and research.

The overwhelming emphasis of contemporary sociological accounts of the relationship between professional self-interests and the public interest, however, has been critical and it is here that the ultimate irony resides for, as Strong (1979: 202) points out in relation to the now dominant Anglo-American work of neo-Weberian and Marxist contributors to the professions: 'In criticizing the imperialism of other professions [such] sociologists also advance their own empire and do so under exactly the same banner as other professions – the service of humanity'. On this interpretation, therefore, it is difficult to distinguish the fast-growing band of more cynical sociologists from their subjects not just in terms of self-interests, but also in relation to the ideological rationale for their actions, as both professional groups and their sociological critics are held to be pursuing their own interests under the guise of advancing the public interest (Saks 1990).

The main reason for highlighting this apparently intensified contemporary paradox – which itself awaits more stringent examination using the frame of reference set out in this book for evaluating the altruism of professional groups – is that it has potentially significant implications for future research in this area. Admittedly, even if Strong's claims about the influence of interests on sociologists of professions are accepted, this does not make their work invalid. But, as Strong (1979: 205) observes, unless sociologists 'understand themselves and their position within society, they are unlikely fully to grasp the social role of those whom they investigate, particularly when the latter have a position which is very similar to their own'. In so far as a lack of such self-awareness is liable to perpetuate the flow of strident and less adequately researched work on the balance struck between self-interests and the public interest in the professions, it is crucial that the sociologists concerned ensure that they are conscious of their own group interests and guard against unduly restrictive thinking from the perspectives within which they operate. The theoretical and methodological framework developed in this book for investigating the extent to which the altruistic ideologies of professions are translated into practice at the macro-level in Britain and the United States, of course, provides an even more direct means of cultivating analytical and empirical rigour in this field. The use of this framework, together with a modicum of self-reflection, should therefore enable sociologists to make greater inroads into the academically important and practically relevant issue of how far professional groups follow their own interests at the expense of the public good and thereby expand existing knowledge of the nature and role of professions in society.

Appendices

APPENDIX 1: RESEARCH INTO THE RESPONSE OF THE MEDICAL PROFESSION TO ACUPUNCTURE IN BRITAIN

The relationship between medical orthodoxy and alternative medicine in general and acupuncture in particular has been relatively rarely studied by sociologists and other social scientists in either the historical or contemporary context in Britain. It is therefore more necessary than usual to set out the means employed in carrying out the research underpinning the case study of the response of the British medical profession to acupuncture in the nineteenth and twentieth centuries. The main methods used are set out below.

Library study

The research is heavily based on the analysis of primary and secondary source material drawn from a range of libraries – spanning from general medical libraries like the Clinical Sciences Library at Leicester Royal Infirmary to specialist centres such as the Wellcome Institute for the History of Medicine in London. Given the focus of this study, particular mention should be made of the fact that this included careful scrutiny of references to acupuncture appearing in mainstream British medical journals from 1800 to the present day (see Saks 1985), which centred on a detailed content analysis of items in the *British Medical Journal* and the *Lancet* from the time of their first appearance in the nineteenth century to the contemporary era (a summary of the results is given in Saks 1991b).

Interviews/correspondence

Interviews/correspondence with many relevant organizations and individuals in the health field over the period from the mid-1970s onwards have formed an integral part of the research underpinning the case study. This work can best be outlined under the following broad categories.

Acupuncture

The research has involved interviewing/corresponding with a broad range of medically and non-medically qualified acupuncturists, with different levels of training and experience. Since the aim of this part of the inquiry was primarily to gain an overview of the general pattern of developments in the acupuncture world, a significant number of respondents were prominent figures in British acupuncture – including, at the various stages when the research was carried out, the Principal of the British Academy of Western Acupuncture, the Chairman of the British Acupuncture Association, the Chairman of the Traditional Acupuncture Society, the founder and President of the Medical Acupuncture Society and a representative of the reconstituted British Medical Acupuncture Society. In addition, contact was established with the more recently formed Council for Acupuncture, which currently represents the International Register of Oriental Medicine, the Register of Traditional Chinese Medicine and the Chung San Acupuncture Society, as well as the British Acupuncture Association and the Traditional Acupuncture Society.

Alternative medicine

In order to situate the study of acupuncture within a wider perspective, discussions were also conducted with high-profile medical and non-medical representatives from a number of other fields of alternative medicine, including chiropractic, herbalism, homoeopathy, naturopathy, osteopathy and spiritual healing. Communications have also taken place with a range of generic bodies associated with unorthodox medicine such as Health for the New Age, the Institute for Complementary Medicine, the Research Council for Complementary Medicine, the Scientific and Medical Network and the Threshold Foundation Bureau.

Orthodox medicine

Apart from many informal discussions with doctors and other orthodox health personnel about acupuncture in particular and alternative medicine in general throughout the duration of the research, formal correspondence has been exchanged with a range of orthodox medical bodies on this subject, not least being the British Medical Association, the General Medical Council, the Medical Defence Union, the Medical Research Council, the Royal College of General Practitioners, the Royal College of Obstetricians and Gynaecologists, the Royal College of Physicians, the Royal College of Psychiatrists and the Royal College of Surgeons. In addition, the help of the editorial staff of the *British Medical Journal* and the *Lancet* should be acknowledged in this context.

Other organizations/individuals

The research has also involved corresponding about acupuncture with the following privately funded bodies involved in medical research: Action Research for the Crippled Child, the Arthritis and Rheumatism Council, the Asthma Research Council, the British Diabetic Association, the British Digestive Foundation, the British Heart Foundation, the Cancer Research Campaign, the Chest, Heart and Stroke Association, the Foundation for Age Research, the Imperial Cancer Research Fund, the Leukemia Research Fund, the Mental Health Foundation, the Migraine Trust, the Multiple Sclerosis Society, the Muscular Distrophy Group, the National Back Pain Association, the Smith and Nephew Foundation, the Spastics Society and the Wellcome Trust. In addition, personal communications have been received on this subject from the Association of the British Pharmaceutical Industry, the British Insurance Association, the British Union Provident Association, the Department of Health and Social Security, the Patients Association, the University Grants Committee and the Western Provident Association. Finally, gratitude should be expressed to the range of other unnamed individuals and organizations directly or indirectly associated with the research – including the practising barrister who provided legal advice on the position of acupuncture in Britain under the common law.

Since it is impossible fully to do justice to this research base without interrupting the flow of the text in the case study, unreferenced points relating to acupuncture should be assumed to be based on the work outlined above, unless otherwise indicated.

APPENDIX 2: ITEMS ON ACUPUNCTURE APPEARING IN THE *BRITISH MEDICAL JOURNAL* AND THE *LANCET*, 1820–1989

Year	BMJ*	Lancet	Combined
1820–29	–	7	7
1830–39	–	13	13
1840–49	1	–	1
1850–59	1	2	3
1860–69	–	–	–
1870–79	1	2	3
1880–89	3	1	4
1890–99	1	1	2
1900–09	–	–	–
1910–19	–	–	–
1920–29	–	–	–
1930–39	1	–	1
1940–49	2	–	2
1950–59	1	–	1
1960–69	2	–	2
1970–79	33	26	59
1980–89	28	29	57
Total	74	81	155

* The *British Medical Journal* was entitled the *Provincial Medical and Surgical Journal* up until 1857.

Reproduced from Saks (1991b) with permission from *Complementary Medical Research*.

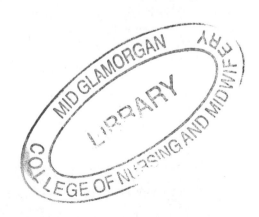

Bibliography

GENERAL SOURCES

Abbott, A. (1983) 'Professional ethics', *American Journal of Sociology* 88(5): 855–85.

—— (1988) *The System of Professions: An Essay on the Division of Expert Labour*, Chicago: University of Chicago Press.

Abbott, P. and Sapsford, R. (1990) 'Health visiting: policing the family', in Abbott, P. and Wallace, C. (eds) *The Sociology of the Caring Professions*, London: Falmer.

Abel-Smith, B. (1976) *Value for Money in Health Services*, London: Heinemann.

Aday, L., Andersen, R. and Fleming, G. (1980) *Health Care in the United States. Equitable for Whom?*, Beverly Hills: Sage.

Alaszewski, A. and Manthorpe, J. (1992) 'Restructuring the professions in the UK: the impact of internal markets on the legal, medical and social work professions', paper presented at ISA Conference on Professions in Transition, University of Leicester/De Montfort University, Leicester, 21–23 April.

Allsop, J. (1984) *Health Policy and the National Health Service*, London: Longman.

Anderson, O.W. (1989) 'Issues in the health services of the United States', in Field, M. (ed.) *Success and Crisis in National Health Systems: A Comparative Approach*, London: Routledge.

Aron, R. (1970) *Main Currents in Sociological Thought* Vols I and II, Harmondsworth: Penguin.

Arrow, K. (1973) 'The welfare economics of medical care', in Cooper, M. and Culyer, A. (eds) *Health Economics*, Harmondsworth: Penguin.

Ashmore, M., Mulkay, M. and Pinch, T. (eds) (1989) *Health and Efficiency: A Sociology of Health Economics*, Milton Keynes: Open University Press.

Ashton, J. and Seymour, H. (1988) *The New Public Health*, Buckingham: Open University Press.

Atkinson, P. and Delamont, S. (1990) 'Professions and powerlessness: female marginality in the learned professions', *Sociological Review* 38(1): 90–110.

Austoker, J. and Bryder, L. (eds) (1989) *Historical Perspectives on the Role of the MRC. Essays in the History of the Medical Research Council of the United Kingdom and Its Predecessor, the Medical Research Committee, 1913–53*, Oxford: Oxford University Press.

Bachrach, P. and Baratz, M. (1962) 'The two faces of power', *American Political Science Review* 56: 947–52.

—— (1963) 'Decisions and non-decisions: an analytical framework', *American Political Science Review* 57: 632–42.

Badhwar, N.K. (1993) 'Altruism versus self interest: sometimes a false dichotomy', *Social Philosophy and Policy* 10(1): 90–117.

Baggott, R. (1994) *Health and Health Care in Britain*, London: Macmillan.

Bakx, K. (1991) 'The "eclipse" of folk medicine in Western society', *Sociology of Health and Illness* 13(1): 20–38.

Baran, P. (1973) *The Political Economy of Growth*, Harmondsworth: Penguin.

Barber, B. (1963) 'Some problems in the sociology of professions', *Daedalus* 92(4): 669–88.

Barnes, B. (1974) *Scientific Knowledge and Sociological Theory*, London: Routledge & Kegan Paul.

Barnes, B. and Mackenzie, D. (1979) 'On the role of interests in scientific change', in Wallis, R. (ed.) *On the Margins of Science*, Sociological Review Monograph No. 27, Keele: University of Keele.

Barry, B. (1965) *Political Argument*, London: Routledge & Kegan Paul.

—— (1967a) 'The public interest', in Quinton, A. (ed.) *Political Philosophy*, London: Oxford University Press.

—— (1967b) 'Justice and the common good', in Quinton, A. (ed.) *Political Philosophy*, London: Oxford University Press.

Bartrip, P. (1990) *Mirror of Medicine: A History of the British Medical Journal*, Oxford: Oxford University Press.

Bechhofer, F. (1981) 'Substantive dogs and methodological tails: a question of fit', *Sociology* 15(4): 495–505.

Becker, H. (1962) 'The nature of a profession', in National Society for the Study of Education *Education for the Professions*, Chicago: University of Chicago Press.

Bell, D. (1974) *The Coming of Post-industrial Society: A Venture in Social Forecasting*, London: Heinemann.

Ben-David, J. (1963) 'Professions in the class system of present-day societies', *Current Sociology* 12(3): 247–98.

Benn, S. and Peters, R. (1959) *Social Principles and the Democratic State*, London: Allen & Unwin.

Bennell, P. (1983) 'The professions in Africa: a case study of the engineering profession in Kenya', *Development and Change* 14: 61–81.

Bennett, W. and Hokenstad, M. (1973) 'Full-time people workers and conceptions of the professional', in Halmos, P. (ed.) *Professionalization and Social Change*, Sociological Review Monograph No. 20, Keele: University of Keele.

Berlant, J. (1975) *Profession and Monopoly: A Study of Medicine in the United States and Great Britain*, Berkeley: University of California Press.

Berliner, H. (1985) *A System of Scientific Medicine: Philanthropic Foundations in the Flexner Era*, London: Tavistock.

Berliner, H. (1993) 'Bills, bills and buttons', *Health Service Journal* 21 October: 21.

Blaikie, N. (1974) 'Altruism in the professions: the case of the clergy', *Australian and New Zealand Journal of Sociology* 10(2): 84–9.

Blalock, H. (1968) 'Theory building and causal inferences', in Blalock, H.

and Blalock, A. (eds) *Methodology in Social Research*, New York: McGraw-Hill.

Blane, D. (1991) 'Inequality and social class', in Scambler, G. (ed.) *Sociology as Applied to Medicine*, third edition, London: Ballière Tindall.

Boadway, R. and Bruce, N. (1984) *Welfare Economics*, Oxford: Basil Blackwell.

Bodenheimer, E. (1966) 'The public interest: the present and future of the concept', in Friedrich, C. (ed.) *The Public Interest*, New York: Atherton Press.

Bodenheimer, T. (1985) 'The transnational pharmaceutical industry and the health of the world's people', in McKinlay, J. (ed.) *Issues in the Political Economy of Health Care*, London: Tavistock.

Bossert, T. (1984) 'Health policy making in a revolutionary context: Nicaragua 1979–81', in Black, N., Boswell, D., Gray, A., Murphy, S. and Popay, J. (eds) *Health and Disease: A Reader*, Milton Keynes: Open University Press.

Bottomore, T. (1965) *Classes in Modern Society*, London: Allen & Unwin.

Bouchayer, F. (1991) 'Alternative medicines: a general approach to the French situation', in Lewith, G. and Aldridge, D. (eds) *Complementary Medicine and the European Community*, Saffron Walden: C. W. Daniel.

Bowers, J. (1974) 'Imperialism and medical education in China', *Bulletin of the History of Medicine* 48(4): 449–64.

—— (1978) 'Reception of acupuncture by the scientific community: from scorn to a degree of interest', *Comparative Medicine East and West* 6(2): 89–96.

Bowles, N. (1993) *The Government and Politics of the United States*, London: Macmillan.

Bradshaw, A. (1976) 'A critique of Steven Lukes' "Power: A Radical View"', *Sociology* 10(1): 121–7.

Brake, M. and Bailey, R. (eds) (1980) *Radical Social Work and Practice*, London: Edward Arnold.

Braverman, H. (1974) *Labor and Monopoly Capital: The Degradation of Work in the Twentieth Century*, New York: Monthly Review Press.

Braybrooke, D. (1966) 'The public interest: the present and future of the concept', in Friedrich, C. (ed.) *The Public Interest*, New York: Atherton Press.

Breckon, W. (1972) *The Drug Makers*, London: Eyre Methuen.

Brelet, C., Forbes, A., Velimirovic, H. and Velimirovic, B. (1983) 'The European region', in Bannerman, R., Burton, J. and Wen-Chieh, C. (eds) *Traditional Medicine and Health Care Coverage*, Geneva: World Health Organization.

Brown, C. (1973) 'The division of laborers: allied health professions', *International Journal of Health Services* 3(3): 435–44.

Brown, P. (1985) 'The vicissitudes of herbalism in late nineteenth and early twentieth century Britain', *Medical History* 29: 71–92.

Burrage, M. (1990) 'Introduction: the professions in sociology and history', in Burrage, M. and Torstendahl, R. (eds) *Professions in Theory and History: Rethinking the Study of the Professions*, London: Sage.

—— (1992) 'Mrs Thatcher versus the professions: ideology, impact and ironies of an eleven year confrontation', Working Paper, University of California: Institute of Governmental Studies.

Burrow, J.G. (1963) *AMA: Voice of American Medicine*, Baltimore: Johns Hopkins Press

Butler, J. and Vaile, M. (1984) *Health and Health Services: An Introduction to Health Care in Britain*, London: Routledge & Kegan Paul.

Butler, J., Bevan, J. and Taylor, R. (1973) *Family Doctors and Public Policy*, London: Routledge & Kegan Paul.

Butler, T. (1990) 'Care out of control', *The Health Service Journal* 23 August: 1250–1.

Bynum, W. and Porter, R. (1987) 'Introduction', in Bynum, W. and Porter, R. (eds) *Medical Fringe and Medical Orthodoxy 1750–1850*, London: Croom Helm.

Calnan, M. (1987) *Health and Illness: The Lay Perspective*, London: Tavistock.

Camp, J. (1973) *Magic, Myth and Medicine*, London: Priory Press.

Camp, V. (1986) 'Acupuncture in the NHS', *Acupuncture in Medicine* 3(1): 4–5.

Campbell, A.V. (1975) *Moral Dilemmas in Medicine*, second edition, Edinburgh: Churchill Livingstone.

—— (1978) *Medicine, Health and Justice: The Problem of Priorities*, Edinburgh: Churchill Livingstone.

Cannan, C. (1972) 'Social workers: training and professionalism', in Pateman, T. (ed.) *Counter Course*, Harmondsworth: Penguin.

Cant, S. and Calnan, M. (1991) 'On the margins of the medical marketplace? An exploratory study of alternative practitioners' perceptions', *Sociology of Health and Illness* 13(1): 39–57.

Carchedi, G. (1975) 'On the economic identification of the new middle class', *Economy and Society* 4(1): 1–86.

Carr-Saunders, A. and Wilson, P. (1933) *The Professions*, Oxford: Clarendon Press.

Cassedy, J. (1974) 'Early uses of acupuncture in the United States, with an Addendum (1826) by Franklin Bache, MD', *Bulletin of New York Academy of Medicine* 50(8): 892–906.

Castells, M. (1978) *City, Class and Power*, London: Macmillan.

Chalmers, A. (1982) *What Is This Thing Called Science? An Assessment of the Nature and Status of Science and Its Methods*, second edition, Milton Keynes: Open University Press.

Chandra, J. and Kakabadse, A. (1985) *Privatisation and the National Health Service*, Aldershot: Gower.

Charles, N. (1993) *Gender Divisions and Social Change*, Hemel Hempstead: Harvester Wheatsheaf.

Child, J. and Fulk, J. (1982) 'Maintenance of occupational control: the case of professions', *Sociology of Work and Occupations* 9(2): 155–92.

Chossudovsky, M. (1986) *Towards Capitalist Restoration? Chinese Socialism after Mao*, Macmillan: London.

Chow, E. (1985) 'Traditional Chinese medicine: a holistic system', in Salmon, J.W. (ed.) *Alternative Medicines: Popular and Policy Perspectives*, London: Tavistock.

Cochrane, A. (1972) *Effectiveness and Efficiency: Random Reflections on the Health Services*, Nuffield Provincial Hospitals Trust.

Cockburn, A. (1993) 'Clinton's health plan', *New Statesman and Society*, 10 October.

Cockburn, C. (1977) *The Local State: Management of Cities and People*, London: Pluto Press.

Cohen, J. (1966) 'A lawman's view of the public interest', in Friedrich, C. (ed.) *The Public Interest*, New York: Atherton Press.

Cohen, P. (1968) *Modern Social Theory*, London: Heinemann.

Collier, J. (1989) *The Health Conspiracy*, London: Century.

Collins, H. and Pinch, T. (1979) 'The construction of the paranormal: nothing unscientific is happening', in Wallis, R. (ed.) *On the Margins of Science*, Sociological Review Monograph No. 27, Keele: University of Keele.

Collins, R. (1990a) 'Changing conceptions in the sociology of the professions', in Torstendahl, R. and Burrage, M. (eds) *The Formation of Professions: Knowledge, State and Strategy*, London: Sage.

—— (1990b) 'Market closure and the conflict theory of the professions', in Burrage, M. and Torstendahl, R. (eds) *Professions in Theory and History: Rethinking the Study of the Professions*, London: Sage.

Colm, G. (1966) 'The public interest: essential key to public policy', in Friedrich, C. (ed.) *The Public Interest*, New York: Atherton Press.

Colombotos, J. (1969) 'Physicians and medicare: a before-after study of the effect of legislation on attitudes', *American Sociological Review* 34: 318–34.

Consumers Association (1972) 'Acupuncture', *Which?* February: 49–51.

—— (1981) 'Alternative medicine', *Which?* August: 473–7.

—— (1986) 'Magic or medicine?', *Which?* October: 443–7.

Cooter, R. (1987) 'Bones of contention? Orthodox medicine and the mystery of the bone-setter's craft', in Bynum, W.F. and Porter, R. (eds) *Medical Fringe and Medical Orthodoxy 1750–1850*, London: Croom Helm.

—— (1988) 'Introduction: the alternations of past and present', in Cooter, R. (ed.) *Studies in the History of Alternative Medicine*, London: Macmillan.

Coulter, H.L. (1985) 'Homoeopathy', in Salmon, J.W. (ed.) *Alternative Medicines: Popular and Policy Perspectives*, London: Tavistock.

Coward, R. (1989) *The Whole Truth: The Myth of Alternative Medicine*, London: Faber & Faber.

Cox, D. (1991) 'Health service management – a sociological view: Griffiths and the non-negotiated order of the hospital', in Gabe, J., Calnan, M. and Bury, M. (eds) *The Sociology of the Health Service*, London: Routledge.

Crenson, M. (1971) *The Un-politics of Air Pollution*, Baltimore: Johns Hopkins Press.

Crompton, R. (1990) 'Professions in the current context', *Work, Employment and Society*, Special Issue: The 1980s: A Decade of Change?

Cuff, E.C., Sharrock, W.W. and Francis, D.W. (1990) *Perspectives in Sociology*, third edition, London: Unwin Hyman.

Culyer, A. (1975) 'The social cost of doctors' discretion', *New Society* 27 February.

Currer, C. and Stacey, M. (eds) (1986) *Concepts of Health, Illness and Disease: A Comparative Perspective*, Leamington Spa: Berg.

Dahl, R. (1961) *Who Governs?*, New Haven: Yale University Press.

—— (1973) 'A critique of the ruling elite model', in Urry, J. and Wakeford, J. (eds) *Power in Britain*, London: Heinemann.

Dahrendorf, R. (1959) *Class and Class Conflict in Industrial Society*, London: Routledge & Kegan Paul.

Daniels, A. (1975) 'Professionalism in formal organizations', in McKinlay, J.

(ed.) *Processing People: Cases in Organizational Behaviour*, London: Holt, Rinehart & Winston.

Daniels, N. (1984) *Just Health Care*, Cambridge: Cambridge University Press.

Davies, P. (1984) *Report on Trends in Complementary Medicine*, London: Institute for Complementary Medicine.

Davis, C. (1989) 'The Soviet health system: a National Health Service in a socialist society', in Field, M. (ed.) *Success and Crisis in National Health Systems: A Comparative Approach*, London: Routledge.

Davis, D. (1975) 'The history and sociology of the scientific study of acupuncture', *American Journal of Chinese Medicine* 3(1): 5–26.

Davis, H. and Scase, R. (1985) *Western Capitalism and State Socialism: An Introduction*, Oxford: Basil Blackwell.

De Santis, G. (1980) 'Medical work: accommodating a body of knowledge to practice', *Sociology of Health and Illness* 2(2): 133–50.

De Swaan, A. (1990) *In Care of the State*, Cambridge: Polity Press.

Deacon, B. (1992) 'The future of social policy in Eastern Europe', in Deacon, B., Castle-Kanerova, M., Manning, N., Millard, F., Orosz, E., Szalai, J. and Vidinova, A. (eds) *The New Eastern Europe*, London: Sage.

Dearlove, J. and Saunders, P. (1984) *Introduction to British Politics*, Cambridge: Polity Press.

Dingwall, R. and Fenn, P. (1987) '"A respectable profession"? Sociological and economic perspectives on the regulation of professional services', *International Review of Law and Economics* 7: 51–64.

Dolby, R. (1979) 'Reflections on deviant science', in Wallis, R. (ed.) *On the Margins of Science*, Sociological Review Monograph No. 27, Keele: University of Keele.

Donabedian, A. (1973) *Aspects of Medical Care Administration: Specifying Requirements for Health Care*, Cambridge: Harvard University Press.

Doyal, L. (1979) *The Political Economy of Health*, London: Pluto Press.

—— (1985) 'Women and the National Health Service: the carers and the careless', in Lewin, E. and Olesen, V. (eds) *Women, Health and Healing: Toward a New Perspective*, London: Tavistock.

Drake, D. (1972) 'The debate continues: Americans are intrigued', in Editors of Enterprise Scientific News (eds) *Acupuncture: What Can It Do for You?*, UPD Special Edition.

Dryberg, T. B. (1992) 'The politics of the individual and public interests', Essex Papers in Politics and Government No. 91, University of Essex: Department of Government.

Dubos, R. (1968) *Man, Medicine and Environment*, London: Pall Mall Press.

Duin, N. and Sutcliffe, J. (1992) *A History of Medicine: From Prehistory to the Year 2020*, London: Simon & Schuster.

Duke, M. (1972) *Acupuncture: The Chinese Art of Healing*, New York: Pyramid House.

Duman, D. (1979) 'The creation and diffusion of a professional ideology in nineteenth century England', *Sociological Review* 27(1): 113–38.

Duncan, S. (1974) 'The isolation of scientific discovery: indifference and resistance to a new idea', *Science Studies* 4: 109–34.

Dunleavy, P. and O'Leary, B. (1987) *Theories of the State: The Politics of Liberal Democracy*, London: Macmillan.

Durkheim, E. (1938) *The Rules of Sociological Method*, New York: Free Press.

—— (1952) *Suicide: A Study in Sociology*, London: Routledge & Kegan Paul.
—— (1964) *The Division of Labour in Society*, New York: Free Press.
—— (1992) *Professional Ethics and Civic Morals*, London: Routledge.
Dworkin, R. (1975) 'The original position', in Daniels, N. (ed.) *Reading Rawls*, Oxford: Basil Blackwell.
Eagle, R. (1978) *Alternative Medicine*, London: Futura.
Eckstein, H. (1960) *Pressure Group Politics: The Case of the British Medical Association*, London: Allen & Unwin.
Editors of the Yale Law Journal (1966) 'The American Medical Association: power, purpose and politics in organized medicine', in Scott, W. and Volkart, E. (eds) *Medical Care*, New York: John Wiley & Sons.
Ehrenreich, B. and Ehrenreich, J. (1979) 'The professional-managerial class', in Walker, P. (ed.) *Between Capital and Labour*, Brighton: Harvester Press.
Eisenberg, D.M., Kessler, R.C., Foster, C., Norlock, F.E., Calkins, D.R. and Delbanco, T.L. (1993) 'Unconventional medicine in the United States: prevalence, cost and patterns of use', *New England Journal of Medicine* 328(4): 246–52.
Elliott, P. (1972) *The Sociology of Professions*, London: Macmillan.
Elston, M.A. (1991) 'The politics of professional power: medicine in a changing health service', in Gabe, J., Calnan, M. and Bury, M. (eds) *The Sociology of the Health Service*, London: Routledge.
Enthoven, A. (1984) 'Reforming US health care: the consumer choice health plan', in Black, N., Boswell, D., Gray, A., Murphy, S. and Popay, J. (eds) *Health and Disease: A Reader*, Milton Keynes: Open University Press.
Esland, G. (1980a) 'Diagnosis and therapy', in Esland, G. and Salaman, G. (eds) *The Politics of Work and Occupations*, Milton Keynes: Open University Press.
—— (1980b) 'Professions and professionalism', in Esland, G. and Salaman, G. (eds) *The Politics of Work and Occupations*, Milton Keynes: Open University Press.
Evan, W. (1969) 'The engineering profession: a cross-cultural analysis', in Perrucci, R. and Gerstl, J. (eds) *The Engineers and the Social System*, New York: John Wiley & Sons.
Ewart, C. (1972) *The Healing Needles: The Story of Acupuncture and Its Pioneer Practitioner, Dr Louis Moss*, London: Elm Tree Books.
Fairfoot, P. (1987) 'Alternative therapies: the BMA knows best?', *Journal of Social Policy* 16(3): 383–90.
Feyerabend, P. (1975) *Against Method: Outline of an Anarchistic Theory of Knowledge*, London: New Left Books.
Field, M. (1957) *Doctor and Patient in Soviet Russia*, Cambridge: Harvard University Press.
—— (1967) *Soviet Socialized Medicine: An Introduction*, New York: Free Press.
—— (1992) 'The Soviet medical profession: impact of perestroika', paper presented at ISA Conference on Professions in Transition, University of Leicester/De Montfort University, Leicester, 21–23 April.
Fielding, S. (1984) 'Organizational impact on medicine: the HMO concept', *Social Science and Medicine* 18(8): 615–20.
Finer, S. (1974) *Comparative Government*, Harmondsworth: Penguin.
Fisher, M. (1973) 'The use of acupuncture as an alternative medicine', MA dissertation, The American University, Washington.

Fisk, M. (1975) 'History and reason in Rawls' moral theory', in Daniels, N. (ed.) *Reading Rawls*, Oxford: Basil Blackwell.

Flexner, A. (1915) 'Is social work a profession?', *Proceedings of the National Conference of Charities and Correction* 62: 576–90.

Forsyth, G. (1966) *Doctors and State Medicine: A Study of the British Health Service*, London: Pitman Medical.

Frankel, J. (1970) *National Interest*, London: Pall Mall.

Franklin, D. (1992) 'Medical practitioners' attitudes to complementary medicine', *Complementary Medical Research* 6(2): 69–71.

Fraser, J. (1981) *The Medicine Men: A Guide to Natural Medicine*, London: Methuen.

Freddi, G. and Björkman, J. (eds) (1989) *Controlling Medical Professionals: The Comparative Politics of Health Governance*, London: Sage.

Freidson, E. (1970) *Profession of Medicine: A Study in the Sociology of Applied Knowledge*, New York: Dodd, Mead & Co.

—— (1973) 'Professions and the occupational principle', in Freidson, E. (ed.) *The Professions and Their Prospects*, Beverly Hills: Sage.

—— (1983) 'The theory of professions: state of the art', in Dingwall, R. and Lewis, P. (eds) *The Sociology of Professions*, London: Macmillan.

—— (1986) *Professional Powers: A Study of the Institutionalization of Formal Knowledge*, Chicago: University of Chicago Press.

Friedman, M. (1962) *Capitalism and Freedom*, Chicago: University of Chicago Press.

Friedrich, C. (ed.) (1966) *The Public Interest*, New York: Atherton Press.

Fry, J. (1969) *Medicine in Three Societies: A Comparison of Medical Care in the USSR, USA and UK*, Aylesbury: MTP.

Fulder, S. (1988) *The Handbook of Complementary Medicine*, second edition, Oxford: Oxford University Press.

—— (1991) *How To Be a Healthy Patient: A Holistic Guide to Medical Treatment*, London: Hodder & Stoughton.

Fulder, S. and Monro, R. (1981) *The Status of Complementary Medicine in the United Kingdom*, London: Threshold Foundation.

Furtak, R. (1986) *The Political Systems of the Socialist States: An Introduction to Marxist-Leninist Regimes*, Brighton: Wheatsheaf.

George, V. and Wilding, P. (1985) *Ideology and Social Welfare*, revised edition, London: Routledge & Kegan Paul.

Giddens, A. (1978) *Durkheim*, Glasgow: Fontana.

—— (1981) *The Class Structure of the Advanced Societies*, second edition, London: Hutchinson.

Gilb, C. (1966) *Hidden Hierarchies: The Professions and Government*, New York: Harper & Row.

Gill, D. (1975) 'The British National Health Service: professional determinants of administrative structure', in Cox, C. and Mead, A. (eds) *A Sociology of Medical Practice*, London: Collier-Macmillan.

Goldthorpe, J. (1982) 'On the service class, its formation and future', in Giddens, A. and Mackenzie, G. (eds) *Social Class and the Division of Labour*, Cambridge: Cambridge University Press.

Goode, W. (1960) 'Encroachment, charlatanism and the emerging profession: psychology, sociology and medicine', *American Sociological Review* 25: 902–14.

Gould, C. (1981) 'Socialism and democracy', *Praxis International* 1(1): 49–63.

Gould, D. (1985) *The Medical Mafia*, London: Sphere.

Gouldner, A. (1971) *The Coming Crisis of Western Sociology*, London: Heinemann.

Greenfield, L. (1992) *Nationalism: Five Routes to Modernity*, Cambridge: Harvard University Press.

Greenwood, E. (1957) 'Attributes of a profession', *Social Work* 2(3): 45–55.

Gregory, P. (1990) 'The Stalinist command economy', *Annals of the American Academy of Political and Social Science* 507: 18–25.

Griffith, B., Iliffe, S. and Rayner, G. (1987) *Banking on Sickness: Commercial Medicine in Britain and the USA*, London: Lawrence & Wishart.

Griffith, J. (1985) *The Politics of the Judiciary*, third edition, London: Fontana.

Gross, E. (1969) 'Change in technological and scientific developments and its impact on occupational structure', in Perrucci, R. and Gerstl, J. (eds) *The Engineers and the Social System*, New York: John Wiley & Sons.

Habermas, J. (1976) *Legitimation Crisis*, London: Heinemann.

Hage, J. and Meeker, B.F. (1988) *Social Causality*, Boston: Unwin Hyman.

Hague, R. and Harrop, M. (1987) *Comparative Government: An Introduction*, second edition, London: Macmillan.

Haller, J. (1973) 'Acupuncture in nineteenth century Western medicine', *New York State Journal of Medicine* 73: 1213–21.

Halmos, P. (1970) *The Personal Service Society*, London: Constable.

—— (1973) 'Introduction', in Halmos, P. (ed.) *Professionalization and Social Change*, Sociological Review Monograph No. 20, Keele: University of Keele.

Halpern, S. (1985) 'What the public thinks of the NHS', *Health and Social Services Journal* 6 June.

Ham, C. (1990) *The New National Health Service: Organization and Management*, Oxford: Radcliffe Medical Press.

—— (1992) *Health Policy in Britain: The Politics and Organisation of the National Health Service*, third edition, London: Macmillan.

Hane, M. (1992) *Modern Japan: A Historical Survey*, second edition, Oxford: Westview Press.

Harris, N. (1989) *Professional Codes of Conduct in the United Kingdom: A Directory*, London: Mansell.

Harrison, S., Hunter, D. and Pollitt, C. (1990) *The Dynamics of British Health Policy*, London: Unwin Hyman.

Hart, N. (1985) *The Sociology of Health and Medicine*, Ormskirk: Causeway Press.

Haug, M. (1973) 'Deprofessionalization: an alternative hypothesis for the future', in Halmos, P. (ed.) *Professionalization and Social Change*, Sociological Review Monograph No. 20, Keele: University of Keele.

Heitlinger, A. (1992) 'The medical profession in Czechoslovakia: legacies of state socialism, prospects for the capitalist future', paper presented at ISA Conference on Professions in Transition, University of Leicester/De Montfort University, Leicester, 21–23 April.

Held, V. (1970) *The Public Interest and Individual Interests*, New York: Basic Books.

Helman, C. (1990) *Culture, Health and Illness: An Introduction for Health Professionals*, second edition, London: Butterworth-Heinemann.

Hemminki, E. (1982) 'Problems of clinical trials as evidence of therapeutic effectiveness', *Social Science and Medicine* 16: 711–12.

Heywood, A. (1992) *Political Ideologies: An Introduction*, London: Macmillan.

Hickson, D. and Thomas, M. (1969) 'Professionalization in Britain: a preliminary measurement', *Sociology* 3(1): 37–53.

Higgins, J. (1988) *The Business of Medicine: Private Health Care in Britain*, London: Macmillan.

Hill, M. and Bramley, G. (1986) *Analysing Social Policy*, Oxford: Basil Blackwell.

Hillier, S. (1988) 'Health and medicine in the 1980s', in Benewick, R. and Wingrove, P. (eds) *Reforming the Revolution: China in Transition*, London: Macmillan.

Hillier, S. and Jewell, J. (1983) 'Chinese traditional medicine and modern Western medicine: integration and separation in China', in Hillier, S. and Jewell, J. (eds) *Health Care and Traditional Medicine in China 1800–1982*, London: Routledge & Kegan Paul.

Hillman, D. and Christianson, J. (1985) 'Health care expenditure containment in the United States: strategies at the state and local level', *Social Science and Medicine* 20(12): 1319–30.

Hoffman, L. (1989) *The Politics of Knowledge: Activist Movements in Medicine and Planning*, New York: SUNY.

Holloway, S. (1964) 'Medical education in England 1830–1858: a sociological analysis', *History* 49: 299–324.

Horn, J. (1971) *Away With all Pests: An English Surgeon in People's China 1954–1969*, New York: Monthly Review Press.

Horrobin, D. (1978) *Medical Hubris: A Reply to Ivan Illich*, Edinburgh: Churchill Livingstone.

Hu, T. (1984) 'Health services in the People's Republic of China', in Raffle, M. (ed.) *Comparative Health Systems*, University Park: Pennsylvania State University Press.

Huard, P. and Wong, M. (1962) 'Present-day trends in acupuncture', *World Medical Journal* September: 335–6.

—— (1968) *Chinese Medicine*, London: Weidenfeld & Nicholson.

Huggon, T. and Trench, A. (1992) 'Brussels post-1992: protector or persecutor?', in Saks, M. (ed.) *Alternative Medicine in Britain*, London: Routledge.

Hughes, E. (1951) 'Work and the self', in Rohrer, J. and Sherif, M. (eds) *Social Psychology at the Crossroads*, New York: Harper & Row.

—— (1963) 'Professions', *Daedalus* 92(4): 655–68.

Humphrey, M. (1989) *Back Pain*, London: Routledge.

Hyman, R. (1984) *Strikes*, third edition, London: Fontana.

Illich, I. (1973) 'The professions as a form of imperialism', *New Society* 13 September.

—— (1975) *Medical Nemesis: The Expropriation of Health*, London: Calder & Boyars.

—— (1976) *Limits to Medicine*, Harmondsworth: Penguin.

Inglis, B. (1964) *Fringe Medicine*, London: Faber & Faber.

—— (1980) *Natural Medicine*, Glasgow: Fontana.

Inkster, I. (1977) 'Marginal men: aspects of the social role of the medical community in Sheffield 1790–1850', in Woodward, J. and Richards, D. (eds)

Health Care and Popular Medicine in Nineteenth Century England, London: Croom Helm.

Jameson, E. (1961) *The Natural History of Quackery*, London: Michael Joseph.

Jamous, H. and Peloille, B. (1970) 'Professions or self-perpetuating systems? Changes in the French university-hospital system', in Jackson, J. (ed.) *Professions and Professionalization*, Cambridge: Cambridge University Press.

Jewson, N. (1974) 'Medical knowledge and the patronage system in eighteenth century England', *Sociology* 8(3): 369–85.

—— (1976) 'The disappearance of the sick-man from medical cosmology 1770–1870', *Sociology* 10(2): 225–44.

Johnson, T. (1972) *Professions and Power*, London: Macmillan.

—— (1977) 'The professions in the class structure', in Scase, R. (ed.) *Industrial Society: Class, Cleavage and Control*, London: Allen & Unwin.

—— (1980) 'Work and power', in Esland, G. and Salaman, G. (eds) *The Politics of Work and Occupations*, Milton Keynes: Open University Press.

Jones, P. (1981) *Doctors and the BMA: A Case Study in Collective Action*, Farnborough: Gower.

Kaiser, R. (1977) *Russia: The People and the Power*, Harmondsworth: Penguin.

Kao, F. (1973) 'China, Chinese medicine and the Chinese medical system', *American Journal of Chinese Medicine* 1(1): 1–59.

King, D. (1987) *The New Right: Politics, Markets and Citizenship*, London: Macmillan.

Klegon, D. (1978) 'The sociology of professions: an emerging perspective', *Sociology of Work and Occupations* 5(3): 259–83.

Klein, R. (1973) *Complaints Against Doctors: A Study in Professional Accountability*, London: C. Knight.

—— (1975) 'Private practice', *New Society* 23 October.

—— (1989) *The Politics of the National Health Service*, second edition, London: Longman.

Krause, E. (1971) *The Sociology of Occupations*, Boston: Little, Brown & Co.

—— (1992) 'Capitalism, state action and the collapse of professional power', paper presented at ISA Conference on Professions in Transition, University of Leicester/De Montfort University, Leicester, 21–23 April.

Kuhn, T. (1970) *The Structure of Scientific Revolutions*, second edition, Chicago: University of Chicago Press.

Kumar, K. (1978) *Prophecy and Progress: The Sociology of Industrial and Post-industrial Society*, Harmondsworth: Penguin.

Kun, K. (1983) 'The Western Pacific region', in Bannerman, R., Burton, J. and Wen-Chieh, C. (eds) *Traditional Medicine and Health Care Coverage*, Geneva: World Health Organization.

Lane, D. (1982) *The End of Social Inequality? Class, Status and Power Under State Socialism*, London: Allen & Unwin.

—— (1985) *State and Politics in the USSR*, Oxford: Basil Blackwell.

Lane, J. and Ersson, S.O. (1991) *Politics and Society in Western Europe*, second edition, London: Sage.

Langan, M. and Lee, P. (1989) 'Whatever happened to radical social work', in Langan, M. and Lee, P. (eds) *Radical Social Work Today*, London: Unwin Hyman.

Langford, M. (1992) 'BCMA – the way forward?', *Journal of Alternative and Complementary Medicine* 10(9): 14.

Larkin, G. (1978) 'Medical dominance and control: radiographers in the division of labour', *Sociological Review* 26(4): 843–58.

—— (1983) *Occupational Monopoly and Modern Medicine*, London: Tavistock.

—— (1988) 'Medical dominance in Britain: image and historical reality', *The Milbank Quarterly* 66 (supp. 2): 117–32.

—— (1992) 'Orthodox and osteopathic medicine in the inter-war years', in Saks, M. (ed.) *Alternative Medicine in Britain*, Oxford: Clarendon Press.

Larner, C. (1992) 'Healing in pre-industrial Britain', in Saks, M. (ed.) *Alternative Medicine in Britain*, Oxford: Clarendon Press.

Latourette, K. (1975) *A History of Christianity* Vols I and II, London: Harper & Row.

Lear, P. (1989) 'Caring for the 1990s in the USSR', *Health Services Management* August: 164–8.

Lee, D. and Newby, H. (1983) *The Problem of Sociology*, London: Hutchinson.

Lee, J. (1976) 'Social change and marginal therapeutic systems', in Wallis, R. and Morley, P. (eds) *Marginal Medicine*, London: Peter Owen.

Lees, D. (1965) 'Health through choice. An economic study of the British National Health Service', in Harris, R. (ed.) *Freedom or Free-for-all? Essays in Welfare, Trade and Choice*, London: Institute of Economic Affairs.

Leeson, J. and Gray, J. (1978) *Women and Medicine*, London: Tavistock.

Levitt, R. and Wall, A. (1992) *The Reorganized National Health Service*, fourth edition, London: Chapman & Hall.

Light, D. (1990) 'Learning from their mistakes', *Health Service Journal* 4 October: 1470–2.

Lindsay, C. (1973) 'Medical care and equality', in Cooper, M. and Culyer, A. (eds) *Health Economics*, Harmondsworth: Penguin.

Linton, R. (1936) *The Study of Man*, New York: Appleton-Century.

Lloyd, W. (1971) *A Hundred Years of Medicine*, London: Duckworth.

Locke, R. (1972) 'The history of acupuncture and its relation to dentistry', *Bulletin of the History of Dentistry* 20: 66–75.

Lonsdale, S. (1991) 'Sharp practice pricks reputation of acupuncture', *Observer* 15 December.

Lorber, J. (1984) *Women Physicians*, London: Tavistock.

Lu Gwei-Djen and Needham, J. (1980) *Celestial Lancets: A History and Rationale of Acupuncture and Moxa*, Cambridge: Cambridge University Press.

Luh, C. and Wilson, D. (1978) 'Acupuncture: politics and medicine', *Bulletin of Concerned Asian Scholars* 10(1): 67–72.

Lukes, S. (1974) *Power: A Radical View*, London: Macmillan.

—— (1985) *Marxism and Morality*, Oxford: Oxford University Press.

McCauley, M. (1986) 'Introduction', in McCauley, M. (ed.) *The Soviet Union Under Gorbachev*, London: Macmillan.

McCreadie, C. (1978) 'Rawlsian justice and the financing of the National Health Service', *Journal of Social Policy* 5(2): 113–31.

MacDonald, K. (1985) 'Social closure and occupational registration', *Sociology* 19(4): 541–56.

MacEoin, D. (1990) 'The myth of clinical trials', *Journal of Alternative and Complementary Medicine* 8(8): 15–18.

Macfarlane, A. (1990) 'Official statistics and women's health and illness', in Roberts, H. (ed.) *Women's Health Counts*, London: Routledge.

McGuire, A., Henderson, J. and Mooney, G. (1988) *The Economics of Health Care: An Introductory Text*, London: Routledge & Kegan Paul.

MacIver, R. (1964) *Social Causation*, New York: Harper & Row.

McKay, D. (1985) 'Domestic policy and the Reagan administration', in Robins, L. (ed.) *The American Way: Government and Politics in the United States*, London: Longman.

McKeown, T. (1979) *The Role of Medicine: Dream, Mirage or Nemesis?*, Oxford: Basil Blackwell.

—— (1984) 'The medical contribution', in Black, N., Boswell, D., Gray, A., Murphy, S. and Popay, J. (eds) *Health and Disease: A Reader*, Milton Keynes: Open University Press.

McKinlay, J. (1977) 'The business of good doctoring or doctoring as good business: reflections on Freidson's view of the medical game', *International Journal of Health Services* 7(3): 459–83.

McKinlay, J. and Arches, J. (1985) 'Towards the proletarianization of physicians', *International Journal of Health Services* 15(2): 161–95.

McKinlay, J. and Stoeckle, J. (1988) 'Corporatization and the transformation of doctoring', *International Journal of Health Services* 18(2): 191–205.

MacLaren, A. (1976) 'The development of medical knowledge and institutions under nineteenth century industrialism', paper presented at the BSA Annual Conference on Sociology, Health and Illness, University of Manchester, 6–9 April.

Mancall, M. (1984) *China at the Center: 300 Years of Foreign Policy*, New York: Free Press.

Mann, M. (1982) 'The social cohesion of liberal democracy', in Giddens, A. (ed.) *Classes, Power and Conflict: Classical and Contemporary Debates*, London: Macmillan.

Marcuse, H. (1991) *One-Dimensional Man*, second edition, London: Routledge.

Marks, F., Leswing, K. and Fortinsky, B. (1972) *The Lawyers, the Public and Professional Responsibility*, Chicago: American Bar Foundation.

Marshall, T. (1963a) 'Citizenship and social class', in Marshall, T. *Sociology at the Crossroads and Other Essays*, London: Heinemann.

Marshall, T. (1963b) 'The recent history of professionalism in relation to social structure and social policy', in Marshall, T. *Sociology at the Crossroads and Other Essays*, London: Heinemann.

Martin, M. (1969) *Colleagues or Competitors? A Study of the Role of Five of the Professions Supplementary to Medicine*, London: G. Bell & Sons.

Means, J. (1963) 'Homus medicus Americanus', *Daedalus* 92(4): 701–23.

Mennell, S. (1980) *Sociological Theory: Uses and Unities*, second edition, London: Nelson.

Merton, R, (1968) *Social Theory and Social Structure*. New York: Free Press.

Miles, A. (1991) *Women, Health and Medicine*, Buckingham: Open University Press.

Millerson, G. (1964) *The Qualifying Associations*, London: Routledge & Kegan Paul.

Mishra, R. (1981) *Society and Social Policy: Theories and Practice of Welfare*, second edition, London: Macmillan.

Mohan, J. (1991) 'Privatization in the British health sector: a challenge to the

NHS?', in Gabe, J., Calnan, M. and Bury, M. (eds) *The Sociology of the Health Service*, London: Routledge.

Mooney, G. (1986) *Economics, Medicine and Health Care*, Brighton: Harvester.

Moore, J., Phipps, K., Marcer, R. and Lewith, G. (1985) 'Why do people seek treatment by alternative medicine?', *British Medical Journal* 5 January: 28–9.

Moore, W. (1970) *The Professions: Roles and Rules*, New York: Russell Sage Foundation.

Moran, M. and Wood, B. (1993) *States, Regulation and the Medical Profession*, Buckingham: Open University Press.

Morgan, M., Calnan, M. and Manning, N. (1985) *Sociological Approaches to Health and Medicine*, London: Croom Helm.

Mowbray, R. (1959) 'Historical aspects of electric convulsant therapy', *Scottish Medical Journal* 4: 373–8.

Mulkay, M. (1972) *The Social Process of Innovation: A Study in the Sociology of Science*, London: Macmillan.

—— (1979) *Science and the Sociology of Knowledge*, London: Allen & Unwin.

—— (1991) *Sociology of Science: A Sociological Pilgrimage*, Milton Keynes: Open University Press.

Mungham, G. and Thomas, P. (1983) 'Solicitors and clients: altruism or self-interest?', in Dingwall, R. and Lewis, P. (eds) *The Sociology of the Professions*, London: Macmillan.

Murphy, R. (1990) 'Proletarianization or bureaucratization: the fall of the professional?', in Torstendahl, R. and Burrage, M. (eds) *The Formation of Professions*, London: Sage.

Musgrave, R. (1966) 'The public interest: efficiency in the creation and maintenance of material welfare', in Friedrich, C. (ed.) *The Public Interest*, New York: Atherton Press.

Navarro, V. (1974) 'A critique of the present and proposed strategies for redistributing resources in the health sector and a discussion of alternatives', *Medical Care* 12(9): 721–42.

—— (1976) *Medicine Under Capitalism*, London: Croom Helm.

—— (1977) *Social Security and Medicine in the USSR: A Marxist Critique*, Lexington: Lexington Books.

—— (1978) *Class Struggle, the State and Medicine: An Historical and Contemporary Analysis of the Medical Sector in Great Britain*, London: Martin Robertson.

—— (1986) *Crisis, Health and Medicine: A Social Critique*, London: Tavistock.

Nicholls, P. (1988) *Homoeopathy and the Medical Profession*, London: Croom Helm.

Nicholls, P. and Luton, J. (1986) 'Doctors and complementary medicine: a survey of general practitioners in the Potteries', Occasional Paper No. 2, Department of Sociology, North Staffordshire Polytechnic.

Niemeyer, G. (1966) 'Public interest and private utility', in Friedrich, C. (ed.) *The Public Interest*, New York: Atherton Press.

Novak, L. (1990) 'USSR: perestroika hits the health service', *Health Matters* September: 20–1.

Novarra, V. (1980) *Women's Work, Men's Work: The Ambivalence of Equality*, London: Marion Boyars.

Nove, A. (1964) *Was Stalin Really Necessary? Some Problems of Soviet Political Economy*, London: Allen & Unwin.

Nudelman, A. (1976) 'The maintenance of Christian Science in scientific society', in Wallis, R. and Morley, P. (eds) *Marginal Medicine*, London: Peter Owen.

Oakley, A. (1992) 'The wisewoman and the doctor', in Saks, M. (ed.) *Alternative Medicine in Britain*, Oxford: Clarendon Press.

Oppenheimer, M. (1973) 'The proletarianization of the professional', in Halmos, P. (ed.) *Professionalization and Social Change*, Sociological Review Monograph No. 20, Keele: University of Keele.

Palfreman, J. (1979) 'Between scepticism and credulity: a study of Victorian scientific attitudes to modern spiritualism', in Wallis, R. (ed.) *On the Margins of Science*, Sociological Review Monograph No. 27, Keele: University of Keele.

Papineau, D. (1976) 'Why ethnomethodology may not be the last word', *Times Higher Education Supplement* 16 April.

Parkin, F. (1979) *Marxism and Class Theory: A Bourgeois Critique*, London: Tavistock.

—— (1992) *Durkheim*, Oxford: Oxford University Press.

Parry, N. and Parry, J. (1976) *The Rise of the Medical Profession*, London: Croom Helm.

—— (1977) 'Social closure and collective social mobility', in Scase, R. (ed.) *Industrial Society: Class, Cleavage and Control*, London: Allen & Unwin.

Parsons, T. (1949) 'The professions and social structure', in Parsons, T. *Essays in Sociological Theory*, Glencoe: Free Press.

—— (1952) *The Social System*, London: Tavistock.

—— (1968) 'Professions', in Sills, D. (ed.) *International Encyclopaedia of the Social Sciences* Vol. 12, New York: Macmillan and Free Press.

Parssinen, T. (1992) 'Medical mesmerists in Victorian Britain', in Saks, M. (ed.) *Alternative Medicine in Britain*, Oxford: Clarendon Press.

Pei, W. (1983) 'Traditional Chinese medicine', in Bannerman, R., Burton, J. and Wen-Chieh, C. (eds) *Traditional Medicine and Health Care Coverage*, Geneva: World Health Organization.

Pentol, A. (1983) 'Cost-benefit analysis in health care', in Allen, D. and Hughes, J. (eds) *Management for Health Service Administrators*, London: Pitman.

Perkin, H. (1989) *The Rise of Professional Society: England Since 1800*, London: Routledge.

Perrucci, R. (1973) 'In the service of man: radical movements in the professions', in Halmos, P. (ed.) *Professionalization and Social Change*, Sociological Review Monograph No. 20, Keele: University of Keele.

Phillips, M. and Dawson, J. (1985) *Doctors' Dilemmas: Medical Ethics and Contemporary Science*, Brighton: Harvester Press.

Picciotto, S. (1979) 'The theory of the state, class struggle and the rule of law', in Fine, B., Kinsey, R., Lea, J., Picciotto, S. and Young, J. (eds) *Capitalism and the Rule of Law*, London: Hutchinson.

Pietroni, P. (1991) *The Greening of Medicine*, London: Victor Gollancz

Plamenatz, J. (1971) *Ideology*, London: Macmillan.

Plant, R. (1991) *Modern Political Thought*, Oxford: Basil Blackwell.

Popper, K. (1963) *Conjectures and Refutations*, London: Routledge & Kegan Paul.
Porter, R. (1987) *Disease, Medicine and Society in England 1550–1860*, London: Macmillan.
—— (1989) *Health for Sale: Quackery in England 1660–1850*, Manchester: Manchester University Press.
Portwood, D. and Fielding, A. (1981) 'Privilege and the professions', *Sociological Review* 29(4): 749–73.
Poulantzas, N. (1973a) *Political Power and Social Classes*, London: New Left Books.
—— (1973b) 'The problem of the capitalist state', in Urry, J. and Wakeford, J. (eds) *Power in Britain*, London: Heinemann.
—— (1975) *Classes in Contemporary Capitalism*, London: New Left Books.
Powell, M. and Anesaki, M. (1990) *Health Care in Japan*, London: Routledge.
Powles, J. (1973) 'On the limitations of modern medicine', *Science, Medicine and Man* 1(1): 1–30.
Poynter, N. (1971) *Medicine and Man*, London: Watts & Co.
Quen, J. (1975a) 'Acupuncture and Western medicine', *Bulletin of the History of Medicine* 49(2): 196–205.
—— (1975b) 'Case studies in nineteenth century scientific rejection: mesmerism, perkinism and acupuncture', *Journal of the History of the Behavioural Sciences* 11(2): 149–56.
Raffel, M. (1984) 'Health services in the Union of Soviet Socialist Republics', in Raffel, M. (ed.) *Comparative Health Systems*, University Park: Pennsylvania State University Press.
Raphael, D. (1990) *Problems of Political Philosophy*, second edition, London: Macmillan.
Raskin, M. (1986) *The Common Good. Its Politics, Policies and Philosophy*, London: Routledge & Kegan Paul.
Rawls, J. (1973) *A Theory of Justice*, London: Oxford University Press.
—— (1993) *Political Liberalism*, New York: Columbia University Press.
Rayner, G. (1988) 'America's curious case for treatment', *Times Higher Education Supplement* 29 July.
Reid, N. and Boore, J. (1987) *Research Methods and Statistics in Health Care*, London: Edward Arnold.
Reilly, D. (1983) 'Young doctors' views on alternative medicine', *British Medical Journal* 30 July: 337–9.
Rex, J. (1970) *Key Problems of Sociological Theory*, London: Routledge & Kegan Paul.
Richman, J. (1987) *Medicine and Health*, London: Longman.
Riddell, P. (1991) *The Thatcher Era and Its Legacy*, Oxford: Blackwell.
Riska, E. and Wegar, K. (1992) 'Medical uncertainty: the gender basis of work within the medical profession', paper presented at ISA Conference on Professions in Transition, University of Leicester/De Montfort University, Leicester, 21–22 April.
—— (eds) (1993) *Gender, Work and Medicine: Women and the Medical Division of Labour*, London: Sage.
Ritzer, G. (1973) 'Professionalism and the individual', in Freidson, E. (ed.) *The Professions and Their Prospects*, Beverly Hills: Sage.

Roberts, H. (1985) *The Patient Patients: Women and Their Doctors*, London: Pandora Press.

Robinson, R. (1990) *Competition and Health Care*, London: King's Fund Institute.

Robson, J. (1973) 'The NHS Company Inc? The social consequences of the professional dominance in the National Health Service', *International Journal of Health Services* 3(3): 413–26.

Roccia, L. (1974) 'Chinese acupuncture in Italy', *American Journal of Chinese Medicine* 2(1): 49–52.

Rocher, G. (1974) *Talcott Parsons and American Sociology*, London: Nelson.

Rodwin, V.C. (1989) 'New ideas for health policy in France, Canada and Britain', in Field, M. (ed.) *Success and Crisis in National Health Systems*, London: Routledge.

Roebuck, J. and Quan, R. (1976) 'Health care practices in the American Deep South', in Wallis, R. and Morley, P. (eds) *Marginal Medicine*, London: Peter Owen.

Roemer, M. (1977) *Comparative National Policies on Health Care*, New York: Marcel Dekker.

Rogers, E. (1962) *The Diffusion of Innovations*, Glencoe: Free Press.

Rosenau, J. (1968) 'National interest', in Shills, D. (ed.) *International Encyclopaedia of the Social Sciences* Vol. 11, New York: Macmillan and Free Press.

Rosenberg, D. (1977) 'Acupuncture and US medicine: a socio-historical study of the response to the availability of knowledge', PhD thesis, University of Pittsburgh.

Rosenthal, M. (1981) 'Political process and the integration of traditional and Western medicine in the People's Republic of China', *Social Science and Medicine* 15A: 599–613.

Roth, J. (1974) 'Professionalism: the sociologist's decoy', *Sociology of Work and Occupations* 1(1): 6–23.

Rothstein, W. (1973) 'Professionalization and employer demands', in Halmos, P. (ed.) *Professionalization and Social Change*, Sociological Review Monograph No. 20, Keele: University of Keele.

Rueschemeyer, D. (1983) 'Professional autonomy and the social control of expertise', in Dingwall, R. and Lewis, P. (eds) *The Sociology of the Professions*, London: Macmillan.

—— (1986) *Power and the Division of Labour*, Cambridge: Polity Press.

Runciman, W. (1970a) 'Games, justice and the general will', in Runciman, W. *Sociology In Its Place and Other Essays*, Cambridge: Cambridge University Press.

—— (1970b) 'False consciousness', in Runciman, W. *Sociology In Its Place and Other Essays*, Cambridge: Cambridge University Press.

Ryan, A. (1970) *The Philosophy of the Social Sciences*, London: Macmillan.

—— (1980) 'R. H. Tawney: a socialist saint', *New Society* 27 November.

Ryan, M. (1978) *The Organization of Soviet Medical Care*, Oxford: Basil Blackwell.

Saks, M. (1983) 'Removing the blinkers? A critique of recent contributions to the sociology of professions', *Sociological Review* 31(1): 1–21.

—— (1985) 'Professions and the public interest: the response of the medical profession to acupuncture in nineteenth and twentieth century Britain', PhD thesis, London School of Economics, University of London.

—— (1987) 'The politics of health care', in Robins, L. (ed.) *Politics and Policy-making in Britain*, London: Longman.

—— (1990) 'Sociology, professions and the public interest: professional ideology and public responsibility', paper presented at ISA Conference on Professions and Public Authority, Northeastern University, Boston, 21–22 April.

—— (1991a) 'Power, politics and alternative medicine', *Talking Politics* 3(2): 68–72.

—— (1991b) 'The flight from science? The reporting of acupuncture in mainstream British medical journals from 1800 to 1990', *Complementary Medical Research* 5(3): 178–82.

—— (1992a) 'Introduction', in Saks, M. (ed.) *Alternative Medicine in Britain*, Oxford: Clarendon Press.

—— (1992b) 'The paradox of incorporation: acupuncture and the medical profession in modern Britain', in Saks, M. (ed.) *Alternative Medicine in Britain*, Oxford: Clarendon Press.

—— (1994) 'The alternatives to medicine', in Gabe, J., Kelleher, D. and Williams, G. (eds) *Challenging Medicine*, London: Routledge.

Saltman, R. and von Otter, C. (1992) *Planned Markets and Public Competition: Strategic Reform in North European Health Systems*, Buckingham: Open University Press.

Saunders, P. (1983) *Urban Politics: A Sociological Interpretation*, London: Hutchinson.

Schubert, G. (1960) *The Public Interest: A Critique of the Theory of a Political Concept*, Glencoe: Free Press.

—— (1966) 'Is there a public interest theory?', in Friedrich, C. (ed.) *The Public Interest*, New York: Atherton Press.

Senior, P. (1989) 'Radical probation: surviving in a hostile climate', in Langan, M. and Lee, P. (eds) *Radical Social Work Today*, London: Unwin Hyman.

Shao, Y. (1988) *Health Care in China*, London: Office of Health Economics.

Shapin, S. (1979) 'The politics of observation: cerebral anatomy and social interests in the Edinburgh phrenology disputes', in Wallis, R. (ed.) *On the Margins of Science*, Sociological Review Monograph No. 27, Keele: University of Keele.

Shapiro, A. (1971) 'Placebo effects in medicine, psychotherapy and psycho-analysis', in Bergin, A. and Garfield, S. (eds) *A Handbook of Psychotherapy*, New York: John Wiley.

Sharma, U. (1992a) *Complementary Medicine Today: Practitioners and Patients*, London: Routledge.

—— (1992b) 'Professionalisation in complementary medicine today: an over-view', paper presented at ISA Conference on Professions in Transition, University of Leicester/De Montfort University, Leicester, 21–23 April.

Shaw, G.B. (1946) *The Doctor's Dilemma*, Harmondsworth: Penguin.

Shaw, K. (1987) 'Skills, control and the mass professions', *Sociological Review* 35(4): 775–94.

Sibeon, R. (1990) 'Social work knowledge, social actors and de-professional-ization', in Abbott, P. and Wallace, C. (eds) *The Sociology of the Caring Professions*, London: Falmer.

Sidel, V. and Sidel, R. (1974) *Serve the People: Observations on Medicine in the People's Republic of China*, Boston: Beacon Press.
—— (1983) *The Health of China: Current Conflicts in Medical and Human Services for One Billion People*, London: Zed Press.
Silverlight, J. (1983) 'The point of the needle', *Observer* 3 April.
Simmie, J. (1974) *Citizens in Conflict: The Sociology of Town Planning*, London: Hutchinson.
Sjöström, H. and Nilsson, R. (1972) *Thalidomide and the Power of the Drug Companies*, Harmondsworth: Penguin.
Smelser, N. (1976) *Comparative Methods in the Social Sciences*, Engelwood Cliffs: Prentice-Hall.
Stacey, M. (1980) 'Charisma, power and altruism', *Sociology of Health and Illness* 2(1): 64–90.
—— (1985) 'Women and health: the United States and the United Kingdom compared', in Lewin, E. and Olesen, V. (eds) *Women, Health and Healing: Towards a New Perspective*, London: Tavistock.
—— (1988) *The Sociology of Health and Healing*, London: Unwin Hyman.
—— (1992) *Regulating British Medicine: The General Medical Council*, Chichester: John Wiley & Sons.
Standen, C.S. (1993) 'The implications of the Osteopaths Act', *Complementary Therapies in Medicine* 1: 208–10.
Starr, P. (1982) *The Social Transformation of American Medicine*, New York: Basic Books.
Stern, B. (1927) *Social Factors in Medical Progress*, New York: Columbia University Press.
Stevens, R. (1966) *Medical Practice in Modern England*, New Haven: Yale University Press.
—— (1971) *American Medicine and the Public Interest*, New Haven: Yale University Press.
—— (1983) 'Comparisons in health care: Britain as contrast to the United States', in Mechanic, D. (ed.) *Handbook of Health, Health Care and the Health Professions*, New York: Free Press.
Strong, P. (1979) 'Sociological imperialism and the profession of medicine: a critical examination of the thesis of medical imperialism', *Social Science and Medicine* 13A: 199–215.
Strong, P. and Robinson, J. (1990) *The NHS: Under New Management*, Milton Keynes: Open University Press.
Sugden, R. (1981) *The Political Economy of Public Choice: An Introduction to Welfare Economics*, Oxford: Martin Robertson.
Tawney, R. (1921) *The Acquisitive Society*, London: Bell & Sons.
Taylor, R. (1985) 'Alternative medicine and the medical encounter in Britain and the United States', in Salmon, J.W. (ed.) *Alternative Medicines: Popular and Policy Perspectives*, London: Tavistock.
Taylor-Gooby, P. (1985) *Public Opinion, Ideology and State Welfare*, London: Routledge & Kegan Paul.
Thomas, K., Carr, J., Westlake, L. and Williams, B. (1991) 'Use of non-orthodox and conventional health care in Great Britain', *British Medical Journal* 26 January: 207–10.
Thomson, A. (1973) *Half a Century of Medical Research: Origins and Policy of the Medical Research Council (UK)* vol. I, London: HMSO.

Tivey, L. and Wright, A. (eds) (1989) *Party Ideology in Britain*, London: Routledge.

Tomasic, R. (1985) *The Sociology of Law*, London: Sage.

Townsend, P., Davidson, N. and Whitehead, M. (1988) *Inequalities in Health: The Black Report and the Health Divide*, Harmondsworth: Penguin.

Turner, B. (1987) *Medical Power and Social Knowledge*, London: Sage.

Unschuld, P. (1987) 'Traditional Chinese medicine: some historical and epistemological reflections', *Social Science and Medicine* 24(12): 1023–9.

Vaskilampi, T. (1991) 'The role of alternative medicine: the Finnish experience', in Lewith, G. and Aldridge, D. (eds) *Complementary Medicine and the European Community*, Saffron Walden: C.W. Daniel.

Vaughan, P. (1959) *Doctors' Commons: A Short History of the British Medical Association*, London: Heinemann.

Venediktov, D. (1973) 'USSR', in Douglas-Wilson, I. and MacLachlan, G. (eds) *Health Service Prospects*, London: Lancet and Nuffield Provincial Hospitals Trust.

Vickers, A.J. (1994) 'Complementary therapies on the NHS: the NAHAT survey', *Complementary Therapies in Medicine* 2: 48–50.

Victor, C. (1991) *Health and Health Care in Later Life*, Milton Keynes: Open University Press.

Visser, J. (1991) 'Alternative medicine in the Netherlands', in Lewith, G. and Aldridge, D. (eds) *Complementary Medicine and the European Community*, Saffron Walden: C.W. Daniel.

Vohra, R. (1990) *China: The Search for Social Justice and Democracy*, Harmondsworth: Penguin.

Waddington, I. (1984) *The Medical Profession in the Industrial Revolution*, Goldenbridge: Gill & Macmillan.

Wallis, R. (1979) 'Introduction', in Wallis, R. (ed.) *On the Margins of Science*, Sociological Review Monograph No. 27, Keele: University of Keele.

Wallis, R. and Morley, P. (1976) 'Introduction', in Wallis, R. and Morley, P. (eds) *Marginal Medicine*, London: Peter Owen.

Wardwell, W. (1966) 'Chiropractic', in Vollmer, H. and Mills, D. (eds) *Professionalization*, Englewood Cliffs: Prentice-Hall.

—— (1976) 'Orthodox and unorthodox practitioners: changing relationships and the future status of chiropractors', in Wallis, R. and Morley, P. (eds) *Marginal Medicine*, London: Peter Owen.

Watkins, J., Drury, L. and Preddy, D. (1992) *From Evolution to Revolution: The Pressures on Professional Life in the 1990s*, Bristol: University of Bristol/ Clerical Medical Investment Group.

Watkins, S. (1987) *Medicine and Labour: The Politics of a Profession*, London: Lawrence & Wishart.

Watson, T. (1987) *Sociology, Work and Industry*, second edition, London: Routledge & Kegan Paul.

Weber, M. (1949) *The Methodology of the Social Sciences*, New York: Free Press.

—— (1968) *Economy and Society: An Outline of Interpretative Sociology* vol. I, New York: Bedminster Press.

Webster, A. (1976) 'The theory and practice of medicine: the case of acupuncture', paper presented at the BSA Annual Conference on Sociology, Health and Illness, University of Manchester, 6–9 April.

—— (1979) 'Scientific controversy and socio-cognitive metonomy: the case of acupuncture', in Wallis, R. (ed.) *On the Margins of Science*, Sociological Review Monograph No. 27, Keele: University of Keele.

—— (1991) *Science, Technology and Society*, London: Macmillan.

West, R. (1992) 'Alternative medicine: prospects and speculations', in Saks, M. (ed.) *Alternative Medicine in Britain*, Oxford: Clarendon Press.

West, R. and Inglis, B. (1985) 'Taking the alternative road to health', *The Times* 13 March.

Wharton, R. and Lewith, G. (1986) 'Complementary medicine and the general practitioner', *British Medical Journal* 7 June: 1497–1500.

Wheelwright, E. and McFarlane, B. (1973) *The Chinese Road to Socialism*, Harmondsworth: Penguin.

White, S., Gardner, J., Schöpflin, G. and Saich, T. (1990) *Communist and Postcommunist Political Systems: An Introduction*, third edition, London: Macmillan.

Widgery, D. (1988) *The National Health: A Radical Perspective*, London: Hogarth Press.

Wilding, P. (1982) *Professional Power and Social Welfare*, London: Routledge & Kegan Paul.

Wilensky, H. (1964) 'The professionalization of everyone?', *American Journal of Sociology* 70(2): 137–58.

Williams, R. (1983) 'Concepts of health: an analysis of lay logic', *Sociology* 7(2): 185–205.

Witz, A. (1990) 'Patriarchy and professions: the gendered politics of occupational closure', *Sociology* 24(4): 675–90.

Wilson, B. (1966) *Religion in a Secular Society*, London: Watts & Co.

Wright, P. (1979) 'A study in the legitimisation of knowledge: the "success" of medicine and the "failure" of astrology', in Wallis, R. (ed.) *On the Margins of Science*, Sociological Review Monograph No. 27, Keele: University of Keele.

Young, M. (1963) *The Rise of Meritocracy*, London: Penguin.

Youngson, A. (1979) *The Scientific Revolution in Victorian Medicine*, London: Croom Helm.

Zander, M. (1978) *Legal Services for the Community*, London: Temple Smith.

MEDICO-SCIENTIFIC SOURCES

Andersson, S., Ericson, T., Holmgren, E. and Lindqvist, G. (1973) 'Electro-acupuncture and pain threshold', Letters, *Lancet* 8 September: 564.

Aust-Lawrence, A. (1889) 'Acupuncture in chronic pelvic inflammations', *British Medical Journal* 16 November: 1093–4.

Austin, M. (1972) *Acupuncture Therapy*, New York: ASI Publishers.

Ballantyne, J. (ed.) (1906) *Green's Encyclopaedia and Dictionary of Medicine and Surgery* vol. 1, London: William Green & Sons.

Banks, J. (1831) 'Observations on acupuncturation', *Edinburgh Medical and Surgical Journal* 35: 323.

—— (1856) 'On the treatment of some forms of rheumatism and neuralgic affections by acupuncture', *Lancet* 14 June: 652–3.

Bannerman, R. (1979) 'Acupuncture: the WHO view', *World Health* December: 24–9.

Baptiste, R. (1962) *L'Acupuncture et Son Histoire: Avantages et Inconvenients d'Une Thérapeutique Millénaire*, Paris: Maloine.

Beecher, H. (1955) 'The powerful placebo', *Journal of the American Medical Association* 159(1): 602–6.

Belcombe, H. (1852) 'Cases of sciatica and neuralgia treated by acupuncture', *Medical Times and Gazette* 4: 85.

Bischko, J. (1973) 'The activities of the Ludwig Boltzmann Institute for acupuncture', Letters, *American Journal of Chinese Medicine* 1(2): 375–8.

Bowers, J. and Carrubba, R. (1970) 'The doctoral thesis of Engelbert Kaempfer on tropical diseases, oriental medicine, and exotic natural phenomena', *Journal of the History of Medicine* 25(3): 270–310.

Bradbury, P. (1969) *Adventures in Healing*, London: Neville Spearman.

BMJ (1863) 'The puff professional: new cures', *British Medical Journal* 3 October: 375.

—— (1945) 'Acupuncture', Any Questions?, *British Medical Journal* 7 July: 34.

—— (1953) 'Acupuncture', Any Questions?, *British Medical Journal* 4 July: 56.

—— (1966) 'Chinese system of medicine on show', *British Medical Journal* 9 April: 930.

—— (1968) 'BMA clinical meeting', Cheltenham 24–27 October. *British Medical Journal* 2 November: 320.

—— (1973a) 'Tests of acupuncture', *British Medical Journal* 2 June: 502.

—— (1973b) 'When acupuncture came to Britain', *British Medical Journal* 22 December: 687–8.

—— (1977) 'Acupuncture-related hepatitis in the West Midlands in 1977', *British Medical Journal* 17 December: 1610

—— (1978) 'Pneumothorax after acupuncture', *British Medical Journal* 26 August: 602–3.

—— (1980) 'The flight from science', *British Medical Journal* 5 January: 1–2.

—— (1981) 'How does acupuncture work?', *British Medical Journal* 19 September: 746–8.

—— (1983) 'Alternative medicine', *British Medical Journal* 30 July: 307–8.

—— (1985) 'A false phoenix', *British Medical Journal* 21/28 December: 1744–5.

—— (1989) 'WHO adopts international nomenclature for acupuncture', *British Medical Journal* 16 December: 1483–4.

Brown, P. (1972) 'Use of acupuncture in major surgery', *Lancet* 17 June: 1328.

Bull, G. (1973) 'Acupuncture anaesthesia', *Lancet* 25 August: 417–18.

Cahn, A., Carayon, P., Hill, C. and Flamant, R. (1978) 'Acupuncture in gastroscopy', *Lancet* 28 January: 182–3.

Campbell, A.V. (1987) *Acupuncture: The Modern Scientific Approach*, London: Faber & Faber.

Capperauld, I. (1972) 'Anaesthesia by acupuncture', Correspondence, *British Medical Journal* 28 October: 232–3.

Capperauld, I., Cooper, E. and Saltoun, D. (1972) 'Acupuncture anaesthesia in China', *Lancet* 25 January: 1136.

Carraro, A. (1841) 'Acupuncture of the heart in apparent death', *Provincial Medical and Surgical Journal* 22 May 1841: 140.

Carrubba, R. and Bowers, J. (1974) 'The Western world's first detailed treatise on acupuncture: Willem Ten Rhijne's "De Acupunctura"', *Journal of the History of Medicine* 29(4): 371–97.

Chung, S. and Dickenson, A. (1980) 'Pain, enkephalin and acupuncture', *Nature* 283: 243–4.

Churchill, J. (1822) *A Treatise on Acupuncturation*, London: Simpkin & Marshall.

—— (1823) 'On acupuncturation', *London Medical, Surgical and Pharmaceutical Repository* 19: 372–4.

—— (1828) *Cases Illustrative of the Immediate Effects of Acupuncturation*, London: Callow & Wilson.

Clement-Jones, V., Lowry, P., McLoughlin, L., Besser, G., Rees, L. and Wen, H. (1979) 'Acupuncture in heroin addicts: changes in met-enkephalin and β-endorphin in blood and cerebrospinal fluid', *Lancet* 25 August: 380–2.

Clement-Jones, V., McLoughlin, L., Tomlin, S., Besser, G., Rees, L. and Wen, H. (1980) 'Increased β-endorphin but not met-enkephalin levels in human cerebrospinal fluid after acupuncture for recurrent pain', *Lancet* 1 November: 946–8.

Coley, W. (1802a) 'A case of tympanites in an infant', *Medical and Physical Journal* 7: 223–34.

—— (1802b) 'On acupuncturation', *Medical and Physical Journal* 7: 235–8.

Craig, W. (1869) 'Acupuncture in a case of cancer', *Edinburgh Medical Journal* 14: 617–20.

Doctor (1974) 'If acupuncture works, how do you prove it?', *Doctor* 17 October: 14.

Donkin, H. (1880) 'Thoughts on ignorance and quackery', *British Medical Journal* 9 October: 577–80.

Downey, S. (1988) 'Acupuncture', in Rankin-Box, D. (ed.) *Complementary Health Therapies: A Guide for Nurses and the Caring Professions*, London: Croom Helm.

Druitt, R. (1859) *Surgeon's Vade-mecum*, eighth edition, London: Renshaw.

Dudgeon, J. (1872) 'Report of the Peking Hospital', *Medical Times and Gazette* 8 May: 509.

Dundee, J. and McMillan, C. (1991) 'Positive evidence of P6 acupuncture antiemesis', *Postgraduate Medical Journal* 67: 417–22.

Dundee, J., Chestnutt, W., Ghaly, R. and Lynas, A. (1986) 'Traditional Chinese acupuncture: a potentially useful antiemetic?', *British Medical Journal* 6 September: 583–4.

Elliotson, J. (1850) 'Acupuncture', in Forbes, J., Tweedie, A. and Conolly, J. (eds) *The Cyclopedia of Practical Medicine* vol. 1, London: Sherwood, Gilbert & Piper.

Fernandez-Herlihy, L. (1972) 'Osler, acupuncture and lumbago', Correspondence, *New England Journal of Medicine* 287(6): 314.

Fergusson, W. (1842) *A System of Practical Surgery*, London: J. Churchill.

Filshie, J. and Abbot, P. (1991) 'Acupuncture for chronic pain: a review', *Acupuncture in Medicine* 9(1): 4–14.

Finch, F. (1824) 'Acupuncture in tetanic trismus', *Medical Repository* 8: 334.

Flood, S. (1845a) 'On the power, nature and evil of popular medical superstition', *Lancet* 16 August: 179–81.

—— (1845b) 'On the power, nature and evil of popular medical superstition' *Lancet* 23 August: 201–4.

Furnivall, J. (1837) 'Ascites treated by acupuncture', Letters, *Lancet* 25 December: 313.

Gee, D.J. (1984) 'Fatal pneumothorax due to acupuncture', *British Medical Journal* 14 January: 114.

Gibson, V. (1893) 'An analysis of one thousand cases of primary sciatica, with special reference to the treatment of one hundred cases by acupuncture', *Lancet* 15 April: 860–1.

Gould, D. (1972) 'The yang, the yin and the consumer', *New Scientist* 10 February: 309.

Grant, A. (1986) 'Editorial', *Acupuncture in Medicine* 3(1): 2–3.

Grant, B. (1993) *Alternative Health: A–Z of Natural Health Care*, London: Optima.

Greene, N. (1972) 'This is no humbug – or is it?', *Journal of Anaesthesiology* 36(2): 101–2.

Gustafsson, L. (1973) 'Acupuncture anaesthesia', Letters, *Lancet* 20 January: 154.

Hacket, W. (1837) 'Cure of hydrocele by acupuncture', Letters, *Lancet* 25 February: 787.

Hamilton, S. (1972) 'Anaesthesia by acupuncture', Correspondence, *British Medical Journal* 28 October: 232.

Hashimoto, M. (1968) *Japanese Acupuncture*, New York: Liveright.

Ho, V. and Bradley, P. (1992) 'Acupuncture for resistant temporo-mandibular joint pain dysfunction syndrome', *Acupuncture in Medicine* 10(2): 53–5.

Hooper, R. (1848) *Medical Dictionary*, eighth edition, London.

Hsü, E. (1992) 'The history and development of auriculotherapy', *Acupuncture in Medicine* 10(supp.): 109–18.

Jefferys, D.B., Smith, S., Brennard-Roper, D.A. and Curry, P.V.L. (1983) 'Acupuncture needles as a cause of bacterial endocarditis', *British Medical Journal* 30 July: 326–7.

Jobst, K., Chen, J., McPherson, K., Arrowsmith, J., Brown, V., Efthimiou, J., Fletcher, H., Maciocia, G., Mole, P., Shifrin, K. and Lane, D. (1986) 'Controlled trial of acupuncture for disabling breathlessness', *Lancet* 20/27 December: 1416–18.

Karols, K. (1972) 'Acupuncture anaesthesia', Letters, *Lancet* 30 December: 1417.

Lancet (1827) 'Case of chronic rheumatism cured by acupuncture', *Lancet* 18 August: 636–7.

—— (1833) 'London Medical Society: rheumatism – elaterium acupuncture', *Lancet* 23 March: 817–18.

—— (1840) 'Progress of medical reform', *Lancet* 4 January: 537–40.

—— (1845) 'Who are the chief quack-fanciers?', *Lancet* 20 September: 328.

—— (1864) 'Quackery', *Lancet* 12 October: 554–5.

—— (1871) 'Quackery', *Lancet* 21 October: 598.

—— (1880) 'Consultations with homoeopaths', *Lancet* 5 June: 888–9.

—— (1889) 'How quackery is supported', *Lancet* 6 July: 51.

—— (1934) 'Psychology of quackery', *Lancet* 3 February: 246.

—— (1938) 'Herbalist and diabetes', *Lancet* 8 October: 849.

—— (1972) 'Twentieth century acupuncture', *Lancet* 17 June: 1321.

—— (1981) 'Endorphins through the eye of a needle', *Lancet* 28 February: 480–2.

—— (1987) 'Acupuncture and AIDS', *Lancet* 30 May: 1275.

—— (1990) 'Many points to needle', *Lancet* 6 January: 20–1.

Lawson-Wood, D. and Lawson-Wood, J. (1959) *Chinese System of Healing: An Introductory Handbook to Chinese Massage Treatment at the Chinese Acupuncture Points for Influencing the Psyche*, Grayshott: Health Science Press.

—— (1964) *Acupuncture Handbook*, Rustington: Health Science Press.

—— (1974) *The Incredible Healing Needles: A Layman's Guide to Chinese Acupuncture*, Wellingborough: Thorsons.

Lavier, J. (1965) *Points of Chinese Acupuncture*, Rustington: Health Science Press.

—— (1966) *Histoire, Doctrine et Practique de l'Acupuncture Chinoise*, Geneva: C. Tohou.

Lever, R. (1987) *Acupuncture for Everyone*, Harmondsworth: Penguin.

Lewis, D. (1836) 'New method of treating hydrocele', Letters, *Lancet* 7 May: 206.

Lewith, G. (1982) *Acupuncture: Its Place in Western Medical Science*, Wellingborough: Thorsons.

—— (1985) 'Acupuncture and TENS', in Lewith, G. (ed.) *Alternative Therapies: A Guide to Complementary Medicine for the Health Professional*, London: Heinemann.

Lewith, G. and Machin, D. (1983) 'On the evaluation of the clinical effects of acupuncture', *Pain* 16: 111–27.

Loh, L., Nathan, P., Schott, G. and Zilkha, K. (1984) 'Acupuncture versus medical treatment for migraine and muscle tension headaches', *Journal of Neurology, Neurosurgery and Psychiatry* 47: 333–7.

London Medical Gazette (1844) 'On the absurdities of mesmerism', *London Medical Gazette* 23 August: 704–6.

Lorimer, G. (1885) 'Acupuncture and its application in the treatment of certain forms of chronic rheumatism', *British Medical Journal* 21 November: 956–8.

Macdonald, A. (1982) *Acupuncture: From Ancient Art to Modern Medicine*, London: Allen & Unwin.

MacIntosh, R. (1973) 'Tests of acupuncture', Correspondence, *British Medical Journal* 25 August: 454–5.

Mann, F. (1962a) *Acupuncture: The Ancient Chinese Art of Healing*, London: Heinemann.

—— (1962b) *Anatomical Charts of Acupuncture Points, Meridians and Extra Meridians*, Barnet: Barnet Publications.

—— (1963) *The Treatment of Disease by Acupuncture*, London: Heinemann.

—— (1964) *The Meridians of Acupuncture*, London: Heinemann.

—— (1966) *Atlas of Acupuncture*, London: Heinemann.

—— (1971) *Acupuncture: The Ancient Chinese Art of Healing*, second edition, London: Heinemann.

—— (1973) *Acupuncture: Cure of Many Diseases*, London: Pan Books.

Mann, F. and Halfhide, A. (1963) 'Treatment of headaches by acupuncture', *Medical World* 98: 284–7.

Mann, F., Bowsher, D., Mumford, J., Lipton, S. and Miles, J. (1973) 'Treatment of intractable pain by acupuncture', *Lancet* 14 July: 57–60.

Marcus, P. (1992) 'Acupuncture in modern medicine', *Acupuncture in Medicine* 10(supp.): 101–8.

Meade, T., Dyer, S., Browne, W., Townsend, J. and Frank, A. (1990) 'Low back pain of mechanical origin: randomised comparison of chiropractic and hospital outpatient treatment', *British Medical Journal* 2 June: 1431–6.

Melzack, R. (1975) 'Prolonged relief of pain by brief intense transcutaneous somatic stimulation', *Pain* 1: 357–74.

Melzack, R. and Wall, P. (1965) 'Pain mechanisms: a new theory', *Science* 150: 971–9.

Mole, P. (1992) *Acupuncture: Energy Balancing for Body, Mind and Spirit*, Longmead: Element.

Monod, G. (1932) 'Treatment by acupuncture', *British Medical Journal* 23 April: 767–8.

Moss, L. (1964) *Acupuncture and You*, London: Paul Alek Books.

Mumford, J. and Bowsher, D. (1973) 'Electro-acupuncture and pain threshold', Letters, *Lancet* 22 September: 667.

Munro, W. (1874) 'Case of dropsy: treatment by acupuncture', *British Medical Journal* 23 May: 679.

Myers, C. (1991) 'Acupuncture in general practice: effect on drug expenditure', *Acupuncture in Medicine* 9(2): 71–2.

Oliver, T. (1889) 'Acute tympanies of the abdomen treated by acupuncture', *Lancet* 6 July: 13–14.

Olsen, K. (1991) *The Encylopaedia of Alternative Health Care*, London: Piatkus.

O'Sullivan, D. (1875) 'Prevention of quacks', Correspondence, *British Medical Journal* 17 April: 534.

Parker, F. (1921) 'Successful quackery', Letters, *Lancet* 10 December: 1256.

Peacher, W. (1975) 'Adverse reactions, contraindicators and complications of acupuncture and moxibustion', *American Journal of Chinese Medicine* 3: 35–46.

Pomeranz, B. (1977) 'Brain's opiates at work in acupuncture?', *New Scientist* 6 January: 12–13.

PMSJ (1843) 'Quackery and its pretensions', *Provincial Medical and Surgical Journal* 9 September: 490–2.

Ramsay, M. (1972) 'Anaesthesia by acupuncture', Correspondence, *British Medical Journal* 16 September: 703.

Renton, J. (1830) 'Observations on acupuncture', *Edinburgh Medical and Surgical Journal* 34: 100–7.

Rice, L. (1972) 'Acupuncture inquiry', Letters, *New Scientist* 3 August: 261–2.

Richardson, P. (1992) 'Pain and the placebo effect', *Acupuncture in Medicine* 10(1): 9–12.

Richardson, P. and Vincent, C. (1986) 'Acupuncture for the treatment of pain: a review of evaluative research', *Pain* 24: 15–40.

Riddle, J. (1974) 'Report of the New York State Commission on Acupuncture', *American Journal of Chinese Medicine* 2(3): 289–318.

Riscalla, L. (1979) 'Towards establishing scientific credibility in acupuncture', *Medical Hypotheses* 5: 221–4.

Roberts, M. (1981) *Acupuncture Therapy: Its Mode of Action*, Leicester: Eresus Publications.

Rose-Neil, S. (1972) 'Acupuncture (continued)', Letters, *New Scientist* 10 August: 309.

Rudolfi, R. (1990) *Shiatsu*, London: Macdonald Optima.

Saltoun, D. (1973) 'What is the truth about acupuncture?', *World Medicine* 13 June: 7–8.

Selly, E. (1991) 'Use of acupuncture in a general practice: the first two years', *Acupuncture in Medicine* 9(2): 72–4.

Skrabanek, P. (1984) 'Acupuncture and the age of unreason', *Lancet* 26 May: 1169–71.

—— (1986) 'Demarcation of the absurd', *Lancet* 26 April: 960–1.

Snell, S. (1880) 'Remarks on acupuncture', *Medical Times and Gazette* 19 June: 661–2.

Stacey-Wilson, T. (1945) 'Acupuncture', Letters, *British Medical Journal* 28 July: 144.

Stanway, A. (1986) *Alternative Medicine: A Guide to Natural Therapies*, Harmondsworth: Penguin.

Stephens, W. (1983) 'Personal view', *British Medical Journal* 24 September: 906.

—— (1989) 'Consultant attitudes to acupuncture in a district general hospital', *Acupuncture in Medicine* 6(1); 20–3.

Stewart, D., Thomson, J. and Oswald, I. (1977) 'Acupuncture analgesia: an experimental investigation', *British Medical Journal* 8 January: 67–70.

Stovickova, D. (1961) 'What is acupuncture?', *New Orient* 15–19.

Tai, P. (1973) 'Revival of an ancient medicine – acupuncture', *Journal of the American Podiatry Association* 63(11): 618–25.

Teale, T. (1871) 'On the relief of pain and muscular disability by acupuncture', *Lancet* 29 April: 507–8.

Tweedale, J. (1823) 'Case of anasarca successfully treated by acupuncture', *Lancet* 5 October: 19–20.

Veith, I. (1962) 'Acupuncture therapy – past and present: verity or delusion', *Journal of the American Medical Association* 180: 478–84.

—— (1972) 'Acupuncture: ancient enigma to East and West', *American Journal of Psychiatry* 129: 109–12.

Vincent, C. (1989) 'The methodology of controlled trials of acupuncture', *Acupuncture in Medicine* 7(1): 9–13.

Vincent, C. and Richardson, P. (1986) 'The evaluation of therapeutic acupuncture: concepts and methods', *Pain* 24: 1–13.

Vowell, J. (1838) 'Acupuncture of ganglions', Letters, *Lancet* 25 August: 769–70.

Wall, P. (1972) 'An eye on the needle', *New Scientist* 20 July: 129–31.

—— (1974) 'Acupuncture revisited', *New Scientist* 3 October: 31–4.

Wansbrough, T. (1826) 'Acupuncturation', *Lancet* 30 September: 846–8.

—— (1827) 'Case of rheumatism successfully treated by acupuncturation', *Lancet* 21 June: 366.

Ward, T. (1858) 'On acupuncture', *British Medical Journal* 28 August: 728–9.

Wei-kang, F. (1975) *The Story of Chinese Acupuncture and Moxibustion*, Peking: Foreign Languages Press.

Wensel, L. (1980) *Acupuncture in Medical Practice*, Reston: Reston Publishing.

OFFICIAL PUBLICATIONS

American Association of Engineering Societies (1987) *Directory of Engineering Societies and Related Organizations*.

British Acupuncture Association (1982) *Register and Year Book*.

British Acupuncture Association and Register (1985) *Handbook*.

British Medical Association (1986) *Report of the Board of Science and Education on Alternative Medicine*, London: BMA.

—— (1993) *Complementary Medicine: New Approaches to Good Practice*, Oxford: Oxford University Press.

Committee of Enquiry into the Cost of the National Health Service (1956) *Report*, London: HMSO.

Council of the Law Society (1974) *A Guide to the Professional Conduct of Solicitors*.

Council for Acupuncture (1987) *Fact Sheet*.

Department of Health (1989) *Working for Patients*, London: HMSO.

—— (1991a) *The Patient's Charter*, London: HMSO.

—— (1991b) 'Stephen Dorrell Clarifies the Position on Alternative and Complementary Therapies', Press Release, 3 December.

—— (1992) *The Health of the Nation*, London: HMSO.

Department of Health and Social Security (1977) *Prevention and Health: Everybody's Business*, London: HMSO.

—— (1979) *Working Group on Back Pain*, London: HMSO.

General Medical Council Education Committee (1980) *Recommendations on Basic Medical Education*.

Hansard (1977) 'Acupuncturists' *Hansard (House of Commons)* 16 December: 1174–85.

Report as to the Practice of Medicine and Surgery by Unqualified Persons in the United Kingdom (1910) London: HMSO.

Royal Commission on the National Health Service (1979) *Report*, London: HMSO.

United Kingdom Central Council for Nursing, Midwifery and Health Visiting (1992) *Code of Professional Conduct*, London.

Working Party of the Royal College of Surgeons (1990) *Report on Pain after Surgery*, London.

Author index

Subject index

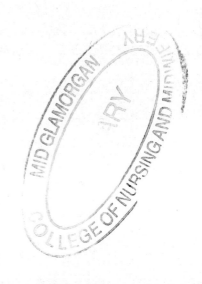